Lymphoma and Leukemia of the Nervous System

Tracy Batchelor · Lisa M. DeAngelis
Editors

Lymphoma and Leukemia of the Nervous System

Foreword by James O. Armitage and Franco Cavalli

Springer

Editors
Tracy Batchelor
Stephen E. and Catherine Pappas Center for Neuro-Oncology
Departments of Neurology and Radiation Oncology
Division of Hematology and Oncology
Massachusetts General Hospital
Harvard Medical School
55 Fruit Street
Boston, MA 02114, USA
tbatchelor@partners.org

Lisa M. DeAngelis
Department of Neurology
Memorial Sloan-Kettering Cancer Center
1275 York Avenue
New York, NY 10021-6007, USA
deangell@mskcc.org

ISBN 978-1-4419-7667-3 e-ISBN 978-1-4419-7668-0
DOI 10.1007/978-1-4419-7668-0
Springer New York Dordrecht Heidelberg London

Library of Congress Control Number: 2011928786

Printed on acid-free paper

Springer is part of Springer Science+Business Media (www.springer.com)

Foreword

A major step in learning to treat any disease is the ability to place patients into groups that are similar clinically, biologically, and in response to therapy. In a complex group of diseases like the immune system malignancies, this is absolutely vital if we are to develop effective therapies for each subgroup. The history of the management of patients with lymphoma is a story of our ability to understand and coherently group these tumors. This work began at the start of the twentieth century with the recognition of the Reed Sternberg cell (i.e. dividing what we now call Hodgkin lymphoma from the other lymphomas), and has continued through new histological classifications, immune studies, and, more recently, genetic studies including gene expression arrays. Over the years, it has become clear that lymphomas originating in certain, perhaps all, extranodal sites have unique characteristics and might require specific treatment approaches. This is true even though we do not always understand the biological explanation for these differences. Perhaps the most unique such subgroup of lymphomas is represented by those that originate in the central nervous system.

It has been known for some time that primary central nervous system lymphoma presents unique challenges. How does such a malignancy arise in the only organ system that is devoid of lymphatics? We know that normal B-cells can move into the CNS, but does such a cell become transformed during this passage, or does it transform in the periphery and find its way later into the CNS where it will proliferate? We have no real answers to this fundamental question, although new genetic and immunological studies are giving insights into the biology of this tumor. It has been highly associated with human immunodeficiency virus (HIV) infection, but today, it is seen increasingly in immunocompetent patients. Although only a small minority of patients will relapse with clinically apparent systemic disease, surgery and cranial irradiation have been demonstrated to be, alone or in combination, suboptimal treatments for CNS lymphoma. The increasingly effective use of systemic chemotherapy agents, such as high doses of methotrexate and cytarabine, often used in combination, is changing this previously dismal prognosis.

In addition to the increasing problem of primary central nervous system lymphoma, other lymphoid malignancies and leukemias, along with their treatments, can have important effects on the nervous system. Many of these malignancies metastasize to the central nervous system, while others can affect neurological function by more complex mechanisms. In addition, a variety of the treatments used to manage patients with lymphoma and leukemia can have adverse effects on neurological function.

Drs. Batchelor and DeAngelis have developed this text to be the best single source of information regarding lymphomas and leukemias of the nervous system. This text has the advantage of being clear, concise, and authoritative. It will be an important reference for neurologists, hematologists, medical oncologists, radiation therapists, neurosurgeons, neuropathologists, neuroradiologists, and hematopathologists who all work for the benefit of patients suffering from these disorders. This book not only teaches the status of current knowledge, but provides direction for how we can improve the outcome for these patients.

James O. Armitage, MD Omaha, NE, USA
Franco Cavalli, MD Bellinzona, Switzerland

Preface

Lymphoma and leukemia of the nervous system may be defined as direct or indirect involvement of the central or peripheral nervous systems by these malignancies. The diagnosis and management of these conditions is the subject of this book. In the first part of the book the focus is on primary central nervous system lymphoma (PCNSL), an uncommon type of non-Hodgkin lymphoma confined to the nervous system. The first two chapters of the book are an overview of the lymphoid malignancies and leukemias for non-oncologists. This introduction is followed by chapters on the pathology, epidemiology, diagnosis and management of PCNSL. These chapters review PCNSL in "immunocompetent" hosts as well as in the setting of immunosuppression. The management of patients with PCNSL involves treatment regimens that are different than the typical approaches used in patients with primary brain tumors or with systemic forms of non-Hodgkin lymphoma. The optimal treatment for patients with PCNSL has yet to be defined and several fundamental therapeutic questions, including the optimal role of radiation and other consolidation therapies, are unresolved. In the final chapters of this section a number of special topics including ocular lymphoma, neurolymphomatosis and intravascular lymphoma of the nervous system are reviewed.

In the second part of the book the neurological complications of the lymphoid malignancies and leukemias are reviewed. The neurotoxicity of therapies for lymphoma and leukemia are also covered in this section of the book. Brain, epidural and leptomeningeal metastases are examples of direct involvement of the nervous system while paraneoplastic complications are an example of indirect involvement of the nervous system. Although exceptions exist the prognosis is usually poor once lymphoma or leukemia involves the nervous system. Prevention of neurological complications with better systemic therapy and, possibly, prophylactic intrathecal chemotherapy are areas of active investigation.

The diagnosis and management of patients with lymphoma and leukemia of the nervous system involves an interdisciplinary team of hematologists, oncologists, radiation oncologists, neurologists, neurosurgeons and pathologists. A single source of information regarding this group of diseases and complications will hopefully serve as a useful resource for these physicians.

Tracy Batchelor, MD — Boston, MA
Lisa DeAngelis, MD — New York, NY

Acknowledgments

The second edition of this book would not have been possible without the collective wisdom and diligent effort of the contributing authors, to whom we owe a deep debt of gratitude. We are especially grateful for the enduring patience and support of our families, Lucy, Adam, and Emily (TB) and Peter, Daniel and Stephen (LDeA). We dedicate this edition of the book to our patients and their families.

Tracy Batchelor, MD
Lisa DeAngelis, MD

Contents

Contributors

Oussama Abla Division of Hematology/Oncology, Department of Pediatrics, The Hospital for Sick Children, Toronto, ON M5G1X8, Canada, oussama.abla@sickkids.ca

Eyal C. Attar Bone Marrow Transplant Unit, Massachusetts General Hospital Cancer Center, Boston, MA 02114, USA, eattar@partners.org

Batia Avni Department of Hematology, Hadassah Hebrew-University Medical Center, Jerusalem, Israel, batiaa@hadassah.org.il

Mark M. Awad Department of Medicine, Wang Ambulatory Care Center, Massachusetts General Hospital, Boston, MA 02114, USA, mawad1@partners.org

Joachim M. Baehring Departments of Neurology, Medicine and Neurosurgery, Yale University School of Medicine, New Haven, CT 06520-8082, USA, joachim.baehring@yale.edu

Tracy Batchelor Stephen E. and Catherine Pappas Center for Neuro-Oncology, Departments of Neurology and Radiation Oncology, Division of Hematology and Oncology, Massachusetts General Hospital, Harvard Medical School, 55 Fruit Street, Boston, MA 02114, USA, tbatchelor@partners.org

Jacoline E.C. Bromberg Department of Epidemiology and Biostatistics, Erasmus University Medical Center, 3015 GE Rotterdam, The Netherlands, j.bromberg@erasmusmc.nl

Marc C. Chamberlain Department of Neurology and Neurological Surgery, University of Washington, Seattle, WA, USA; Division of Neuro-Oncology, Department of Neurology, Fred Hutchinson Research Cancer Center, Seattle Cancer Care Alliance, Seattle, WA 98109-1023, USA, chambemc@uw.edu

Denise D. Correa Department of Neurology, Memorial Sloan-Kettering Cancer Center, New York, NY 10021, USA, corread@mskcc.org

Josep Dalmau Division of Neuro-Oncology, Department of Neurology, Hospital of the University of Pennsylvania, Philadelphia, PA 19104, USA, josep.dalmau@uphs.upenn.edu

Lisa M. DeAngelis Department of Neurology, Memorial Sloan-Kettering Cancer Center, 1275 York Avenue, New York, NY 10021-6007, USA, deangell@mskcc.org

Jan Drappatz Department of Neurology, Harvard Medical School, Center for Neuro-Oncology, Dana Farber Cancer Institute, Brigham and Women's Hospital, Boston, MA 02115, USA, jan_drappatz@dfci.harvard.edu

Andrés J.M. Ferreri Unit of Lymphoid Malignancies, Medical Oncology Unit, Department of Oncology, San Raffaele Scientific Institute, Milan, Italy, andres.ferreri@hsr.it

Judith A. Ferry Department of Pathology, Massachusetts General Hospital, Boston, MA 02114, USA, jferry@partners.org

David C. Fisher Division of Hematologic Malignancies, Department of Medicine, Dana Farber Cancer Institute, Brigham and Women's Hospital, Boston, MA 02115, USA, david_c_fisher@dfci.harvard.edu

Elizabeth R. Gerstner Department of Neurology, Massachusetts General Hospital and Harvard Medical School, Boston, MA, USA, egerstner@partners.org

Mark Gilbert Department of Neuro-Oncology, The University of Texas M.D. Anderson Cancer Center, Houston, TX 77030, USA, mrgilbert@mdanderson.org

Jon Glass Departments of Neurology and Neurological Surgery, Thomas Jefferson University, Philadelphia, PA, USA, jon.glass@jefferson.edu; jglassmd@gmail.com

R. Gilberto Gonzalez Department of Radiology, Massachusetts General Hospital and Harvard Medical School, Boston, MA 02114, USA, rggonzalez@partners.org

Silvia Govi Unit of Lymphoid Malignancies, Medical Oncology Unit, Department of Oncology, San Raffaele Scientific Institute, Milan, Italy, govi.silvia@hsr.it

Andrew Grigg Royal Melbourne Hospital, Melbourne, Australia, andrew.grigg@mh.org.au

Sigal Grisariu Department of Hematology, Hadassah Hebrew-University Medical Center, Jerusalem, Israel, rsigag@hadassah.org.il

Ingfrid Salvesen Haldorsen Department of Radiology, Haukeland University Hospital, Bergen, Norway, 5021, ingfrid.haldorsen@helse-bergen.no

Nancy L. Harris Department of Pathology, Massachusetts General Hospital and Harvard Medical School, Boston, MA 02114, USA, nlharris@partners.org

Gerald Illerhaus Department of Haematology and Oncology, University Medical Center Freiburg, Freiburg, Germany, gerald.illerhaus@uniklinik-freiburg.de

Samar Issa Clinical Head, Lymphoma Service, Middlemore Hospital, Auckland, New Zealand, samar.issa@middlemore.co.nz

Kurt A. Jaeckle Departments of Oncology and Neurology, Mayo Clinic Jacksonville, Jacksonville, FL 32224, USA, jaeckle.kurt@mayo.edu

Kristoph Jahnke Department of Hematology and Oncology, Charité-Universitätsmedizin Berlin, D-12200 Berlin, Germany, kristoph.jahnke@charite.de

Patrick Johnston Division of Hematology, Department of Medicine, Mayo Clinic Graduate School of Medicine, Rochester, MN, USA, johnston.patrick@mayo.edu

Mustafa Khasraw Department of Neurology, Memorial Sloan-Kettering Cancer Center, New York, NY 10065, USA, khasrawm@mskcc.org

Jill Lacy Section of Medical Oncology, Yale University School of Medicine, New Haven, CT 06520-8032, USA, jill.lacy@yale.edu

M. Beatriz S. Lopes Division of Neuropathology, Department of Pathology, University of Virginia School of Medicine, Charlottesville, VA 22908-0214, USA, msl2e@virginia.edu

Warren P. Mason Department of Medicine, Princess Margaret Hospital and University of Toronto, Toronto, ON M5G 2M9, USA, warren.mason@uhn.on.ca

Silvia Montoto CR-UK Medical Oncology Unit, Barts and the London School of Medicine and Dentistry, St Bartholomew's Hospital, EC1A 7BE London, UK, s.montoto@qmul.ac.uk

Maciej M. Mrugala Departments of Neurology and Neurosurgery, Medical School, Fred Hutchinson Cancer Research Center, University of Washington, Seattle, WA, USA, mmrugala@u.washington.edu

Edward Neuwelt Blood Brain Barrier and Neuro-Oncology Program, Departments of Neurology and Neurosurgery, Oregon Health Sciences University, Portland, OR 97239, USA, neuwelte@ohsu.edu

Ariela Noy Department of Medicine, Memorial Sloan-Kettering Cancer Center, New York, NY 10065, USA, noya@mskcc.org

Brian Patrick O'Neill Department of Neurology, Mayo Medical School, Mayo Clinic Cancer Center, Rochester, MN 55905, USA, boneill@mayo.edu

Antonio Omuro Department of Neurology, Memorial Sloan-Kettering Cancer Center, New York, NY 10065, USA, omuroa@mskcc.org

Rolf Pfannl Department of Pathology, Tufts Medical Center, Boston, MA 02111, USA, rpfannl@tuftsmedicalcenter.org

Nikolai Podoltsev Section of Hematology, Yale University School of Medicine, New Haven, CT 06520-8032, USA, nikolai.podoltsev@yale.edu

Maurilio Ponzoni Pathology Unit, Unit of Lymphoid Malignancies, Scientific Institute, San Raffaele Hospital, Milan, Italy, ponzoni.maurilio@hsr.it

José S. Pulido Department of Ophthalmology, Mayo Clinic, Rochester, MN, USA, pulido.jose@mayo.edu

Eudocia C. Quant Division of Neuro-Oncology, Department of Neurology, Dana Farber Cancer Institute, Center for Neuro-Oncology, Brigham and Women's Hospital, Boston, MA 02115, USA, equant@partners.org

Myrna R. Rosenfeld Division of Neuro-Oncology, Department of Neurology, Hospital of the University of Pennsylvania, Philadelphia, PA 19104, USA, myrna.rosenfeld@uphs.upenn.edu

James L. Rubenstein Division of Hematology/Oncology, Department of Medicine, University of California, San Francisco, CA 94143-1270, USA, jamesr@medicine.ucsf.edu

David Schiff Departments of Neurology, Neurological Surgery and Medicine, School of Medicine, University of Virginia, Charlottesville, VA 22908-0214, USA, davidschiff@virginia.edu

Tamara N. Shenkier Division of Medical Oncology, University of British Columbia, British Columbia Cancer Agency, Vancouver, BC, V5Z 4E6, Canada, tshenkier@bccancer.bc.ca

Tali Siegal Gaffin Center for Neuro-Oncology, Hadassah Hebrew-University Medical Center, Jerusalem, Israel, siegal@hadassah.org.il

Harshabad Singh Keen Postdoctoral Research Scholar, Center for Regenerative Medicine, Massachusetts General Hospital Cancer Center, Boston, MA 02114, USA, hsingh3@partners.org

Carole Soussain Service d'Hématologie, Centre de Lutte Contre le Cancer René Huguenin, Saint-Cloud, France, soussain@crh1.org

Eckhard Thiel Department of Hematology and Oncology, Charité-Universitätsmedizin Berlin, Berlin, Germany, eckhard.thiel@charite.de

Julie Vose Section of Hematology and Oncology, University of Nebraska Medical Center, Omaha, NE 68198-7680, USA, jmvose@unmc.edu

Daphne L. Wang Department of Neurology, Stephen E. and Catherine Pappas Center for Neuro-Oncology, Massachusetts General Hospital and Harvard Medical School, Boston, MA 02114, USA, dlwang@partners.org

Patrick Y. Wen Division of Neuro-Oncology, Department of Neurology, Dana Farber Cancer Institute, Center for Neuro-Oncology, Brigham and Women's Hospital, Boston, MA 02115, USA, pwen@partners.org

Joachim Yahalom Department of Radiation Oncology, Memorial Sloan-Kettering Cancer Center, New York, NY 10065, USA, yahalomj@mskcc.org

Emanuele Zucca Lymphoma Unit, IOSI – Oncology Institute of Southern Switzerland, Ospedale San Giovanni, Bellinzona, Switzerland, emanuelezucca@yahoo.com

Part I
Introduction

Chapter 1
Overview of the Lymphoid Neoplasms

Nikolai Podoltsev, Jill Lacy, and Julie Vose

Introduction

Lymphomas comprise a diverse array of neoplasms that arise from lymphoid cells. Our current understanding of the pathogenesis of lymphomas derives from our knowledge of the immune system. Specifically, the molecular and genetic analysis of B- and T-lymphocyte development and maturation is linked directly to our conceptual framework of lymphomagenesis. It is now widely accepted that distinct subtypes of lymphoma arise from and correlate with subsets of normal lymphocytes at discrete points in lymphocyte development or maturation. Moreover, lymphomas are often associated with superimposed molecular genetic abnormalities that involve the B-cell or T-cell receptor genes and oncoproteins. Given the intimate relationship between the basic concepts of immunobiology and lymphomagenesis, the first portion of this chapter is devoted to an overview of the fundamentals of the immune system. The second portion of this chapter discusses the clinical aspects of lymphoma and includes brief descriptions of the common subtypes of lymphoma.

The Immune System

Function of the Immune System

The central role of the immune system is: (1) to detect the presence of foreign antigens derived from bacteria, viruses, fungi, parasites or tumor cells and (2) to eliminate the source of these antigens. This function is dependent on several

J. Lacy (✉)
Section of Medical Oncology, Yale University School of Medicine, New Haven, CT 06520-8032, USA
e-mail: jill.lacy@yale.edu

T. Batchelor, L.M. DeAngelis (eds.), *Lymphoma and Leukemia of the Nervous System*, DOI 10.1007/978-1-4419-7668-0_1,

highly choreographed responses of the innate and adaptive immune systems that are mediated by cytokines and specific cell–cell interactions. The phagocytic cells of the innate immune system (macrophages, neutrophils, NK cells) detect and rapidly destroy pathogenic microorganisms by defense mechanisms that do not require antigenic specificity, such as phagocytosis and release of cytokines that evoke inflammatory responses. The phagocytic cells of the innate immune system respond to a limited repertoire of foreign antigens comprised primarily of common constituents of the cell surface of bacteria, such as lipopolysaccharides. Innate immunity provides the first line of defense against common microorganisms, plays a critical role in controlling bacterial infections, and recruits the adaptive immune response via cytokine release and antigen presentation [1–5].

In contrast to the phagocytic cells of the innate immune system, B- and T-lymphocytes of the adaptive immune response bear receptors of unique antigenic specificity that are generated by genetic recombination events during lymphocyte development in the bone marrow and thymus. Genetic recombination of the immune receptor molecules generates a vast repertoire of lymphocytes with unique antigenic specificities. T- and B-cells are stimulated to differentiate into immune effector cells, proliferate, and undergo clonal expansion when foreign antigen binds to the immune receptor molecule. Clonal selection of lymphocytes, in response to specific antigens and memory for specific antigens such that subsequent exposure results in more rapid and vigorous responses, are fundamental principles of the adaptive immune response [1, 2, 4, 5].

The antigen receptor of B-cells is the surface immunoglobulin (Ig) molecule, a membrane-bound form of the soluble antibody that is produced in large quantities upon B-cell activation. Antibodies bind to foreign antigens in plasma and extracellular fluids, mediating an array of antibody-dependent immune processes, classically regarded as the humoral immune response. The antigen receptor of T-cells is structurally similar to the immunoglobulin. In contrast to surface immunoglobulins, the T-cell receptor (TCR) recognizes foreign antigens only when the antigenic peptide is complexed to proteins of the major histocompatibility complex (MHC) and displayed on the cell surface of specialized antigen-presenting cells after intra-cellular processing. The recognition of foreign antigen as a peptide fragment bound to an MHC molecule displayed at the cell surface is a unique feature of the T-cell response. T-cells perform an array of functions in the adaptive immune response, including those that are classically regarded as cellular immune responses [1, 2, 4–6].

Components of the Immune System

The immune system is comprised of lymphoid organs where lymphocyte development, activation, and proliferation occur within a highly organized framework of non-lymphoid stromal cells. The *bone marrow* and *thymus* are classified as *central* (*primary*) *lymphoid organs*, where precursor lymphocytes originate and mature. The *lymph nodes*, *spleen*, and *mucosa-associated lymphoid tissues* (*MALT*) comprise the *peripheral* (*secondary*) *lymphoid organs*, where mature lymphocytes engage antigens and undergo activation and proliferation. Lymphocytes circulate continuously through the peripheral lymphoid tissues via the vascular and lymphatic systems.

The *bone marrow* compartment is the site of lymphopoiesis and hematopoiesis. Pluripotent hematopoietic stem cells reside in the bone marrow and give rise to lymphoid and myeloid progenitors (Fig. 1.1). The bone marrow stroma, comprised of mesenchymal and epithelial cells, provides the growth factors and cell–cell interactions essential for hematopoietic stem cell survival and differentiation. B-and T-lymphocyte precursors originate in the bone marrow, but only B-cells undergo maturation in the bone marrow microenvironment. Precursor T-cells migrate from the bone marrow to the *thymus* where T cell maturation occurs in proximity to the thymic epithelial stroma in the outer (cortical) region of the thymus. The thymus reaches its peak weight during adolescence and thereafter, begins to atrophy.

Mature lymphocytes localize to *peripheral lymphoid organs* (lymph nodes, spleen, MALT). Within the microenvironment of the peripheral lymphoid tissue,

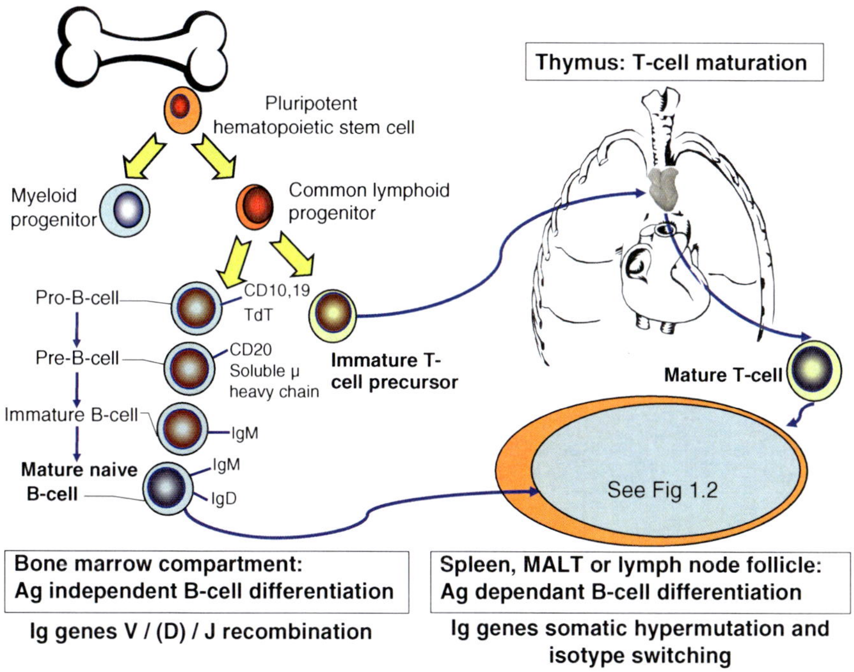

Fig. 1.1 B and T-cell development. MALT, mucosa-associated lymphoid tissue

lymphocytes encounter antigen and interact with stromal cells. These interactions orchestrate the complex processes of antigen-specific lymphocyte activation, differentiation, selection, and proliferation. Continuous circulation of lymphocytes, through these tissues via the vascular and lymphatic systems, is essential for adaptive immune surveillance.

Lymph nodes are sites of convergence of the extensive lymphatic drainage system that delivers lymph carrying soluble microbial antigens and antigen-presenting cells from peripheral tissues to the nodes. Lymph is delivered via afferent lymphatic vessels to the subcapsular sinus overlying the outer cortex, and is collected in efferent lymphatics via inter-connecting sinuses localized within the inner medulla. The cortex is organized into lymphoid follicles composed predominantly of B-cells, whereas T-cells are distributed in the surrounding para-cortical area. At the height of an immune response, lymphoid follicles develop central reactive areas, called *germinal centers*, comprised of activated and proliferating B-cells that undergo somatic hypermutation, positive antigen selection, and immunoglobulin isotype switching (Fig. 1.2). Unstimulated B-cells are pushed to the peripheral *mantle zone*. The *marginal zone* appears in the outer mantle zone and is comprised of antigen-specific B-cells with monocytoid features. The lymphoid tissue of *the spleen* traps antigens in blood rather than lymph. The spleen is comprised of red pulp, which is the site of senescent red blood cell disposal, interspersed with lymphoid areas, described as the white pulp, which surround a central arteriole. As in lymph nodes, B and T-cells are segregated within the white pulp into a periarteriolar lymphoid sheath,

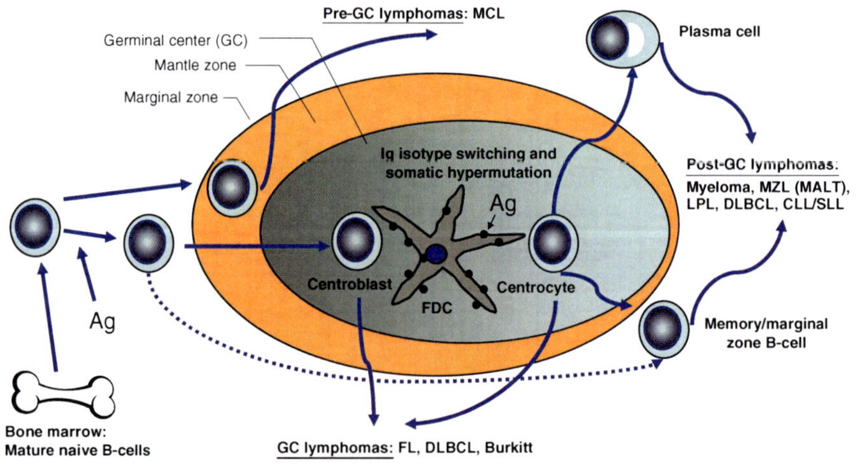

Fig. 1.2 Schematic structure of a lymph node follicle showing B-cell differentiation and its relationship with the origin of B-cell lymphomas. Ag, antigen; FDC, follicular dendritic cell; Ig, immunoglobulin; CLL/SLL, chronic lymphocytic leukemia/small lymphocytic lymphoma; DLBCL, diffuse large B-cell lymphoma; FL, follicular lymphoma; MCL, mantle cell lymphoma; MZL, marginal zone lymphoma; LPL, lymphoplasmacytic lymphoma

composed of T-cells and flanking follicles, or corona, composed of B-cells. *Mucosa-associated lymphoid tissues (MALT)* collect antigens from epithelial surfaces, and include the gut-associated lymphoid tissues (tonsils, adenoids, Peyer patches of the small intestine), as well as more diffusely organized aggregates of lymphocytes at other mucosal sites.

Lymphocytes circulate continuously in the lymphatic and vascular systems. In peripheral blood, lymphocytes comprise 20–40% of leukocytes; the proportion is higher in newborns and children. Approximately 80% of peripheral blood lymphocytes are T-cells, and the remainder is largely B-cells. The majority of peripheral blood lymphocytes are mature, resting lymphocytes that morphologically appear small with scant cytoplasm and inconspicuous nucleoli. A small percentage of peripheral blood lymphoid cells represent a third category of cells referred to as natural killer (NK) cells. NK cells do not bear the characteristic cell surface molecules of B- or T-cells, and their immunoglobulin, or TCR genes, have not undergone rearrangement. Morphologically, NK cells are described as large, granular lymphocytes, and functionally, they are part of the innate immune system.

Cells of the Immune System: Lymphocyte Development, Function, and Localization

B-Cell Development and Function

B-, or bone marrow derived, lymphocytes undergo maturation in the bone marrow compartment [7]. The earliest B-cells are derived from pluripotent, hematopoietic stem cells committed to lymphoid differentiation. Lymphoid progenitor cells are stimulated to differentiate from early pro-B cells to mature B-cells in a series of highly coordinated steps that involve sequential rearrangement of the heavy- and light-chain immunoglobulin gene segments and expression of B-cell–specific cell surface proteins (Fig. 1.1) [7]. Rearrangement of the immunoglobulin genes through recombination of the VDJ segments results in the generation of a huge repertoire of B cells that are each characterized by a surface immunoglobulin receptor molecule with unique antigenic specificity [2, 7]. The expression of B-cell specific surface proteins (e.g., CD10 or CALLA, CD19, CD20), as well as the expression of cytoplasmic and surface immunoglobulin, mark the developmental stages of B-cell maturation. Mature B-cells migrate from the bone marrow to peripheral lymphoid tissue throughout the body and are characterized by co-expression of surface IgM and IgD, as well as the presence of the B-cell specific surface proteins CD19, CD20, and CD21.

Within peripheral lymphoid tissues, mature B-cells undergo activation and proliferation after interacting with their specific antigen and helper T-cells [7]. Transition of the mature B-cell through the germinal center is accompanied by random mutations of the V regions of the heavy and light chain genes. This process, known as somatic hypermutation, generates variant surface immunoglobulins, some of which bind antigen with high affinity. When high affinity antigen binding occurs, those mature B-cells are positively selected for maturation and proliferation. In the absence of positive selection, B-cells undergo spontaneous cell death. The final steps of differentiation in the germinal center are completed with isotype switching, resulting in B-cells capable of producing a high affinity antibody of the IgM, IgG, IgA, or IgE class. B-cells exiting the germinal center, designated memory B-cells, return to the peripheral circulation. If the host is re-challenged with the same antigenic stimulus, memory B-cells, with high antigenic affinity, are rapidly activated. The activated B-cell proliferates and terminally differentiates into a mature plasma cell capable of producing large quantities of soluble antibodies. Terminal B-cell differentiation to plasma cells is marked by the loss of B-cell specific markers and surface Ig, and acquisition of plasma cell-specific markers (e.g., CD38).

Malignant lymphomas of B-cell origin appear to arise from pointed interruptions in B-cell growth and development during its course of maturation (Fig. 1.2). Thus, B-cell lymphomas are highly varied in their morphology and expression of B-cell antigens.

T-Cell Development and Function

T-cell precursors migrate from the bone marrow to the thymus where further maturation occurs [6]. In the thymus, T-cell precursors differentiate into mature T-cell subsets and undergo selection; initially, to eliminate cells without a self-recognized MHC and secondly, to eliminate autoreactive T-cells that respond to self-peptides. T-cell maturation is a highly coordinated process that involves rearrangement and expression of the T-cell receptor (TCR) genes and acquisition of cell surface proteins unique to T-cells, including CD2, CD3, CD4, CD7, and CD8. As T-cells mature in the thymus, they ultimately lose either the CD4 or CD8 protein, and thus mature T cells are composed of two major subsets: $CD4^+$ and $CD8^+$ cells. Mature CD4 and CD8 T-cells leave the thymus and migrate to peripheral lymphoid tissues, constituting 40 and 25% of lymph node and splenic lymphocytes, respectively.

Mature CD4 and CD8 T-cells subsets mediate distinct immune functions [1, 2, 6]. $CD8^+$ cells kill virus-infected or foreign cells, and thus are designated cytotoxic T-cells (CTLs). $CD4^+$ cells activate other immune response cells, such as B-cells and macrophages, by production of cytokines, and thus are considered helper T-cells. Like B-cells, T-cells express unique TCR molecules that recognize specific peptide antigens. In contrast to B-cells, T-cells only respond to peptides that are processed intracellularly and bound to, or presented by, MHC molecules. Furthermore, CD4 and CD8 T-cells are MHC-class restricted in their response to peptide/MHC complexes. CD4 cells recognize antigenic peptide fragments only when they are presented by MHC class II molecules, whereas CD8 cells only recognize antigens presented by MHC class I molecules. Antigenic peptides, complexed with MHC class I and class II molecules, originate from different sources. MHC class I molecules generally present intra-cellular, or endogenous, antigens found within the cytosol and processed through the endoplasmic reticulum. MHC class II molecules generally present antigens derived from extra-cellular sources taken up via endocytosis and processed in intra-cellular vesicles. Binding of the TCR by a specific peptide/MHC complex, triggers activation signals that leads to the expression of gene products that mediate the wide diversity of helper functions in $CD4^+$ cells or cytotoxic effector functions in $CD8^+$ cells [1, 2, 5, 6].

Neoplasia of Lymphoid Origin

Malignant transformation of lymphocytes leads to a diverse group of lymphoid malignancies that arise from T-cells or B-cells at different stages of lymphocyte maturation and differentiation [8]. Although lymphoid malignancies usually involve the lymphoid organs (described above), they can arise in or spread to virtually any site. The major clinical groupings of lymphoid malignancies include *non-Hodgkin lymphomas* (NHL), *Hodgkin lymphomas* (HL), and *plasma cell neoplasms*. Each is discussed in separate sections below.

Diagnosis of Lymphomas

Although the clinical presentation of lymphoma varies with specific subtypes, the majority of patients with a lymphoid malignancy present with painless enlargement of lymph nodes, or lymphadenopathy. There are many non-neoplastic causes of lymphadenopathy, and thus a thorough history and careful physical examination should always precede a lymph node biopsy. Cervical lymphadenopathy is often due to infections of the upper respiratory tract, including viral syndromes, infectious mononucleosis, and bacterial pharyngitis. Skin infections of the extremities can cause unilateral axillary, inguinal, or femoral adenopathy (e.g., cat-scratch fever). Generalized lymphadenopathy can result from systemic infections (e.g., human immunodeficiency virus or cytomegalovirus infection), drug reactions (e.g., phenytoin), autoimmune diseases (e.g., systemic lupus erythematosus), granulomatous and inflammatory disorders (e.g., sarcoidosis), or metabolic and storage disorders (e.g., amyloidosis, Gaucher disease). If the etiology of persistent lymphadenopathy is not apparent after a careful evaluation, an excisional lymph node biopsy should be undertaken. An enlarged supraclavicular lymph node is highly suggestive of malignancy and should always be sampled.

The diagnosis of lymphoma usually requires an excisional biopsy of a lymph node or a generous biopsy of involved lymphoid tissue. Fine-needle aspiration, or needle biopsy, is rarely sufficient for the diagnosis of lymphoid malignancy. Analysis of the pathologic specimen routinely includes both histologic examination and immunophenotyping. Immunophenotyping involves the characterization of the antigens expressed on the malignant lymphocyte, using a panel of monoclonal antibodies. Immunophenotyping permits identification of the origin of the tumor cell (B-, T-, NK- or nonlymphoid cell). In the case of B-cell NHLs, immunophenotyping can also reveal whether the process is clonal in origin (i.e., neoplastic) by determining whether the surface immunoglobulin is restricted to either kappa or lambda light chains. Molecular studies to detect TCR gene re-arrangements (e.g., PCR) are required to confirm a clonal T-cell process, although an aberrant immunophenotype is usually adequate to confirm the diagnosis of a T-cell malignancy. Immunophenotyping has become an essential aspect of the diagnosis of lymphomas, accomplished by flow cytometric analysis or by immunohistochemical studies on tissue specimens. In some cases, molecular genetic analysis for chromosomal translocations, presence of viral DNA, or immunohistochemistry (IHC) for oncoprotein expression is required to confirm the pathologic subtype of a lymphoproliferative process. If a lymph node biopsy is nondiagnostic and unexplained lymphadenopathy persists, the biopsy should be repeated.

Classification of Lymphomas

Lymphomas comprise a heterogeneous group of malignancies that differ with respect to their histology, cell of origin, immunophenotype, molecular genetic abnormalities, clinical and epidemiologic features, prognosis, and outcome with therapy. In view of the heterogeneity of lymphoid neoplasms, classification systems have been devised to identify specific pathologic subtypes that correlate with distinct clinical entities [9, 10]. The Revised European American Lymphoma (REAL) classification system, introduced in 1994 [11], incorporated not only histologic features, but also immunophenotype, cytogenetics, and epidemiologic/etiologic factors. The WHO classification finally replaced all previous classification systems in 2001 [12, 13]. In addition to NHL, HL and plasma cell malignancies were included in the WHO classification, as these entities were recognized as B-lymphoid in origin. The WHO classification was updated in 2008 to build upon recent advances and to better define heterogeneous or ambiguous categories of disease (Table 1.1). Some changes included the introduction of provisional borderline categories, the recognition of small clonal lymphoid populations, and the identification of diseases characterized by involvement of specific anatomic sites or by other clinical features such as age [14]. Unresolved issues include defining pathologic predictors of prognosis in common diseases, such as follicular lymphoma (FL), diffuse large B-cell lymphoma (DLBCL), and peripheral T-cell lymphomas (PTCL) [15].

Non-Hodgkin Lymphoma (NHL)

Etiology of NHL

There is no identifiable cause of NHL in the majority of patients. However, genetic, environmental, and epidemiologic factors have been causally linked to some types of NHL. The pathogenesis of NHLs often involves pathognomonic chromosomal

Table 1.1 WHO classification of the B-cell, T-cell, and NK-cell neoplasms [14]

Precursor B-cell neoplasms	*Precursor T-cell neoplasms*
Precursor B lymphoblastic leukemia/lymphoma	Precursor lymphoblastic leukemia/lymphoma
Mature B-cell neoplasms	*Mature T-cell and NK-cell neoplasms*
Chronic lymphocytic leukemia/small lymphocytic lymphoma	T-cell prolymphocytic leukemia
B-cell prolymphocytic leukemia	T-cell large granular lymphocytic leukemia
Splenic marginal zone lymphoma	– Chronic lymphoproliferative disorder of NK cells[a]
Hairy cell leukemia	Aggressive NK cell leukemia
Splenic lymphoma/leukemia, unclassifiable[a]	Systemic EBV$^+$ T-cell lymphoproliferative disease of childhood
– Splenic diffuse red pulp small B-cell lymphoma[a]	Hydroa vacciniforme-like lymphoma
– Hairy cell leukemia-variant[a]	Adult T-cell leukemia/lymphoma
Lymphoplasmacytic lymphoma	Extranodal NK/T-cell lymphoma, nasal type
– Waldenström macroglobulinemia	Enteropathy-associated T-cell lymphoma
Heavy chain diseases	Hepatosplenic T-cell lymphoma
– Alpha heavy chain disease	Subcutaneous panniculitis-like T-cell lymphoma
– Gamma heavy chain disease	Mycosis fungoides
– Mu heavy chain disease	Sézary syndrome
Plasma cell myeloma	Primary cutaneous CD30$^+$ T-cell lymphoproliferative disorders
Solitary plasmacytoma of bone	– Lymphomatoid papulosis
Extraosseous plasmacytoma	– Primary cutaneous anaplastic large cell lymphoma
Extranodal marginal zone lymphoma of mucosa-associated lymphoid tissue (MALT lymphoma)	Primary cutaneous gamma-delta T-cell lymphoma
Nodal marginal zone lymphoma	Primary cutaneous CD8$^+$ aggressive epidermotropic cytotoxic T-cell lymphoma[a]
– Pediatric nodal marginal zone lymphoma[a]	Primary cutaneous CD4$^+$ small/medium T-cell lymphoma[a]
Follicular lymphoma	Peripheral T-cell lymphoma, NOS
– Pediatric follicular lymphoma[a]	Angioimmunoblastic T-cell lymphoma
Primary cutaneous follicle center lymphoma	Anaplastic large cell lymphoma, *ALK*$^+$
Mantle cell lymphoma	Anaplastic large cell lymphoma, ALK$^-$[a]
Diffuse large B-cell lymphoma (DLBCL), NOS	*Hodgkin lymphoma*
– T-cell/histiocyte rich large B-cell lymphoma	Nodular lymphocyte-predominant Hodgkin lymphoma
– Primary DLBCL of the CNS	Classical Hodgkin lymphoma
– Primary cutaneous DLBCL, leg type	– Nodular sclerosis classical Hodgkin lymphoma
– EBV$^+$ DLBCL of the elderly[a]	– Lymphocyte-rich classical Hodgkin lymphoma
DLBCL associated with chronic inflammation	– Mixed cellularity classical Hodgkin lymphoma
Lymphomatoid granulomatosis	– Lymphocyte-depleted classical Hodgkin lymphoma
Primary mediastinal (thymic) large B-cell lymphoma	
Intravascular large B-cell lymphoma	
ALK$^+$ large B-cell lymphoma	
Plasmablastic lymphoma	
Large B-cell lymphoma arising in HHV8-associated multicentric Castleman disease	

Table 1.1 (continued)

Primary effusion lymphoma Burkitt lymphoma B-cell lymphoma, unclassifiable, with features intermediate between diffuse large B-cell lymphoma and Burkitt lymphoma B-cell lymphoma, unclassifiable, with features intermediate between diffuse large B-cell lymphoma and classical Hodgkin lymphoma	*Posttransplantation lymphoproliferative disorders (PTLD)* Early lesions – Plasmacytic hyperplasia – Infectious mononucleosis-like PTLD Polymorphic PTLD Monomorphic PTLD (B- and T/NK-cell types)[b] Classical Hodgkin lymphoma type PTLD[b]

[a]Provisional entities for which the WHO Working Group felt there was insufficient evidence to recognize as distinct diseases at this time.
[b]These lesions are classified according to the leukemia or lymphoma to which they correspond.

Table 1.2 Chromosomal translocations associated with some common NHL types [16]

Lymphoma classification	Translocation	Oncogene (protein)	Oncogene function
Follicular	t(14;18)	*Bcl*-2	Anti-apoptosis
Mantle cell	t(11;14)	*CCND*1 (Cyclin D1)	Cell cycle regulator
Diffuse large B-cell	t(14;18)	*Bcl*-2	Anti-apoptosis
	3q27	*Bcl*-6	Transcription deregulation
Burkitt	t(8;14), t(8;22), t(2;8)	*C-myc*	Transcription deregulation
Anaplastic large T-cell	t(2;5)	*NPM/ALK*	Tyrosine kinase
MALT	t(11;18)	*API2/MLT*	Anti-apoptosis

translocations that juxtapose the immunoglobulin or TCR locus and an oncogene (Table 1.2) [16]; however, the cause of these aberrant chromosomal rearrangements is unknown. Patients with immune dysregulation from congenital immunodeficiency syndromes, autoimmune disorders, or acquired immunodeficiency states (HIV infection, iatrogenic immunsuppression) are at increased risk of developing NHL. Oncogenic human viruses play a causal role in some uncommon NHL variants. Epstein–Barr virus (EBV) is associated with HIV-related aggressive lymphomas, post-transplantation lymphoproliferative disorders (PTLD), and endemic Burkitt lymphoma. Human T-lymphotropic virus 1 (HTLV-1) is causally linked with adult T-cell leukemia/lymphoma that is endemic in southern Japan and in the Caribbean basin. The Kaposi sarcoma herpes virus (HHV-8) has been implicated in a variant of aggressive NHL that arises in serosal cavities (primary effusion lymphoma) and is encountered almost exclusively in HIV-infected patients. Hepatitis C virus (HCV) infection is associated with indolent NHL subtypes, including follicular, lymphoplasmacytic, and marginal zone variants. Bacterial infections have been linked to some marginal zone lymphomas: *Helicobacter pylori* infection is associated with gastric MALT lymphoma, and *Chlamydia psittaci* has been linked to ocular adnexal marginal zone lymphomas.

Clinical Presentation, Initial Evaluation, Staging, and Response Assessment

Most patients with NHL will present with painless lymphadenopathy, involving one or more nodal regions. Additionally, NHL may involve extranodal sites, and thus patients can present with a variety of symptoms related to the site of involvement. The most common sites of extranodal disease are the gastrointestinal tract, bone marrow, liver, and Waldeyer ring, although virtually any site can be involved with NHL. In general, the aggressive subtypes of NHL are more likely than the indolent lymphomas to involve extranodal sites. Central nervous system involvement, including leptomeningeal dissemination, rarely occurs in the indolent subtypes, but does occur in the aggressive variants. The most aggressive NHLs (Burkitt and lymphoblastic) have a particular propensity to disseminate to the leptomeninges. Involvement of brain parenchyma in systemic NHL is rare. However, aggressive NHL can arise in the brain parenchyma as the primary site of disease, and this entity is classified as primary central nervous system lymphoma (discussed in detail in subsequent chapters). Constitutional symptoms such as fevers, weight loss, or night sweats (designated "B" symptoms) occur in 20% of patients with NHL at presentation and are more common in patients with aggressive subtypes.

The diagnosis of NHL requires an adequate biopsy of the involved nodal tissue with immunophenotyping, as described above (Section "Diagnosis of Lymphomas"). In patients with bone marrow and peripheral blood involvement, such as chronic lymphocytic leukemia/small lymphocytic lymphoma (CLL/SLL), it is often possible to make a definitive diagnosis from immunophenotyping of peripheral blood lymphocytes by flow cytometry. Once the diagnosis of NHL is made, patients should undergo a complete staging evaluation to determine the extent of involvement. Staging is important to assess prognosis and may influence the choice of therapy for some subtypes of NHL. In general, the modified Ann Arbor staging classification is used to stage patients with both NHL and HL (Table 1.3). However, for CLL, the Binet or Rai staging systems are used (Table 1.4). The standard staging evaluation includes: (1) a careful history to elicit symptoms referable to the lymphoma including the presence of "B" symptoms, (2) a complete physical examination with documentation of the size and distribution of enlarged lymph nodes, (3) blood tests that include lactate dehydrogenase (LDH), (4) bone marrow aspirate and biopsy, and (5) computed tomography (CT) of chest, abdomen, and pelvis. Positron emission tomography (PET) scans can be helpful in assessing response to therapy in metabolically active NHL subtypes and is included routinely in the staging evaluation of the aggressive and highly aggressive NHLs. A diagnostic lumbar puncture for CSF cytology is necessary only in patients at risk for leptomeningeal involvement, which includes all patients with Burkitt and lymphoblastic lymphoma, and patients with DLBCL with involvement of bone marrow, testes, or structures abutting the central nervous system (e.g., paranasal sinuses, paravertebral, and epidural sites).

Table 1.3 Ann Arbor staging classification for Non-Hodgkin lymphomas

Stage	Area of involvement
I	One lymph node region
IE	Involvement of single extra-nodal site
II	Two or more lymph node regions on the same side of the diaphragm
IIE	NHL in extra-lymphatic site with involved lymph node region on the same side of the diaphragm
III	Two or more lymph node groups on both sides of the diaphragm
IIIE	Two or more lymph node groups on both sides of the diaphragm with an extra-nodal site
IV	One or more lymph node regions with diffuse involvement of one or more extra-nodal sites

Modifiers for NHL and HL:
A – no systemic symptoms present
B – presence of any B symptom: weight loss greater than 10% of body weight over the preceding 6 months; fever higher than 38°C unrelated to any infections; and drenching night sweats
E – extra-nodal involvement adjacent to affected lymph node group
S – spleen involvement
X – bulky disease is present (a mediastinal mass with a maximum width that is equal to or greater than one-third of the internal transverse diameter of the thorax at the level of T5/6 interspace or > 10 cm maximum dimension of a nodal mass)
CS – clinical stage
PS – pathologic stage

Table 1.4 Rai & Binet staging systems for chronic lymphocytic leukemia

Rai stage	*Risk*	*Definition*
0	Low	Lymphocytosis only
I	Intermediate	Lymphocytosis and lymphadenopathy
II	Intermediate	Lymphocytosis, lymphadenopathy with hepatomegaly or splenomegaly
III	High	Lymphocytosis and anemia
IV	High	Lymphocytosis and thrombocytopenia
Binet stage	*Risk*	*Definition*
A	Low	Lymphocytosis with fewer than three areas of lymph node involvement
B	Intermediate	Lymphocytosis with more than three areas of lymph node involvement
C	High	Lymphocytosis with anemia and/or thrombocytopenia

A variety of ancillary tests may be performed in specific situations. For example, a test for HTLV-I or HIV should be performed if adult T-cell leukemia/lymphoma or HIV-associated lymphoma is suspected, respectively. A gastrointestinal series or endoscopic evaluation is warranted in any patient with gastrointestinal symptoms or in those at risk for gastrointestinal tract involvement (lymphomas involving the Waldeyer ring). Serum and urine protein electrophoresis (SPEP, UPEP) and determination of serum free light chains, beta$_2$-microglobulin, and quantitative immunoglobulins should be performed if a plasma cell malignancy is suspected. A laparotomy for the sole purpose of staging is never performed, as it no longer influences therapeutic decisions.

A variety of prognostic variables have been identified for NHL. Consistent predictors for poor survival of patients with aggressive NHLs include advanced stage at presentation (stage III or IV), involvement of multiple extranodal sites of disease, elevated LDH, presence of "B" symptoms, and poor performance status. These variables have been incorporated into the International Prognostic Index (IPI), which is useful for predicting outcome in most subtypes of NHL (Table 1.5) [17, 18].

Table 1.5 Non-Hodgkin Lymphoma International Prognostic Index (IPI)

Standard IPI risk group[a] [17]	*Number of risk factors*	*5-year OS (%)*
Low	0 or 1	73
Low intermediate	2	51
High intermediate	3	43
High	4 or 5	26
Revised IPI risk group[b] [46]	*Number of risk factors*	*4-year OS (%)*
Very good	0	94
Good	1,2	79
Poor	3,4,5	55

Risk factors: age >60 years; ECOG performance status 2–4; LDH > normal; > 1 extranodal site; Ann Arbor stage III/IV. OS – overall survival.
[a]Developed in pre-rituximab era.
[b]DLBCL patients treated with CHOP-R.

Assessment of response to treatment in NHL is based on consensus criteria that include lymph node or tumor mass size as measured by CT scan, metabolic activity on PET scan, and extent of bone marrow involvement as assessed by biopsy, IHC, and flow cytometry. The incorporation of functional (PET) imaging has eliminated the need for a designation of "complete remission unconfirmed" (CRu) category for patients with residual tumor masses on CT scan containing only fibrotic tissue [19].

Natural History, Prognosis, and Treatment of Specific Common Subtypes of NHL

Given the large number of NHL subtypes, it is useful to broadly categorize NHLs into groupings that share common clinical features, such as aggressiveness, potential for cure, and approach to treatment. The clinically useful categories are termed *indolent*, *aggressive,* and *highly aggressive* lymphomas (Table 1.6).

Table 1.6 Common NHL subtypes classified by clinical aggressiveness

The indolent lymphomas	The aggressive lymphomas	The highly aggressive lymphomas
– Follicular lymphoma (grade I and II) – Small lymphocytic lymphoma/B-cell chronic lymphocytic leukemia – Marginal zone B-cell lymphoma – Lymphoplasmacytic lymphoma (Waldenstrom macroglobulinemia) – Plasma cell myeloma/plasmacytoma	– Follicular lymphoma (grade III) – Diffuse large B-cell lymphoma – Mantle cell lymphoma	– Burkitt lymphoma – Precursor B lymphoblastic leukemia/lymphoma – Precursor T lymphoblastic leukemia/lymphoma

Indolent NHLs

The most common indolent NHLs are small B-cell lymphomas, such as follicular lymphoma (FL), chronic lymphocytic leukemia/small lymphocytic lymphoma (CLL/SLL), and marginal zone lymphoma (MZL), including mucosa-associated lymphoid tissue (MALT) lymphoma, splenic and nodal MZL, as well as lymphoplasmacytic lymphoma (LPL).

Clinically, indolent NHLs are generally characterized by an indolent course associated with long survival and responsiveness to a variety of treatments. However, paradoxically, they are rarely curable with standard treatment modalities [20]. These clinical features have led to the practice of deferring treatment in asymptomatic patients with advanced disease until the development of tumor-related symptoms.

Follicular Lymphoma (FL)

FL is the most common indolent NHL sub-type and accounts for 22% of all NHL. The histopathology of FL is characterized by the presence of neoplastic "nodules" in lymph nodes that mimic germinal centers of secondary follicles. The malignant lymphocyte is a mature B-cell that demonstrates the presence of kappa- or lambda-restricted surface Ig, pan B-cell markers (CD19, CD20), and CD10, and absence of CD5. FL is characterized cytogenetically by the t(14;18) that juxtaposes the Ig heavy chain locus with the anti-apoptotic gene *Bcl*-2. Over-expression of Bcl-2 is a hallmark of FL, although Bcl-2 is also expressed in 30% of DLBCL. The WHO classification defines three histologic grades based on the number of follicular centroblasts per high power field; Grades 1 and 2 are designated "low grade," whereas Grade 3 (>15 centroblasts/hpf) is an aggressive NHL similar to DLBCL [15].

Table 1.7 The follicular lymphoma international prognostic index (FLIPI)

Risk group	Number of risk factors	5-year OS (%)[a] [21]	2-year TTF (%)[b] [22]
Low	0 or 1	90.6	92
Intermediate	2	77.6	90
High	≥ 3	53	67

Risk factors: Nodal regions > 4; LDH > normal; age > 60 years; stage III/IV; hemoglobin < 12 g/dL. OS – overall survival; TTF – time to treatment failure.
[a]Developed in pre-rituximab era.
[b]FL patients treated with CHOP-R.

Although FLs are generally indolent neoplasms (median survival approaches 10 years), the majority of patients (70%) present with advanced disease (stage III or IV), often with bone marrow involvement, and such patients cannot be cured with current treatment modalities. The clinical course and outcome of FL can be quite variable, and the Follicular Lymphoma International Prognostic Index (FLIPI) may be useful in determining prognosis (Table 1.7) [21, 22]. Most patients with FL eventually experience transformation of their disease to a more aggressive histology, characterized by rapidly enlarging lymph nodes or tumor masses, rising LDH, and onset of "B" symptoms.

The management of low grade FL is determined by stage and clinical symptoms [23]. For those few patients with early-stage disease (I or non-bulky II), the appropriate treatment is radiation therapy. More than half of the patients with early-stage disease will achieve a durable remission and may be cured with involved field, subtotal, or total lymphoid irradiation. For patients with bulky or advanced-stage disease, multiple systemic treatment options are available, and clinical practices vary widely. Although advanced-stage FL is responsive to a variety of treatments, the long natural history, incurability, and failure to demonstrate survival benefit with immediate treatment has led to the "watch and wait" approach of deferring therapy until the patient develops symptoms. Indications for treatment include cosmetic or mechanical problems caused by enlarging lymph nodes, constitutional symptoms, rapid disease progression, or evidence of organ or bone marrow compromise.

The appropriate initial treatment of advanced-stage FL, when necessary, is chemotherapy in combination with the monoclonal anti-CD20 antibody, rituximab [24–28]. The addition of rituximab to chemotherapy improves response rate and duration and overall survival compared to chemotherapy alone, with little added toxicity, and it is now used routinely in the treatment of FL [26]. Single oral alkylating agents (cyclophosphamide or chlorambucil), alkylator-based, multi-drug regimens (e.g., CVP [cyclophosphamide, vincristine, prednisone]), or fludarabine-based regimens (e.g., fludarabine with mitoxantrone or cyclophosphamide), are all effective, initial regimens. When rapid cytoreduction is desirable, the multi-drug chemotherapy regimens are preferred [24, 25]. Alternatively, rituximab alone may be used in selected patients with low-bulk symptomatic disease. The majority of patients respond to initial treatment, and at least one third achieve a complete remission that lasts 1–3 years. Treatment should be discontinued when the maximum response has been achieved to minimize cumulative toxicity. Maintenance therapy with rituximab after initial treatment has been shown to prolong duration of response, but its impact on survival is uncertain. At relapse, a patient can be re-treated with rituximab alone, or in combination with chemotherapy, using the same regimen, if the initial response was durable, or different agents (e.g., bendamustine) [29–32]; maintenance rituximab, after re-treatment of relapsed disease, improves both progression-free and overall survival [32]. Treatment with anti-CD20 radioimmunoconjugates (ibritumomab or tositumomab) is another effective option for relapsed FL and is associated with a high response rate [31].

The role of high-dose chemotherapy with autologous or allogeneic stem cell transplant in the management of FL remains unclear [33]. Transplantation procedures are not recommended for patients in first remission, but may be considered for selected patients with relapsed FL. Long term follow-up of patients undergoing allogeneic transplant suggests that some patients are cured with this modality, although the associated morbidity has precluded its widespread use in refractory FL.

For patients who have clinical or pathologic evidence of transformation to a higher grade lymphoma, treatment that is appropriate for DLBCL should be offered (discussed below).

Chronic Lymphocytic Leukemia/Small Lymphocytic Lymphoma (CLL/SLL)

CLL and SLL are indolent B-cell lymphoid malignancies characterized by involvement of the bone marrow, peripheral blood, and nodal tissue. In the WHO classification, CLL and SLL are clinically the same disease entities, representing 6% of all NHLs. Tumor cells of CLL/SLL are monomorphic small B-cells that are faintly positive for surface Ig and express pan B-cell antigens (CD19, CD20). CLL/SLL cells characteristically express both CD5, which marks a subset of normal B-cells as well as mature T-cells, and CD23 (the Fc receptor for IgE). CD23 is helpful in distinguishing CLL/SLL from mantle cell lymphoma, which also expresses CD5, but does not express CD23. Approximately 40% of CLL/SLL show somatic hypermutations of immunoglobulin variable regions (IgV_H), indicating exposure to the germinal center and antigenic selection, as well as favorable outcome.

A diagnosis of CLL requires a blood count of > 5,000 CLL-phenotype cells per cubic millimeter. Asymptomatic persons with fewer cells have monoclonal B-cell lymphocytosis (MBL), which evolves to symptomatic CLL at the rate of 1.1% per year [34]. Patients with CLL/SLL typically present with asymptomatic lymphadenopathy or lymphocytosis. Less common presenting features of CLL/SLL include "B" symptoms, recurrent infections related to hypogammaglobulinemia, or hematologic autoimmune diseases (hemolytic anemia or thrombocytopenia) that may accompany CLL/SLL. Staging of CLL is based on the Rai or Binet system endorsed by the International Workshop on CLL (Table 1.4) [35]. Most patients with CLL have early stage disease at diagnosis (Rai 0 or I). Patients with early-stage disease are a heterogeneous group in that 30–50% will have accelerated disease progression, and the remainder may live for decades and possibly never require therapy. Prognostic factors predictive of poor outcome include high lymphocyte count (>40–50 × 10^9/L), short lymphocyte doubling time (<12 months), prolymphocytic morphology, advanced clinical stage, and hypogammaglobulinemia. Unmutated IgV_H and high expression of CD38 or zeta-associated protein 70 (ZAP-70) also predict an unfavorable outcome. Cytogenetic abnormalities are found in approximately 80% of patients and carry prognostic significance. Deletions of 11q and 17p are associated with poor survival and resistance to chemotherapy, whereas deletion of 13q14 as a sole abnormality is associated with a favorable outcome [36].

CLL/SLL is usually an indolent, slowly progressive disorder with a median survival in excess of 7 years. Standard therapies may palliate symptoms and prolong survival, but are not curative. Therefore, treatment should be withheld in asymptomatic patients until the development of tumor-related symptoms (e.g., bulky lymphadenopathy, "B" symptoms, or cytopenias caused by bone marrow infiltration or autoimmune phenomenon). As with FL, when systemic treatment for CLL/SLL is required, there are multiple effective chemotherapy options, including the nucleoside analog fludarabine, a monoclonal antibody to the pan-lymphocyte marker CD52, alemtuzumab, or an alkylating agent, such as chlorambucil or bendamustine. Treatment with fludarabine, bendamustine, or alemtuzumab is associated with superior response rates compared with chlorambucil [37–39]. Combination regimens (e.g., FCR [fludarabine, cyclophosphamide, rituximab]) have shown particularly encouraging results, albeit with greater toxicity compared to single agents. Fludarabine/rituximab combinations can be associated with tumor lysis syndrome and severe infusion reactions in CLL, and appropriate precautions should be taken. The majority of patients respond to initial treatment with significant reductions in tumor burden. Treatment is generally continued as long as patients are responding to and tolerating therapy, but there is no evidence that maintenance therapy is of benefit. Patients with recurrent disease, occurring >6 months after the discontinuation of treatment, often can be successfully re-treated with the initial regimen. Other active agents in recurrent disease include rituximab or alemtuzumab [40–42]. Patients with hypogammaglobulinemia and recurrent infections may benefit from intravenous gamma globulin infusions, and those with autoimmune anemia and thrombocytopenia require corticosteroids. Allogeneic hematopoietic transplantation may provide curative therapy for eligible patients. The development of a rapidly enlarging mediastinal mass, constitutional symptoms, and high serum LDH suggests transformation of disease to a DLBCL, designated the Richter syndrome, which is associated with a poor prognosis.

Extranodal Marginal Zone B-Cell Lymphoma of Mucosa-Associated Lymphoid Tissue (MALT)

MALT lymphomas are low-grade, indolent NHL subtypes that involve mucosa-associated lymphoid tissue in a variety of sites, including stomach, lung, thyroid, salivary gland, and orbit. These lymphomas comprise 5% of NHL. Many patients with MALT lymphoma have an underlying autoimmune disorder, such as Sjogren syndrome or Hashimoto thyroiditis, and the presence of activated antigen-driven T-cells may play a role in the pathogenesis of these lymphomas.

Given the excellent prognosis, localized nature, and long natural history of the MALT lymphomas (>80% of patients survive for more than 8 years), they are generally managed conservatively with local treatment modalities (irradiation or surgery) and avoidance of systemic chemotherapy. Importantly, gastric MALT lymphomas are frequently associated with *H. pylori* infection, and remissions can be achieved with eradication of this infection. Thus, antibiotics are the appropriate first-line treatment for these patients. Patients who fail to respond to antibiotics may be treated with rituximab alone or in combination with chemotherapy, similar to low grade FLs.

Lymphoplasmacytic Lymphoma (LPL)

LPL is an indolent malignancy of plasmacytoid lymphocytes, comprising 1–2% of all NHLs. LPLs arise from the post-germinal center cell that has undergone somatic hypermutation, but not heavy-chain class switch, and is characterized by the presence, both cytoplasmic and surface IgM, pan B-cell antigens (CD19, CD20), and absence of CD5, CD10, and CD23.

LPL usually affects older adults (median age 63). It manifests features of both a low-grade NHL and a plasma cell dyscrasia, with lymphadenopathy, hepatosplenomegaly, bone marrow infiltration, and, in the majority of patients, the presence of an IgM monoclonal paraprotein (Waldenström macroglobulinemia). Less than 5% of LPL patients secrete non-IgM monoclonal paraprotein. The major clinical manifestation of Waldenström macroglobulinemia is the hyperviscosity syndrome caused by the physical properties of IgM. Epistaxis, retinal hemorrhages, neurologic symptoms, and congestive heart failure are common manifestations of hyperviscosity syndrome. Approximately 10% of IgM proteins have properties of cryoglobulins, and these patients present with symptoms of cryoglobulinemia or cold agglutinin syndrome. Non-lymphoid tissues may be involved in LPL by infiltration of malignant cells, deposition of light chains or amyloid fibrils.

Indications for immediate treatment include hyperviscosity syndrome, cytopenias, bulky adenopathy or organomegaly, peripheral neuropathy, cryoglobulinemia, and amyloidosis. The approach to and treatment of LPL is similar to that of CLL/SLL. The use of fludarabine or an alkylating agent, alone or in combination with prednisone, is effective in decreasing the tumor burden and M spike, but is not curative. Rituximab has activity in LPL, as does the proteosome inhibitor bortezomib. Patients who develop hyperviscosity syndrome require plasmapharesis [43]. The median survival of patients with LPL who respond to treatment is 4 years, and some patients survive more than 10 years.

Aggressive NHLs

The aggressive NHLs are characterized pathologically by effacement of lymph node architecture with a diffuse infiltrate of large lymphocytes. They are comprised of several distinct disease entities, including diffuse large B-cell lymphoma

(DLBCL, 31% of NHL), primary mediastinal large B-cell lymphoma (PMLBCL, 2% of NHL), peripheral T-cell lymphoma (PTCL, 6% of NHL), and anaplastic large cell lymphoma (ALCL, 2% of NHL). Mantle cell lymphoma (MCL, 6% of NHL) is characterized by a diffuse infiltration of small- to intermediate-sized lymphocytes, and although MCL is clinically heterogeneous, it often pursues an aggressive clinical course and is discussed herein. Grade 3 FL is considered biologically aggressive and is managed similarly to DLBCL. The aggressive NHLs are usually B-cell in origin (Table 1.6), and are characterized by clonal surface Ig and pan B-cell markers. In contrast to indolent NHLs, the aggressive NHL subtypes generally require immediate treatment and are potentially curable. With the exception of mantle cell lymphoma, the treatment approaches to the distinct subtypes of aggressive NHL subtypes are similar.

Diffuse Large B-Cell Lymphoma (DLBCL)

DLBCL represents a pathogenetically diverse subtype. Several distinct cytogenetic abnormalities have been identified (Table 1.2), including t(14;18) with involvement of *Bcl*-2, and 3q abnormalities with involvement of *Bcl*-6, a zinc finger transcriptional repressor. Molecular profiling has revealed three distinct gene expression groups that correlate with survival after chemotherapy: germinal center B cell-like (GCB), activated B cell-like (ABC), and not-otherwise-specified type 3 [44, 45]. However, it is not clear how this information should be used in selecting treatment. The typical immunophenotype of DLBCL is kappa- or lambda-restricted surface Ig+/CD20+/CD45+. It is important to distinguish DLBCL from other diffuse large cell NHLs, including PTCLs, which carry a worse prognosis, compared with their B-cell counterparts. Primary CNS lymphoma (PCNSL) is a diffuse aggressive B-cell NHL that arises in brain parenchyma and rarely spreads systemically. PCNSL has distinct clinical features and unique management issues, and is discussed separately in subsequent chapters.

DLBCL exhibits clinically aggressive behavior, and if left untreated, the median survival can be measured in months. Compared with the indolent lymphomas, a higher percentage of patients with DLBCL present with a localized extranodal site of involvement (30%), early-stage disease (40–50%), or "B" symptoms (30%). Only 16% of patients with DLBCL have bone marrow involvement. The outcome and likelihood of cure of patients with diffuse aggressive histologies is directly related to the total number of adverse prognostic features present at clinical presentation, as described by the IPI (Table 1.5) [17, 46]. The likelihood of 4-year progression-free survival in the post-rituximab era ranges from 94% in patients with no adverse factors to 53% in patients with three or more adverse factors.

All patients with DLBCL should be offered immediate therapy, as it is a potentially curable lymphoma. Standard initial therapy is a multidrug chemotherapy regimen that includes an anthracycline in combination with the anti-CD20 monoclonal antibody, rituximab. The most widely used regimen is CHOP-R (cyclophosphamide, doxorubicin, vincristine, prednisone, and rituximab), as it is equivalent to more complex and intensive regimens [47]. The addition of rituximab increases survival with almost no increase in toxicity [48, 49]. Patients with early-stage disease (I or II) may be treated with involved field radiation therapy after a minimum of three cycles of CHOP-R. Patients with advanced-stage disease require six to eight cycles of CHOP-R given at 21- or 14-day intervals with growth factor support to maintain dose intensities [50–52]. The role of local radiation to sites of bulky disease in the setting of advanced-stage disease is not established.

Patients who relapse after achieving a remission often can be cured with high-dose chemotherapy with autologous stem cell transplantation if their relapsed disease is chemosensitive (i.e., responsive to standard doses of chemotherapy) [53]. This procedure is superior to conventional salvage chemotherapy and is considered the standard of care for relapsed chemosensitive DLBCL.

Mantle Cell Lymphoma (MCL)

With the advent of routine immunophenotyping, MCL has been recognized with increasing frequency, representing 6% of NHLs. MCLs are mature B-cell neoplasms that arise in the mantle zone of the lymphoid follicle and display a highly characteristic immunophenotype [54, 55]. Like CLL/SLL, mantle cells express CD5, as well as surface Ig and pan B-cell markers (CD19, CD20), but in contrast to CLL/SLL, are negative for CD23 and positive for FMC7. Because MCL can be confused pathologically and clinically with CLL/SLL, absence of CD23 is important for distinguishing these subtypes. MCL is characterized by a pathognomonic translocation, t(11;14), juxtaposing the Ig heavy chain locus and the *cyclin D*1 locus (*CCND*1), resulting in dysregulated expression of cyclin D1. Nuclear staining for cyclin D1 expression by IHC is present in >90% of cases of MCL. Presence of t(11;14) is considered diagnostic of MCL, even in CD5-negative cases, and can be detected by fluorescent in-situ hydridization (FISH) analysis.

MCLs share some similarities with indolent lymphomas, in that patients usually present with advanced-stage disease with frequent bone marrow involvement. These lymphomas have a propensity to involve Waldeyer ring and the gastrointestinal tract, often with diffuse intestinal polyposis. As with the low-grade FLs, MCLs are treatable, but rarely curable. However, unlike indolent lymphomas, MCLs are usually biologically aggressive with a median survival of just 3–5 years. A small subset of patients (10–20%) have an indolent course with longer survival and may not require treatment at diagnosis. Unfortunately, there are no reliable tools to identify these patients prospectively. In contrast, patients with the blastic variant or a high IPI score have a worse prognosis [55–57].

The majority of patients with MCL require treatment at diagnosis. Despite response rates of 60–90%, durable remissions are difficult to achieve, and the optimal treatment program for this challenging NHL subtype remains uncertain. Outside of a clinical trial, patients are treated with a conventional chemotherapy regimen, such as CHOP, or an intensive regimen, such as HyperCVAD (hyperfractionated cyclophosphamide, vincristine, doxorubicin, and dexamethasone alternating with high-dose methotrexate and cytarabine) in combination with rituximab [58–60]. Consolidation with high dose chemotherapy and autologous transplant may be offered to patients who respond to initial therapy, with an improvement in response durability but uncertain survival benefit and curative potential [61]. Patients with refractory or relapsed disease can be treated with a salvage regimen that may include bortezomib or bendamustine [62, 63]. Allogeneic transplantation may be considered for the same group of patients if a suitable donor is available, but its role in the management of this lymphoma subtype has not been established.

Highly Aggressive NHL

Burkitt and lymphoblastic lymphoma represent <1 and 2% of NHLs, respectively, and are the most aggressive subtypes of NHL. Although uncommon, these subtypes are important because they predominantly affect young adults (median age 30) and are potentially curable with appropriate therapy. These lymphomas are characterized by a high degree of cellular proliferation, as determined by the Ki-67 proliferation index. Patients require urgent inpatient treatment at diagnosis because of rapid tumor growth with compromised organ function and the potential for tumor lysis on initiation of therapy. Due to frequent involvement of the leptomeninges, diagnostic lumbar puncture, as well prophylactic intrathecal administration of methotrexate and/or cytarabine is required.

Lymphoblastic lymphomas are highly aggressive lymphoid malignancies that arise from precursor B or T-cells. The majority are T-cell in origin (90%), and in the WHO classification are defined as the same clinical entity as T-cell acute lymphocytic leukemia (designated precursor T-lymphoblastic lymphoma/leukemia). Lymphoblastic lymphoma is readily distinguished from most NHLs by its aberrant T-cell immunophenotype and the presence of the lymphoid precursor marker, terminal deoxynucleotide transferase (TdT). Lymphoblastic lymphoma usually afflicts young adult men, involves the mediastinum and bone marrow, and has a propensity to relapse in the leptomeninges.

Burkitt lymphoma (BL) is a rare B-cell lymphoma in adults. In central Africa, BL is endemic in children and is associated with EBV infection. In the United States and Western Europe, sporadic BL affects both children and young adults, and is usually EBV-negative. HIV testing should be performed in all patients with BL due to the frequency of this association. Like lymphoblastic lymphoma, BL is highly aggressive with a propensity to involve the bone marrow and the central nervous system. A high proliferation rate, as well as a high rate of apoptotic cell death is responsible for two characteristic pathological findings: frequent mitotic figures with the fraction of Ki-67+ (MIB-1+) cells approaching 100% and a "starry-sky" appearance with numerous macrophages that have ingested apoptotic tumor cells (tingible body macrophages). BL is characterized by the presence of pan B-cell markers (CD19, CD20), CD10, bcl-6, kappa- or lambda-restricted surface IgM, and the absence of CD5, CD23, bcl-2, and TdT. BL cells harbor one of the pathognomonic chromosomal translocations, t(8;14) (80% of the patients), t(8;22), or t(2;8), which juxtaposes an *Ig* locus (heavy chain, or kappa or lambda light chain), with the *C-myc* oncogene, located on chromosome 8.

BL and lymphoblastic lymphomas both require specialized treatment with intensive multi-agent systemic chemotherapy and intrathecal chemotherapy to prevent leptomeningeal relapse, with 2-year survival of 70–80% [64–66]. Lymphoblastic lymphoma has been treated with acute lymphoblastic leukemia regimens, with a 3-year survival approaching 70% [67–69]. Since these lymphomas undergo tumor lysis upon initiation of chemotherapy, it is imperative that all patients are hospitalized and receive prophylaxis against tumor lysis syndrome before and during their first course of chemotherapy, including vigorous hydration and the use of allopurinol or rasburicase [70].

Hodgkin Lymphoma (HL)

Diagnosis, Pathology, Natural History, and Staging

Although HL arises from B-lymphoid cells, it is clinically and morphologically distinct from NHL. HL is the most common lymphoma in young adults. In industrialized countries, there is an age-dependent bimodal distribution with the larger peak occurring between ages 15 and 35, and a smaller peak occurring in patients older than age 50. The etiology of HL remains enigmatic. Although EBV is frequently present in the malignant cell of HL, a direct causal link between EBV and HL has not been established. HL does not appear with increased frequency in patients with congenital immunodeficiency syndromes, or in immunosuppressed organ transplant recipients, but there is an increased risk of HL in HIV-infected patients.

The diagnosis of HL is made by identifying the Reed-Sternberg (RS) cell in lymphoid tissue. The classic RS cell is large and binucleated, with each nucleus containing a prominent nucleolus, suggesting the appearance of "owl's eyes". In contrast to NHL, the bulk of the infiltrate in lymph nodes involved with HL is usually composed of benign reactive inflammatory cells, and often the diagnostic RS cells can be difficult to find (often only 2–3% of the total cells in the tumor). Classic RS cells have a distinct immunophenotype that is positive for CD30 (Ki-1), CD15, and CD25 (IL-2 receptor) and negative for CD20, CD45, and cytoplasmic or surface immunoglobulin [71].

The WHO classifies HL as "classical" HL (CHL, 95% of cases) with nodular sclerosis, mixed cellularity, lymphocyte-depleted, and lymphocyte-rich patterns, or nodular lymphocyte predominant HL (NLPHL, 5% of cases) (Table 1.1). The separation of NLPHL from CHL is important, as it has a different natural history, prognosis, and treatment.

The nodular sclerosing pattern (NS) is the most common type of CHL (80% of HL), and is characterized by the presence of fibrous bands separating the node into nodules and the presence of the lacunar type of RS cells. It is the predominant type of HL encountered in adolescents and young adults and typically involves the mediastinum and other supradiaphragmatic nodal sites. In the mixed cellularity (MC) type (15% of HL), band-forming sclerosis is absent, and RS cells are easily identified in a diffuse infiltrate that is more heterogeneous compared with that seen in the NS variant. The MC variant may be encountered in any age group, and advanced-stage disease with subdiaphragmatic involvement is more common in MC than NS HL. The rare lymphocyte-depleted type (<1% of HL) is characterized by sheets of RS cells with a paucity of inflammatory cells. This variant is encountered in older adults and in patients infected with HIV, as well as in patients from nonindustrialized countries. Lymphocyte-rich classical HL (6% of HL) is usually morphologically similar to the NLPHL subtype (below) and contains diagnostic RS cells with a background infiltrate that consists predominantly of lymphocytes. In contrast to NLPHL, it has the classical CD15/CD30-positive immunophenotype. The subtypes of CHL have little prognostic difference and are treated similarly.

The NLPHL type is a distinct entity that may be more closely related to indolent NHL than HL. Pathologically, NLPHL is characterized by a nodular growth pattern with variants of RS cells that have polylobated nuclei ("popcorn cells"); classic RS cells are usually absent. The immunophenotype is distinct from classic RS cells, with expression of B-cell antigens (CD19, CD20) and CD45 and the absence of CD15 and CD30. CD20 expression has allowed the therapeutic use of the monoclonal antibody rituximab, an agent not typically active in other subtypes of HL. NLPHL accounts for 5% of HL cases, has a strong male preponderance, and tends to involve peripheral nodes with sparing of the mediastinum. The prognosis is excellent, although late relapses are more common than they are in the other types of HL.

HL arises in lymph nodes, most commonly in the mediastinum or neck, and spreads to adjacent contiguous or noncontiguous nodal sites, including retroperitoneal nodes and the spleen. As the disease progresses, it spreads hematogenously to extranodal sites, including bone marrow, liver, and lung. In contrast to NHL, HL rarely arises in extranodal sites, although involvement of extranodal sites by contiguous spread from an adjacent lymph node (e.g., involvement of vertebrae from adjacent retroperitoneal lymph nodes or involvement of pulmonary parenchyma from adjacent hilar nodes) does occur.

Patients with HL usually present with painless enlargement of lymph nodes, most often in the neck. Mediastinal adenopathy may be found incidentally in an asymptomatic patient on routine chest radiography. Massive mediastinal or hilar adenopathy, with or without adjacent pulmonary involvement, may cause respiratory symptoms such as cough, dyspnea, wheezing, or stridor. Approximately one third of patients with HL have "B" symptoms. Pruritus is associated with NS HL and may precede the diagnosis for months to years. Rarely, patients with HL experience pain in involved nodal sites following alcohol ingestion. The mechanism of this infrequent (<10%) but highly specific disease manifestation is unknown. Although HL is associated with functional T-lymphocyte defects, manifested as anergy to intradermal skin tests, patients rarely present with opportunistic infections. As the disease advances, patients experience the onset of "B" symptoms, malaise, cachexia, organ failure, and infectious complications. Infection is the most common cause of death in patients with progressive, refractory HL [72].

Accurate staging of patients with newly diagnosed HL is important for treatment planning, prognosis, and response assessment. A modification of the Ann Arbor staging classification is used (Table 1.3). The initial staging evaluation of a patient with newly diagnosed HL is similar to that for patients with NHL (described previously). Bone marrow aspirate and biopsy may be omitted for patients with stage IA or IIA disease. PET scans are useful in assessing early response to treatment, prognosis, and eradication of disease when residual mass is present, and should be performed prior to therapy in all patients [73]. Staging laparotomy to accurately determine pathologic involvement below the diaphragm in the spleen and retroperitoneal lymph nodes is no longer recommended, as therapy for early-stage disease has evolved to include chemotherapy.

A variety of prognostic factors that influence the risk of relapse or survival have been identified in HL. The most important adverse prognostic factors for patients with localized disease (stage I or II) are the presence of "B" symptoms and bulky disease (Table 1.3). Other unfavorable prognostic factors are age $\geq$50, >3 involved nodal sites and a high erythrocyte sedimentation rate [74]. The prognosis of patients with advanced HL can be assessed using the International Prognostic Score (IPS) based on the total number of seven unfavorable features at diagnosis [75]. Using the IPS, progression-free survival at 5 years was 84% with a score of 0 and 42% with a score of 5 or higher (Table 1.8).

Table 1.8 Outcomes for advanced Hodgkin lymphoma based on international prognostic score (IPS) [75]

	5 years	
No. of factors	Freedom from progression (%)	Overall survival (%)
0	84	89
1	77	90
2	67	81
3	60	78
4	51	61
$\geq$ 5	42	56

One point is given for each of the seven factors: albumin < 4 g/dL; hemoglobin < 10.5 g/dL; male sex; age $\geq$ 45 years; stage IV disease; leukocytosis (WBC $\geq$ 15,000/mm^3); lymphocytopenia (< 8% of WBCs and/or lymphocyte count < 600/mm^3).

Treatment of HL

The treatment of HL has evolved considerably in the past few decades. The cure rate exceeds 80% with the use of current treatment modalities. Because most patients with HL are young adults and will experience long survival, the emphasis has shifted toward using therapies that minimize late treatment-related morbidity and mortality, without sacrificing curative potential. Thus, extended-field radiation therapy in standard doses for early stage disease has largely been abandoned due to a substantially increased risk of radiation-induced solid tumors and accelerated coronary artery disease decades after therapy. Similarly, in advanced disease, MOPP chemotherapy (nitrogen mustard, vincristine (Oncovin), procarbazine, and prednisone) [76] is rarely used in current practice due to a high risk of treatment-related acute leukemia and reproductive failure.

The predominant factors that determine the choice of treatment include stage, as well as the presence of "B" symptoms and bulky disease (adverse prognostic factors). Patients are divided into 3 groups: *early stage favorable* (stage I-II without adverse prognostic factors), *early stage unfavorable* (stage I-II with adverse prognostic factors), and *advanced stage* disease (stage III-IV). Most centers favor combined modality treatment for early stage patients using an abbreviated course of chemotherapy with involved-field radiation therapy (IFRT), and a full course of chemotherapy for patients with advanced disease.

To avoid the long-term sequelae of full-dose extended field radiation, patients with *early stage favorable HL* are now generally treated with a short course of chemotherapy (e.g. 2–4 cycles of doxorubicin [Adriamycin], bleomycin, vinblastine, and dacarbazine, designated ABVD, or 2 cycles of doxorubicin, vinblastine, mechlorethamine, vincristine, bleomycin, etoposide, and prednisone, designated Stanford V) followed by low to moderate doses of IFRT [77]. Patients with *early stage unfavorable HL* may be treated with a full course of chemotherapy (6 cycles of ABVD or 3 cycles of Stanford V) followed by IFRT [78].

All patients with *advanced stage HD* should be treated with a full course of chemotherapy. ABVD administered every 2 weeks for 6–8 months is now the most widely used regimen in the United States for the treatment of advanced HL. ABVD is as effective as MOPP, but is less toxic acutely and does not cause sterility or treatment-induced leukemias [79]. Roughly 60% of patients with stage III or IV disease are cured with ABVD. ABVD can cause bleomycin-induced pulmonary fibrosis in a small percentage of patients (<5%), and patients who have underlying lung disease or receive chest radiation are at highest risk for this complication. The inclusion of an anthracycline in ABVD precludes its use in patients who have an underlying cardiomyopathy, and alternate regimens are required in these patients. More recently, the intensive regimen BEACOPP (bleomycin, etoposide, Adriamycin, cyclophosphamide, vincristine, prednisolone and procarbazine) has been associated with higher rates of complete response and freedom from treatment failure in patients with advanced disease compared to ABVD, albeit with increased acute and chronic toxicity including infertility and myelodysplasia, and may be appropriate for selected high risk patients [80]. Radiation therapy in combination with chemotherapy is not generally used to treat advanced HL. However, in patients with bulky mediastinal disease, consolidative radiation to the mediastinum after completion of chemotherapy has been shown to decrease the rate of relapse.

Evaluating response to therapy in HL involves repetition of staging procedures during and at the completion of treatment. An interim PET scan after two cycles of ABVD has been shown to correlate with eventual resistance or relapse of disease [73]. At completion of treatment, patients may have persistent abnormalities on CT scan (e.g., enlarged nodes, residual mediastinal mass) that reflect fibrosis, rather than persistent tumor. A positive PET scan after treatment in patients with residual CT abnormalities is associated with a high rate of subsequent relapse, and these patients should be monitored closely or considered for immediate repeat biopsy.

Despite high cure rates with current treatment modalities, 5–10% of patients with HL will have primary refractory disease, and another 10–30% will relapse after initial complete remission. The majority of patients destined to relapse will do so within 2 years; relapses after 5 years are exceedingly rare. Patients with relapsed or refractory disease should be offered salvage chemotherapy followed by high dose chemotherapy with autologous stem cell transplant as more than 50% of patients with relapsed disease may still be cured [81–83].

Plasma Cell Neoplasms

The monoclonal plasma cell disorders or "dyscrasias" comprise a group of B-cell disorders that are related to each other by virtue of their production and secretion of monoclonal immunoglobulin, or M protein. Plasma cell disorders include multiple myeloma (MM) and closely related solitary plasmacytomas of bone or soft tissue, Waldenström macroglobulinemia (or LPL, discussed above), heavy chain diseases, primary amyloidosis, and light and heavy chain deposition diseases. MGUS (monoclonal gammopathy of undetermined significance) is an asymptomatic pre-neoplastic plasma cell disorder that may precede the development of myeloma.

The neoplastic cell of these disorders exhibits features of a differentiated immunoglobulin-secreting plasma cell. The hallmark of the plasma cell dyscrasias is the presence of an M protein: an immunoglobulin molecule (IgG, IgA, IgD, IgE, or IgM) or its light chain (kappa or lambda) that can be detected in serum or urine by protein electrophoresis (SPEP, UPEP), or the more sensitive immunofixation electrophoresis (IFE) assay. When neoplastic cells produce only light chains (Bence Jones protein), M protein may only be detectable by the above-mentioned methods in the patient's urine or may not be detected at all. The highly sensitive, serum free light chains (FLC) assay is now routinely used for these patients and aids not only in the diagnosis, but also in determining the prognosis, and response assessment of plasma cell dyscrasias [84]. M proteins can be found in benign and malignant conditions other than the plasma cell disorders including autoimmune or infectious disorders, or with other subtypes of NHL (e.g., CLL).

MGUS and Smoldering Myeloma

MGUS is an asymptomatic plasma cell disorder defined by the presence of a low serum M protein level (<3 gm/dL), <10% bone marrow plasma cells, and the absence of clinical manifestations related to myeloma (lytic bone lesions, anemia, hypercalcemia, renal failure), or other B-cell lymphoproliferative disorders. MGUS increases in frequency with age, occurring in >3% of the population over age 50. Although it is considered a pre-malignant condition, progression of MGUS to a frank plasma cell neoplasm only occurs in approximately 1% of patients per year

[85]. Risk of progression is greatest in patients with non-IgG M proteins, initial M protein >1.5 g/dL, and with an abnormal serum free light chain ratio. Although there is no definitive evidence that monitoring patients with MGUS improves survival, annual evaluation to detect progression to multiple myeloma (MM) prior to the onset of overt symptoms or complications is recommended [86]. Smoldering (asymptomatic) myeloma is diagnosed when the M protein is $\geq$3 g/dL or when there are $\geq$10% plasma cells in the bone marrow in the absence of clinical manifestations of MM. Patients with smoldering myeloma do not require treatment until progression to symptomatic disease (median 4.8 years) [87].

Multiple Myeloma (MM)

MM is the most common plasma cell neoplasm. It is characterized by plasma cell infiltration of the bone marrow and bone, and the presence of monoclonal immunoglobulin or light chains in the serum or urine. The diagnosis of MM is made by identifying excess plasma cells in the bone marrow (>30%) and the presence of M protein exceeding 3.5 g/dL for IgG or 2 g/dL for IgA in serum or 1 g/24 h in urine. Patients with lower levels of M protein or bone marrow plasmacytosis may still be diagnosed with myeloma based on the presence of a combination of other features, such as hypogammaglobulinemia, lytic bone lesions, or plasmacytoma. For some patients lacking these features, the distinction between MGUS and myeloma can only be made by longitudinal follow-up for evidence of rising M protein or the development of clinical manifestations of myeloma. Approximately 20% of patients with MM do not have detectable serum M protein but have free light chains (Bence Jones protein) in the serum or urine that can be detected by urine electrophoretic studies, or by serum free light chain measurement ("light chain disease").

The clinical manifestations of MM relate to the direct effects of bone marrow and bone infiltration by malignant plasma cells, the systemic effects of the M protein, or the effects of the concomitant deficiency in humoral immunity that occurs in this disease. The most common symptom in multiple myeloma is bone pain. Bone radiographs typically show pure osteolytic "punched out" lesions, often in association with generalized osteopenia, and pathologic fractures. Bony lesions can present as expansile masses associated with spinal cord compression. Hypercalcemia caused by extensive bony involvement is common in MM. Anemia occurs in the majority of patients as a result of marrow infiltration and suppression of hematopoiesis; granulocytopenia and thrombocytopenia are less common. Patients with MM are susceptible to recurrent bacterial infections because of impaired production and increased catabolism of normal immunoglobulins. Renal insufficiency occurs in approximately 25% of patients with myeloma. The cause of renal failure in these patients is often multifactorial; hypercalcemia, hyperuricemia, infection, and amyloid can contribute. However, direct tubular damage from light chain excretion is often present ("myeloma kidney" or myeloma cast nephropathy). M proteins can also cause a host of diverse problems because of their physicochemical properties, including cryoglobulinemia, hyperviscosity, amyloidosis, and clotting abnormalities resulting from interaction of M protein with platelets or clotting factors.

Staging systems for MM have been developed to predict prognosis. The three-tier Durie–Salmon staging system for myeloma is based on bone radiographs and laboratory tests that correlate with tumor mass and survival [88]. Recently, a simplified prognostic scheme, the International Staging System for Myeloma, identified three stages with distinct prognoses based on only two variables: β_2-microglobulin and albumin levels (Table 1.9) [89]. In addition to stage, other adverse prognostic factors include chromosomal abnormalities (deletion of 13 or 17p, Ig heavy chain translocations t(4;14) or t(14;16), or hypoploidy), and plasma cell labeling index $\geq$3% [90].

Most patients with myeloma exhibit symptomatic, advanced-stage disease and require therapy. However, approximately 10% of patients have stage I disease or smoldering myeloma and an indolent course. These patients do not require immediate therapy, but should be monitored at 3–6 month intervals for disease progression by serial quantification of the M protein. For patients with solitary bone or extramedullary plasmacytomas, local radiation therapy can induce long-term remissions and is the treatment of choice.

Patients with symptomatic, advanced-stage (II or III) MM require systemic chemotherapy, as well as meticulous attention to supportive care. Although MM is

Table 1.9 Myeloma staging systems [77]

Stage	Durie–Salmon criteria [88]	ISS criteria [89]
I	All of the following: – Hemoglobin > 10 g/dL – Serum calcium < 12 mg/dL – Normal bone X-ray or solitary lesion – Low M-component production (a) IgG level < 5 g/dL (b) IgA level < 3 g/dL (c) Urine light chain < 4 g/24 h	Serum beta-2 microglobulin < 3.5 mg/dL Serum albumin ≥ 3.5 g/dL
II	Fitting neither I nor III	Fitting neither I nor III
III	One or more of the following: – Hemoglobin < 8.5 g/dL – Serum calcium > 12 mg/dL – Advanced lytic bone lesions – High M-component production (a) IgG level > 7 g/dL (b) IgA level > 5 g/dL (c) Urine light chains > 12 g/24 h	Serum beta-2 microglobulin ≥ 5.5 mg/dL

Subclassification criteria:
A Serum creatinine < 2 mg/dL
B Serum creatinine > 2 mg/dL

not curable, systemic chemotherapy can significantly prolong survival and improve the quality of life. Treatment of symptomatic MM depends on risk assessment and the patient's eligibility for consolidative high-dose chemotherapy with autologous stem cell transplantation. Multiple initial treatment options have emerged in the past decade due to the availability of thalidomide and lenalidomide (referred to as *immunomodulatory agents or IMiDs*) and bortezomib (a proteosome inhibitor), each of which are typically administered in combination with dexamethasone, in addition to standard chemotherapy options [90]. These newer agents have largely supplanted traditional multi-drug chemotherapy regimens as initial and secondary therapies, as they are highly effective, and generally well tolerated. The combination of IMiD and dexamethasone, with or without melphalan, is the most widely used initial therapy. In contrast to chemotherapy, thalidomide is rarely myelosuppressive, but can cause peripheral neuropathy, constipation, somnolence, and rash. The thalidomide/dexamethasone combination is associated with a high risk of venous thromboembolic disease (25% of patients), and thus prophylaxis is recommended. Lenalidomide is a more potent agent with fewer side effects than thalidomide, although it is myelosuppressive. Bortezomib-based regimens may be used as initial therapy or in recurrent or refractory disease. Alternative initial systemic therapies include dexamethasone as a single agent, alkylator–based combination chemotherapy regimens, and the VAD regimen (vincristine, Adriamycin, dexamethasone). The use of alkylating agents generally should be avoided in patients who are eligible for consolidative stem cell transplantation due to their stem cell depleting properties.

The majority of patients respond to initial therapy with a decline in the M protein and symptomatic improvement. Consolidative high-dose chemotherapy with alkylating agents followed by autologous peripheral stem cell transplantation in responding patients after initial therapy has been shown to improve survival and quality of life compared with standard doses of chemotherapy [90–93]. Although this approach is not curative, it represents an important treatment option for some patients, with an acceptable toxicity profile, even in older patients. Allogeneic bone marrow transplantation may represent the only potentially curative treatment for myeloma, but excessive morbidity and mortality in elderly or heavily pretreated patients have limited its use.

Supportive care directed toward anticipated complications of myeloma is an important aspect of management. Regular injections of bisphosphonates (pamidronate or zoledronic acid) are indicated for all patients who have bone disease, including osteopenia, to reduce bone pain and risk of fractures. Symptomatic hyperviscosity or acute renal failure caused by myeloma cast nephropathy may improve with plasmapheresis. All patients should receive pneumococcal and *H. influenzae* vaccines, and intravenous gamma globulin is useful in preventing recurrent infections in patients with hypogammaglobulinemia. Erythropoiesis-stimulating agents may alleviate anemia and decrease the need for blood transfusions, especially in patients with renal failure. Patients treated with bortezomib have a higher incidence of herpes zoster and should receive prophylactic acyclovir or valacyclovir. Anticoagulation prophylaxis is generally recommended for patients receiving IMiDs in combination with dexamethasone.

Rare Plasma Cell Disorders

Primary Amyloidosis and Light and Heavy Chain Deposition Diseases

Primary amyloidosis (AL) is a systemic illness characterized by deposition of immunoglobulin light chain (kappa or lambda) fragments in organs and tissues in a beta-pleated configuration that has the biochemical properties of amyloid (with Congo Red staining polarized light microscopy reveals apple green color). Congestive heart failure, bleeding diathesis, nephrotic syndrome, and peripheral neuropathy are common complications. AL responds poorly to the treatments used for myeloma. Encouraging results have been reported with high-dose chemotherapy and autologous stem cell transplantation, particularly if patients are treated prior to the development of significant end organ dysfunction, such as cardiomyopathy. Transplant-related mortality rates are in the range of 13–15%, and a risk-adapted approach based on age, renal function, and organ involvement may improve the outcomes [94, 95]. Patients who are not eligible for autologous transplantation may be offered therapy on clinical trials or treated with melphalan/dexamethasone [96].

Light and heavy chain deposition diseases are similar pathogenetically and clinically to primary amyloidosis, with overproduction of a monoclonal light chain (usually kappa) or heavy chain fragments, which are deposited in different organs. Unlike primary amyloidosis, however, the deposits do not have the biochemical characteristics of amyloid fibrils.

Heavy Chain Diseases

Heavy chain diseases are rare lymphoplasmacytoid neoplasms characterized by production of defective Ig heavy chains of the gamma, alpha, or mu type in the absence of light chains. The clinical manifestations vary with the type of heavy chain secreted. Gamma heavy chain disease is associated with lymphadenopathy, Waldeyer ring involvement, palatal edema, and constitutional symptoms. Alpha chain disease, also known as Mediterranean lymphoma, is characterized by lymphoid infiltration of the small intestine and is associated with diarrhea and malabsorption. Mu chain disease is associated with CLL. Data are limited on the treatment of heavy chain diseases, with therapeutic approaches similar to those employed in MM.

Lymphomas in Immunocompromised Patients

HIV-Associated NHL

Patients with acquired immunodeficiency from HIV infection are at a significantly increased risk of developing systemic NHL and primary CNS lymphoma (PCNSL) compared to the general population. Although the risk of developing NHL in the setting of HIV infection has diminished substantially with the widespread use of highly active antiretroviral therapy (HAART), it is estimated that 2–5% of patients with HIV infection develop NHL [97]. The NHL subtypes that are associated with HIV are B-cell in origin and defined in the WHO classification as either DLBCL or Burkitt lymphoma. These entities are considered AIDS-defining illnesses. HL and plasma cell dyscrasia also occur with increased frequency in patients with HIV infection, but are not considered AIDS-defining illnesses. HIV-associated lymphomas are strongly linked to EBV infection; 50% of systemic NHL, 90% of HL, and virtually all PCNSL are EBV-positive.

HIV-associated systemic NHL is characterized by advanced stage at presentation (stage III or IV), involvement of extra-nodal sites, and the presence of "B" symptoms. Primary effusion lymphoma (PEL) is a distinct HIV-associated clinico-pathologic entity characterized by lymphomatous effusions in the pericardial, pleural, and peritoneal cavities. The majority of PELs are positive for both EBV and Kaposi sarcoma associated herpes virus (HHV-8). PEL is often resistant to chemotherapy and associated with a poor prognosis.

HIV-associated NHL is potentially curable using the same multi-drug chemotherapy regimens (e.g., CHOP) that are used for the treatment of aggressive or highly aggressive NHLs (discussed in preceding sections). In addition, treatment of the underlying HIV infection with HAART is an important aspect of management and has substantially improved the outcome and prognosis of patients with HIV-associated NHL [97]. The use of rituximab (in CD20-positive disease) in combination with chemotherapy should be considered in patients with a relatively high CD4 count, recognizing that there is an increased risk of fatal infection associated with rituximab in patients with CD4 counts <50 cells/μL [98]. Patients with advanced HIV infection or a history of opportunistic infections are at an increased risk of developing chemotherapy-related myelosuppression and infection, and thus routine use of prophylactic G-CSF and antibiotics is important in reducing morbidity of treatment. Lumbar puncture at diagnosis is indicated to rule out occult leptomeningeal dissemination in all patients with HIV-associated NHLs. Those patients at highest risk of leptomeningeal spread (Burkitt histology, EBV-positive tumor, paraspinal or paranasal disease) should receive prophylactic intrathecal chemotherapy.

Prior to the widespread use of HAART, the incidence of PCNSL was dramatically increased in patients with HIV infection. PCNSL is an AIDS-defining illness, which typically occurs in profoundly immunodeficient patients with end-stage AIDS and is associated with a dismal outcome. In recent years, the incidence of HIV-associated PCNSL has plummeted while the prognosis may be improving, presumably due to the use of HAART, to restore immune function. (See Chapter 9 for a detailed discussion of HIV-associated PCNSL.)

Posttransplantation Lymphoproliferative Disorder (PTLD)

Patients who have undergone an allogeneic stem cell or solid organ transplant require potent immunosuppressive drugs (cyclosporine, tacrolimus, mycophenolate mofetil, azathioprine, corticosteroids, methotrexate) to prevent graft-versus-host disease (in allogeneic stem cell transplantation) or allograft rejection (in solid organ transplantation). These drugs cause profound defects in T-cell function, with an associated acquired immunodeficiency state, that predisposes transplant recipients to the development of a variety of lymphoproliferative disorders (Table 1.1). PTLD occurs in 1–20% of allograft recipients, and the risk is related primarily to the transplanted organ, the potency of the immunosuppressive regimen, and EBV serological status (sero-positive donor to sero-negative recipient) [99]. Pathogenetically, PTLD in most cases evolves from unrestrained EBV-driven B-cell proliferation, and the histopathology is characterized by a polymorphous or monomorphous population of EBV-positive B-cells that can be monoclonal or polyclonal (Table 1.1) [14]. EBV-negative and T-cell lymphomas are less common. The diagnosis of PTLD requires a high index of suspicion, appropriate imaging including PET/CT scans, and an adequate tissue biopsy of suspicious sites (in some cases the allograft) that will permit full characterization of the lesion, including clonality and EBV status. Serial measurement of EBV viral load can facilitate early detection of PTLD.

Treatment of these disorders must be individualized and is based on the type of PTLD and the risk of organ rejection. The initial management of PTLD usually entails reduction in the immunosuppressive regimen, if possible. This intervention alone will result in regression of PTLD in approximately half of patients, including the majority of polyclonal PTLDs, thus obviating the need for cytotoxic therapy. Patients who are not candidates for withdrawal of immunosuppression because of the risks of allograft rejection, or those who fail to respond to this strategy, can be managed with rituximab alone, or in combination with chemotherapy. Patients who have aggressive or highly aggressive B-cell NHL requiring immediate treatment may be managed with discontinuation of immunosuppression, administration of standard chemotherapy with rituximab (as discussed in the preceding sections), and reintroduction of immunosuppressive medications after discontinuation of chemotherapy.

References

1. Delves PJ, Roitt IM (2000) The immune system-first of two parts. N Engl J Med 343:37–49
2. Delves PJ, Roitt IM (2000) The immune system-second of two parts. N Engl J Med 343:108–117
3. Medzhitov R, Janeway C Jr. (2000) Innate immunity. N Engl J Med 343:338–344
4. Pure E (2000) Overview of the immune system (including compartmentalization of the immune response). In: Hoffman R, Benz EJ, Shattil SJ et al (eds) Hematology: Basic principles and practice, 5th edn. Churchill Livingstone, New York, 74–79
5. Restifo NP, Wunderlich JR (2001) Essentials of immunology. In: Devita VT, Hellman S, Rosenberg SA, (eds) Cancer principles and practice of oncology. Lippincott Williams & Wilkins, Philadelphia, PA, 43–73
6. Clayberger C, Krensky AM (2000) T-cell immunity. In: Hoffman R, Benz EJ, Shattil SJ et al (eds) Hematology: Basic principles and practice. Churchill Livingstone, New York, 90–100
7. Dorshkind K (2000) B-Cell development. In: Hoffman R, Benz EJ, Shattil SJ et al (eds) Hematology principles and practice. Churchill Livingstone, New York, 80–90
8. Kuppers R, Klein U, Hansmann M-L RK (1999) Cellular origin of human B-cell lymphomas. N Engl J Med 341:1520–1529

9. (1982) Non-Hodgkin's Lymphoma pathologic classification project: National Cancer Institute sponsored study of classifications of non-Hodgkin's lymphomas. Summary and description of a working formulation for clinical usage. Cancer 49:2112–2135
10. Pugh WC, McBride A (2000) The pathologic basis for the classification of non-Hodgkin lymphomas. In: Hoffman R, Benz EJ, Shattil SJ et al (eds) Hematology: Basic principles and practice, 5th edn. Churchill Livingstone, New York, 1263–1293
11. Harris NL, Jaffe ES, Stein H, Banks PM, Chan JKC et al (1994) A revised European-American classification of lymphoid neoplasms: a proposal from the International Lymphoma Study Group. Blood 84:1361–1392
12. Harris NL, Jaffe ES, Diebold J et al. (1999) World Health Organization of neoplastic disease of the hematopoietic and lymphoid tissues: report of the Clinical Advisory Committee meeting-Airlie House, Virginia, November 1997. J Clin Oncol 17:3835–3849
13. Jaffe ES, Harris NL, Stein H et al (2001) Pathology and genetics of tumours of haematopoietic and lymphoid tissues. IARC Press, Lyon, France
14. Swerdlow SH, Campo E, Harris NL et al (2008) WHO classification of tumours of haematopoietic and lymphoid tissues, 4th edn. IARC Press, Lyon, France
15. Jaffe ES, Harris NL, Stein H et al (2008) Classification of lymphoid neoplasms: the microscope as a tool for disease discovery. Blood 112:4384–4397
16. Friedberg JW, Mauch PM, Rimsza LM et al (2008) Non-Hodgkin's lymphomas. In: Devita VT, Hellman S, Rosenberg SA, (eds) Cancer principles and practice of oncology. Lippincott Williams & Wilkins, Philadelphia, PA, 2099–2143
17. Shipp M, Harrington D, Anderson J et al (1993) Development of a predictive model for aggressive lymphoma: the international non-Hodgkin's lymphoma prognostic factors project. N Engl J Med 329:987–994
18. Lopez-Guillermo A, Montserrat E, Bosch F, Terol MJ, Campo E, Rozman C (1994) Applicability of the International Index for aggressive lymphomas to patients with low-grade lymphoma. J Clin Oncol 12:1343–1348
19. Cheson BD, Pfistner B, Juweid ME et al (2007) Revised response criteria for malignant lymphoma. J Clin Oncol 25:579–586
20. Horning SJ, Rosenberg SA (1984) The natural history of initially untreated low-grade non-Hodgkins lymphomas. N Engl J Med 311:1471–1475
21. Solal-Celigny P, Roy P, Colombat P et al (2004) Follicular lymphoma international prognostic index. Blood 104:1258–1265
22. Buske C, Hoster E, Dreyling M et al (2006) The follicular lymphoma international prognostic index (FLIPI) separates high-risk from intermediate- or low-risk patients with advanced-stage follicular lymphoma treated front-line with rituximab and the combination of cyclophosphamide, doxorubicin, vincristine, and prednisone (R-CHOP) with respect to treatment outcome. Blood 108:1504–1508
23. Federico M, Vitolo U, Zinzani PL, Chisesi T et al (2000) Prognosis of follicular lymphoma: a predictive model based on a retrospective analysis of 987 cases. Blood 95:783–789
24. McLaughlin P, Hagemeister F, Romaguera JE et al (1996) Fludarabine, mitoxantrone and dexamethasone: An effective new regimen for indolent lymphoma. J Clin Oncol 14: 1262–1268
25. Reiser M, Current DV (2002) Treatment of follicular non-Hodgkin's lymphoma. Eur J Cancer 38:1167–1172
26. Schulz H, Bohlius JF, Trelle S et al (2007) Immunochemotherapy with rituximab and overall survival in patients with indolent or mantle cell lymphoma: a systematic review and meta-analysis. J Natl Cancer Inst 99(9):706–714
27. Colombat P, Salles G, Brousse N et al (2001) Rituximab (anti-CD20 monoclonal antibody) as single first-line therapy for patients with follicular lymphoma with a low tumor burden: Clinical and molecular evaluation. Blood 97:101–106
28. Czuczman M, Grillo-Lopez A, White C et al (1999) Treatment of patients with low-grade B-cell lymphoma with the combination of chimeric anti-CD20 monoclonal antibody and CHOP chemotherapy. J Clin Oncol 17:268–276

29. McLaughlin P, Grillo-Lopez A, Link B et al (1998) Rituximab chimeric anti-CD20 monoclonal antibody therapy of relapsed indolent lymphoma: half of patients respond to a four dose treatment program. J Clin Oncol 16:2825–2833
30. Piro LD, White C, Grillo-Lopez A et al (1999) Extended Rituximab (anti-CD20 monoclonal antibody) therapy for relapsed or refractory low-grade or follicular non-Hodgkin's lymphoma. Ann Oncol 10:655–661
31. Cheson BD, Leonard JP (2008) Therapy for B-cell non-Hodgkin's lymphoma. N Engl J Med 359(6):613–626
32. van Oers MH, Klasa R, Marcus RE et al (2006) Rituximab maintenance improves clinical outcome of relapsed/resistant follicular non-Hodgkin lymphoma in patients both with and without rituximab during induction: results of a prospective randomized phase 3 intergroup trial. Blood 108:3295–3301
33. Hunault-Berger M, Ifrah N, Solal-Celigny P (2002) Intensive therapies in follicular non-Hodgkin lymphomas. Blood 100:1141–1151
34. Rawstron AC, Bennett FL, O'Connor SJ et al (2008) Monoclonal B-cell lymphocytosis and chronic lymphocytic leukemia. N Engl J Med 359:575–583
35. Hallek M, Cheson BD, Catovsky D et al (2008) Guidelines for the diagnosis and treatment of chronic lymphocytic leukemia: a report from the International Workshop on Chronic Lymphocytic Leukemia updating the National Cancer Institute-Working Group 1996 guidelines. Blood 111:5446–5456
36. Shanafelt TD, Byrd JC, Call TG et al (2006) Narrative review: initial management of newly diagnosed, early-stage chronic lymphocytic leukemia. Ann Intern Med 145:435–447
37. Hillmen P, Skotnicki AB, Robak T et al (2007) Alemtuzumab compared with chlorambucil as first-line therapy for chronic lymphocytic leukemia. J Clin Oncol 25:5616–5623
38. Rai KR, Peterson BL, Applebaum FR et al (2000) Fludarabine compared with chlorambucil as primary therapy for chronic lymphocytic leukemia. N Engl J Med 343:1750–1757
39. Knauf WU, Lissichkov T, Aldaoud A et al (2008) Bendamustine versus chlorambucil as first-line treatment in B-cell chronic lymphocytic leukemia (B-CLL): An updated analysis from an international phase III study (abstract). Blood 112:728
40. Keating MJ, Flinn I, Jain V, Binet J, Hillmen P et al (2002) Therapeutic role of alemtuzumab (Campath-1H) in patients who have failed fludarabine: results of a large international study. Blood 100:768–773
41. Byrd JC, Murphy T, Howard RS (2001) Rituximab using a thrice weekly dosing schedule in B-cell chronic lymphocytic leukemia and small lymphocytic lymphoma demonstrates clinical activity and acceptable toxicity. J Clin Oncol 19:2153–2163
42. Obrien S, Kantarjian H, Thomas D (2001) Rituximab dose-escalation trial in chronic lymphocytic leukemia. J Clin Oncol 19:2165–2170
43. Dimopoulos MA, Gertz MA, Kastritis E et al (2009) Update on treatment recommendations from the Fourth International Workshop on Waldenstrom's Macroglobulinemia. J Clin Oncol 27:120–126
44. Rosenwald A, Wright G, Chan WC et al (2002) The use of molecular profiling to predict survival after chemotherapy for diffuse large B-cell lymphoma. N Engl J Med 346:1937–1947
45. Alizadeh A, Eisen MB, Davis R et al (2000) Distinct types of diffuse large B-cell lymphoma identified by gene expression profiling. Nature 403:503–511
46. Sehn LH, Berry B, Chhanabhai M et al (2007) The revised International Prognostic Index (R-IPI) is a better predictor of outcome than the standard IPI for patients with diffuse large B-cell lymphoma treated with R-CHOP. Blood 109:1857–1861
47. Fisher RI, Gaynor E, Dahlberg S et al (1993) Comparison of a standard regimen (CHOP) with three intensive chemotherapy regimens for advanced non-Hodgkin's lymphoma. N Engl J Med 328:1002–1006
48. Coiffer B, Lepage E, Herbrecht R (2002) CHOP chemotherapy plus rituximab compared with CHOP alone in elderly patients with diffuse Large B-cell lymphoma. N Engl J Med 346: 235–242

49. Sehn LH, Donaldson J, Chhanabhai M et al (2005) Introduction of combined CHOP plus rituximab therapy dramatically improved outcome of diffuse large B-cell lymphoma in British Columbia. J Clin Oncol 23:5027–5033
50. Pfreundschuh M, Trumper L, Kloess M et al (2004) Two-weekly or 3-weekly CHOP chemotherapy with or without etoposide for the treatment of elderly patients with aggressive lymphomas: results of the NHL-B2 trial of the DSHNHL. Blood 104:634–641
51. Verdonck LF, Notenboom A, de Jong DD et al (2007) Intensified 12-week CHOP (I-CHOP) plus G-CSF compared with standard 24-week CHOP (CHOP-21) for patients with intermediate-risk aggressive non-Hodgkin lymphoma: a phase 3 trial of the Dutch-Belgian Hemato-Oncology Cooperative Group (HOVON). Blood 109:2759–2766
52. Cunningham D, Smith P, Mouncey P et al (2009) A phase III trial comparing R-CHOP 14 and R-CHOP 21 for the treatment of patients with newly diagnosed diffuse large B-cell non-Hodgkin's lymphoma (abstract). J Clin Oncol 27:abstract 8506
53. Philip T, Guglielmi C, Hagenbeek A et al (1995) Autologous bone marrow transplantation as compared with salvage chemotherapy in relapses of chemotherapy-sensitive non-Hodgkin's lymphoma. N Engl J Med 333:1540–1545
54. Frater JL, Hsi ED (2002) Properties of the mantle cell and mantle cell lymphoma. Curr Opin Hematol 9:56–62
55. Ghielmini M, How ZE (2009) How I treat mantle cell lymphoma. Blood 8:1469–1475
56. Determann O, Hoster E, Ott G et al (2008) Ki-67 predicts outcome in advanced-stage mantle cell lymphoma patients treated with anti-CD20 immunochemotherapy: results from randomized trials of the European MCL Network and the German Low Grade Lymphoma Study Group. Blood 111:2385–2387
57. Hoster E, Dreyling M, Klapper W et al (2008) A new prognostic index (MIPI) for patients with advanced-stage mantle cell lymphoma. Blood 111:558–565
58. Romaguera JE, Fayad L, Rodriguez MA et al (2005) High rate of durable remissions after treatment of newly diagnosed aggressive mantle-cell lymphoma with rituximab plus hyper-CVAD alternating with rituximab plus high-dose methotrexate and cytarabine. J Clin Oncol 23:7013–7023
59. Lenz G, Dreyling M, Hoster E et al (2005) Immunochemotherapy with rituximab and cyclophosphamide, doxorubicin, vincristine, and prednisone significantly improves response and time to treatment failure, but not long-term outcome in patients with previously untreated mantle cell lymphoma: results of a prospective randomized trial of the German Low Grade Lymphoma Study Group (GLSG). J Clin Oncol 23:1984–1992
60. Geisler CH, Kolstad A, Laurell A et al (2008) Long-term progression-free survival of mantle cell lymphoma following intensive front-line immunochemotherapy with in vivo-purged stem cell rescue: A non-randomized phase-II multicenter study by the Nordic Lymphoma Group. Blood 112:2687–2693
61. Dreyling M, Lenz G, Hoster E et al (2005) Early consolidation by myeloablative radiochemotherapy followed by autologous stem cell transplantation in first remission significantly prolongs progression-free survival in mantle cell lymphoma: results of a prospective randomized trial of the European MCL Network. Blood 105:2677–2684
62. Fisher RI, Bernstein SH, Kahl BS et al (2006) Multicenter phase II study of bortezomib in patients with relapsed or refractory mantle cell lymphoma. J Clin Oncol 24:4867–4874
63. Robinson KS, Williams ME, van der Jagt RH et al (2008) Phase II multicenter study of bendamustine plus rituximab in patients with relapsed indolent B-cell and mantle cell non-Hodgkin's lymphoma. J Clin Oncol 26:4473–4479
64. McGrath IT, Adde M, Shad A et al (1996) Adults and children with small non-cleaved cell lymphoma have a similar excellent outcome when treated with the same chemotherapy regimen. J Clin Oncol 14:925
65. Mead GM, Sydes MR, Walewski J et al (2002) An international evaluation of CODOX-M and CODOX-M alternating with IVAC in adult Burkitt lymphoma: results of United Kingdom Lymphoma Group LY06 study. Ann Oncol 13:1264–1274

66. Thomas DA, Faderl S, O'Brien S, Bueso-Ramos C et al (2006) Chemoimmunotherapy with hyper-CVAD plus rituximab for the treatment of adult Burkitt and Burkitt-type lymphoma or acute lymphoblastic leukemia. Cancer 106:1569–1580
67. Larson R, Dodge R, Burns C et al (1995) A five-drug remission induction regimen with intensive consolidation for adults with acute lymphoblastic leukemia: cancer and leukemia group B study 8811. Blood 85:2025–2037
68. Thomas DA, O'Brien S, Cortes J et al (2004) Outcome with the hyper-CVAD regimens in lymphoblastic lymphoma. Blood 104:1624–1630
69. Weiss M, Maslak P, Feldman E et al (1996) Cytarabine with high-dose mitoxantrone induces rapid complete remissions in adult acute lymphoblastic leukemia without the use of vincristine or prednisone. J Clin Oncol 14:2480–2485
70. Coiffier B, Altman A, Pui CH et al (2008) Guidelines for the management of pediatric and adult tumor lysis syndrome: an evidence-based review. J Clin Oncol 26:2767–2778
71. Pileri SA, Falini B, Agostinelli C et al (2008) Pathobiology of Hodgkin lymphoma. In: Hoffman R, Benz EJ, Shattil SJ et al (eds) Hematology: Basic principles and practice, 5th edn. Churchill Livingstone, New York, 1221–1238
72. Ansell SM, Armitage JO (2006) Management of Hodgkin lymphoma. Mayo Clin Proc 81:419–426
73. Gallamini A, Hutchings M, Avigdor A et al (2008) Early interim PET scan in Hodgkin lymphoma: Where do we stand?. Leuk Lymphoma 49:659–662
74. Cosset JM, Henry-Amar M, Meerwaldt JH et al (1992) The EORTC trials for limited stage Hodgkin's disease. The EORTC Lymphoma Cooperative Group. Eur J Cancer 28A: 1847–1850
75. Hasenclever D, Diehl V (1998) A prognostic score for advanced Hodgkin's disease. N Engl J Med 339:1506–1514
76. DeVita VT Jr, Simon RM, Hubbard SM et al (1980) Curability of advanced Hodgkin's disease with chemotherapy. Long-term follow-up of MOPP-treated patients at the National Cancer Institute. Ann Intern Med 92:587–595
77. National Comprehensive Cancer Network (NCCN) Clinical Practice Guidelines in Oncology available at http://www.nccn.org/professionals/physician_gls/f_guidelines.asp. Accessed 14 Aug 2009
78. Horning SJ, Hoppe RT, Breslin S et al (2002) Stanford V and radiotherapy for locally extensive and advanced Hodgkin's disease: mature results of a prospective clinical trial. J Clin Oncol 20:607–609
79. Canellos G, Anderson J, Propert K et al (1992) Chemotherapy of advanced Hodgkin's disease with MOPP, ABVD or MOPP alternating with ABVD. N Engl J Med 327:1478–1484
80. Federico M, Luminari S, Iannitto E et al (2009) ABVD compared with BEACOPP compared with CEC for the initial treatment of patients with advanced Hodgkin's lymphoma: results from the HD2000 Gruppo Italiano per lo Studio dei Linfomi Trial. J Clin Oncol 27:805–811
81. Moskowitz C, Nimmer S, Zelentz A et al (2001) A 2-step comprehensive high-dose chemoradiotherapy second-line program for relapsed and refractory Hodgkin disease:analysis by intent to treat and development of a prognostic model. Blood 97:616–623
82. Yuen A, Rosenberg SA, Hoppe R et al (1997) Comparison between conventional salvage therapy and high-dose therapy with autografting for recurrent or refractory Hodgkin's disease. Blood 89:814–822
83. Armitage JO, Bierman PJ, Vose JM et al (1991) Autologous bone marrow transplantation for patients with relapsed disease. Am J Med 91:605–611
84. Pratt G (2008) The evolving use of serum free light chain assays in haematology. Br J Haematol 141:413–422
85. Kyle R, Therneau T, Rajkumar S et al (2002) A long-term study of prognosis in monoclonal gammopathy of undertermined significance. N Engl J Med 346:564–569
86. Bladé J (2006) Monoclonal gammopathy of undetermined significance. N Engl J Med 355:2765–2770

87. Kyle RA, Remstein ED, Therneau TM et al (2007) Clinical course and prognosis of smoldering (asymptomatic) multiple myeloma. N Engl J Med 356:2582–2590
88. Durie BG, Salmon SE (1975) A clinical staging system for multiple myeloma: correlation of measured myeloma cell mass with presenting clinical features, response to treatment, and survival. Cancer 36:842–854
89. Greipp PR, San Miguel JF, Durie BG et al (2005) International staging system for multiple myeloma. J Clin Oncol 23:3412–3420
90. Kyle RA, Rajkumar SV (2008) Multiple myeloma. Blood 111:2962–2972
91. Harousseau J, Moreau P (2009) Autologous hematopoietic stem-cell transplantation for multiple myeloma. N Engl J Med 360:2645–2654
92. Attal M, Harousseau JL, Facon T et al (2003) Single vs double autologous stem-cell transplantation for multiple myeloma. N Engl J Med 349:2495–2502
93. Cavo M, Tosi P, Zamagni E et al (2007) Prospective, randomized study of single compared with double autologous stem-cell transplantation for multiple myeloma: Bologna 96 Clinical Study. J Clin Oncol 25:2434–2441
94. Cohen AD, Zhou P, Chou J et al (2007) Risk-adapted autologous stem cell transplantation with adjuvant dexamethasone +/– thalidomide for systemic light-chain amyloidosis: results of a phase II trial. Br J Haematol 139:224–233
95. Jaccard A, Moreau P, Leblond V et al (2007) High-dose melphalan versus melphalan plus dexamethasone for AL amyloidosis. N Engl J Med 357:1083–1093
96. Palladini G, Perfetti V, Obici L et al (2004) Association of melphalan and high-dose dexamethasone is effective and well tolerated in patients with AL (primary) amyloidosis who are ineligible for stem cell transplantation. Blood 103:2936–2938
97. Ratner L, Redden D, Hamzeh F et al (1999) Chemotherapy for HIV-NHL in combination with HAART. In: 3rd National AIDS Malignancy meeting, Bethesda, MD, 1999.
98. Kaplan LD, Lee JY, Ambinder RF et al (2005) Rituximab does not improve clinical outcome in a randomized phase 3 trial of CHOP with or without rituximab in patients with HIV-associated non-Hodgkin lymphoma: AIDS-Malignancies Consortium Trial 010. Blood 106:1538–1543
99. Everly MJ, Bloom RD, Tsai DE et al (2007) Posttransplant lymphoproliferative disorder. Ann Pharmacother 41:1850–1858

Chapter 2
Overview of the Leukemias

Mark M. Awad, Harshabad Singh, and Eyal C. Attar

Introduction

The previous chapter described malignant cells that originate in lymphoid organs, such as lymph nodes and the spleen. Leukemias are also cancers of the immune system, but these neoplasms originate within hematopoietic stem and progenitor cells in the blood and bone marrow. Leukemias can arise from lymphoid cells (B cells and T cells), like lymphomas, or from cells of the myeloid lineage. Clonal expansion of one cell line results in underproduction of normal red blood cells, platelets, and other leukocytes. Cytopenias lead to requirement for blood product transfusions. Also, cytopenias result in weakening of the immune system and increased risk of infection, which is the most common cause of death in patients with leukemia. Importantly, leukemias not only occupy the bone marrow space, but can also infiltrate organs such as the liver, spleen, skin, and central nervous system (CNS). Major CNS consequences result from leptomeningeal spread of disease, parenchymal infiltration by leukemia cells, paravertebral masses leading to spinal cord or cauda equina compression, hemorrhage in the setting of disseminated intravascular coagulation, and leukostasis. These CNS complications can cause central and peripheral nerve palsies, seizures, and altered sensorium. Treatment of CNS involvement may involve leukapheresis, radiation, intrathecal chemotherapy, and systemic chemotherapy using agents capable of traversing the blood-brain barrier.

Normal and Malignant Hematopoiesis

Bone Marrow Architecture

Production of hematopoietic cells occurs within the bone marrow, located within the proximal regions of long bones of the body, ribs, sternum, vertebrae, ileum,

---

E.C. Attar (✉)
Bone Marrow Transplant Unit, Massachusetts General Hospital Cancer Center, Boston, MA 02114, USA
e-mail: eattar@partners.org

T. Batchelor, L.M. DeAngelis (eds.), *Lymphoma and Leukemia of the Nervous System*, DOI 10.1007/978-1-4419-7668-0_2,

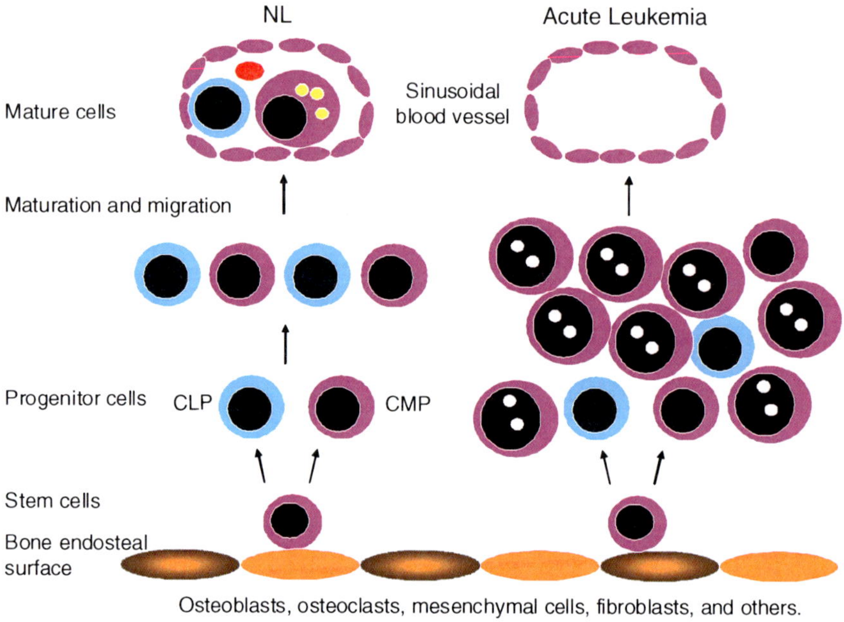

Fig. 2.1 The bone marrow environment is comprised of hematopoietic cells, which include stem, progenitor, and precursor cells, which terminally differentiate to form mature elements of blood. Malignant transformation results in accumulation of lymphoblasts, or myeloblasts, in the bone marrow, which causes a reduction in the normal hematopoietic elements and cytopenias

and calvarium. Bone marrow is comprised of hematopoietic cells that participate in the formation of blood and supportive cells, which provide cytokines and physical support for hematopoietic cells. Osteoblasts and osteoclasts are involved in maintenance of bone structure, but also contribute to hematopoiesis (Fig. 2.1).

Hematopoietic Stem and Progenitor Cells and Differentiation

The adult bone marrow contains approximately 500,000 hematopoietic stem cells (HSCs) and, from these, approximately 10^{10} blood cells are formed hourly. HSCs, like other stem cells, have the property of self-renewal, whereby one of the daughter cells retains stem cell-like function to prevent the depletion of the HSC pool [1]. Hematopoiesis occurs in a unidirectional manner, with cells gradually losing the capacity for self-renewal as they acquire more differentiated characteristics. HSCs divide and differentiate to form hematopoietic progenitor cells (HPCs), comprised of common myeloid and lymphoid progenitors (CMPs, CLPs), respectively. CLPs give rise to lymphoid progenitors. Progenitor cells divide to form precursor cells, which form the bulk of the bone marrow cellularity when viewed by light microscopy. Precursor cells then terminally divide and differentiate to form the mature elements of blood: leukocytes, red blood cells, and platelets. T cells, B cells, and plasma cells are derived from CLPs while RBCs, platelets, granulocytes (neutrophils, eosinophils and basophils), monocytes, dendritic cells, and macrophages are derived from the CMPs.

The differentiation process is guided by several principles. First, hematopoietic cells lose the capacity for self-renewal, with the accumulation of differentiated characteristics. Second, differentiation is considered unidirectional – differentiated cells are unable to "de-differentiate" to a more primitive, stem-like form.

Upon maturation, cells gradually transmigrate to bone marrow sinusoidal vessels and are released into the circulatory system. Even rare HSCs and HPCs transiently leave the bone marrow, circulate, and return to the bone marrow, often at other sites. A large number of these HSCs and HPCs may enter the circulation in response to agents such as G-CSF, CXCR4 inhibitors like AMD3100, and cytotoxic chemotherapy agents like cyclophosphamide. In fact, these agents are used to mobilize HSCs to the blood to facilitate collection for the purpose of allogeneic stem cell transplantation.

Hematopoietic Support Cells

HSCs receive and are dependent on enumerable cues from their microenvironment, or niche. The role of the niche in HSC function was first emphasized by Schofield who proposed that the fate of HSC progeny was dependent on the surrounding niche [2].

The various cells and extracellular macromolecules present in the hematopoietic tissue are collectively referred to as stroma. The stromal cells consist of adipocytes, fibroblast-like cells, endothelial cells, osteoblasts, and mesenchymal stem cells. These stromal cells are important sources of many paracrine and juxtacrine growth factors, which are necessary for self-renewal, and differentiation of HSCs and progenitors [3, 4]. In addition, the stroma plays a role in the homing and trafficking of HSCs to hematopoietic organs via ligand-receptor interactions [5]. This is of great importance for engraftment of HSCs given peripherally during a stem cell transplant.

The cells of the osteoblastic lineage form an integral component of the HSC niche and support hematopoiesis. Periosteal marrow is enriched for HSCs and selective ablation of osteoblasts in mice reduces bone marrow cellularity and promotes extramedullary hematopoiesis, underscoring the contribution of osteoblasts to normal hematopoiesis [6, 7].

Mesenchymal stem cells (MSCs) are pluripotent stem cells found in the marrow, which have the capacity to replicate as undifferentiated multipotent cells and to differentiate into a variety of lineages of mesenchymal origin [8]. MSCs have been shown to support hematopoiesis and regulate immune responses by suppressing T cell activation [9] and hence, are under investigation for treatment of graft versus host disease [10].

Malignant Transformation

Both lymphoid and myeloid cells may undergo malignant transformation. However, the exact cell of origin of a leukemia is unclear. Further complicating the identification of the malignant cell is the observation that some individuals have biphenotypic leukemias, which display both myeloid and lymphoid cell surface markers, or multilineage leukemias, where two or more populations of malignant cells of lymphoid, myeloid, or hybrid immunophenotypes may be identified.

Whether a hematopoietic stem or progenitor cell can undergo transformation is not fully understood. However, leukemias arise from activation of oncogenes, inactivation of tumor suppressor genes, and alterations in transcription factors that block differentiation. Identifying the specific genetic lesions is important as specific cytogenetic and molecular mutations have implications for diagnosis, risk stratification, and treatment.

The concept of a "leukemia stem cell" (LSC) has arisen and describes the capacity for certain populations of bone marrow cells from individuals with leukemia to give rise to leukemia in murine xenotransplant model systems; these LSCs have the capacity for enhanced self-renewal and are likely responsible for the perpetuation of the leukemia while other cells, which may form the bulk of the leukemia, are incapable of perpetuating the disease. This recapitulates the hierarchy found in the normal hematopoietic system where a rare, self-renewing stem cell maintains the entire population of terminally differentiated, non self-renewing cells [11]. The relationship of the LSC to the normal HSC is unclear and different leukemias likely emerge from different cells along the hematopoietic cascade.

Classification of Leukemias

Leukemias represent malignant, clonal leukocyte proliferations, which may be grossly classified based on the myeloid or lymphoid cell of origin. Lymphoid leukemias, such as B-ALL, T-ALL, and Burkitt's leukemia/lymphoma, may involve the CNS in up to 25% of patients, while myeloid malignancies, such as MDS, AML, and myeloproliferative disorders, rarely involve the CNS.

A second distinction is made based upon the chronicity of the leukemias. Acute leukemias, such as AML and ALL, have a rapidly evolving clinical course, with changes in the peripheral blood counts and clinical status occurring over days and weeks. Aggressive treatment is required within days or, sometimes, hours of diagnosis. In contrast, chronic leukemias, like CLL and CML, demonstrate indolent clinical courses, with subacute changes in the blood counts and clinical signs and symptoms. Treatment may be delayed to provide time for accurate diagnosis and, in some cases of CLL for example, treatment may be delayed for years from the time of diagnosis.

Diagnosis of Leukemias

Leukemia is suspected in patients with abnormal peripheral blood counts. Some individuals present with cytopenias, while others have elevated leukocyte counts. It is crucial to obtain a complete blood count (CBC) and differential from individuals suspected of having a bone marrow disorder. Patients with acute leukemia may have "blasts," myelo- or lymphoblasts, evident within the blood differential. However, some individuals simply have cytopenias without abnormal cells evident within the peripheral blood. While myeloblasts differ from lymphoblasts morphologically, the two cell types are very similar and only flow cytometry can reliably distinguish between them. Occasionally, Auer rods can be seen within the cytoplasm of blasts, providing definitive morphologic evidence that a cell is of myeloid origin.

A bone marrow biopsy is required to diagnose leukemia, myelodysplastic syndrome (MDS), and most cases of myeloproliferative disorders. The bone marrow biopsy consists of a liquid aspirate, approximately 5 cc in volume. A portion of the aspirate is spread over a glass slide at the bedside. Some institutions prepare a buffy coat, which is similarly used to prepare slides. The slides are stained with Wright-Giemsa stain and the bone marrow cellular morphology, examined by light microscopy. The percentage of bone marrow blasts is derived from the morphologic analysis of the bone marrow aspirate. The aspirate is also used for flow cytometric analysis, where fluorochrome-labelled antibodies are incubated with the bone marrow cells and the presence or absence of cell surface markers are used to characterize the bone marrow cells. In addition, cytogenetic analysis is performed on the bone marrow and is crucial to the diagnosis and treatment of leukemias. Lastly, molecular analyses may be conducted on the bone marrow aspirate.

The second component of the bone marrow biopsy involves obtaining a 1–2 cm bone core. "Touch preps" are prepared by applying the bone core to a glass slide and depositing a thin layer of cells on the slide. This is particularly useful in patients who have a "dry tap," where a aspirate cannot be obtained due to elevated bone marrow reticulin fibrosis or the presences of a marrow "packed" with leukemia cells. The slide is then stained with Wright-Giemsa and interpreted similarly to an aspirate. The bone core is then placed in a decalcification and fixation solution. Following a period of decalcification, the bone core is sectioned, stained with hematoxylin and eosin, and analyzed by light microscopy. Immunohistochemistry may also be performed on sections of the core. The core provides information on the ratio of bone marrow cellularity to fat in addition to morphology. Proper bone marrow analysis is highly complex and a specialized hematopathologist should be consulted throughout the process.

For patients with CNS symptoms, or patients at high risk of CNS involvement, a lumbar puncture (LP) should be performed for CSF analysis. AML, MDS, and MPDs rarely involve the CNS and an LP is not performed routinely as part of diagnosis and treatment in the absence of CNS symptoms. In contrast, ALL more frequently involves the CNS. In such patients, an LP is performed at diagnosis and several times during treatment, even in the absence of CNS symptoms. Useful diagnostic samples include analysis of the white blood cell count and differential, red blood cells, total protein, glucose, cytology, flow cytometry, and microbiologic studies. In patients who are receiving intrathecal therapy for active disease or who are receiving routine prophylactic intrathecal chemotherapy, a cell count is often the only test sent at the time of these LPs because once the presence or absence of CNS disease is established, repeated flow cytometric analysis of the CSF is not required. Patients with acute leukemias are often treated according to research protocols, and the specific guidelines for timing of diagnostic and therapeutic LPs, and instillation of chemotherapy, are established by the protocol.

Treatment of Leukemias

Appropriate leukemia treatment requires the involvement of a leukemia specialist. Once the diagnosis is established using the techniques outlined above, a treatment plan is developed. For acute leukemias, risk stratification is extremely important in developing the treatment plan. Important risk factors include patient age, WBC count at diagnosis, presence of extramedullary or CNS disease, and cytogenetic and molecular analyses of the leukemia.

Most patients undergo a period of intense therapy oriented toward achieving disease remission. This period, termed "induction," often requires a 4-week inpatient hospitalization. Once a remission is achieved, multiple cycles of consolidation chemotherapy may be employed to lessen the risk of disease recurrence. For patients with lymphoid leukemias, CNS-directed therapy involving intrathecal therapy, radiation, and systemic chemotherapies that traverse the blood-brain-barrier may be incorporated prophylactically or therapeutically.

For patients in remission following induction, stem cell transplantation (SCT) may be recommended. Autologous SCT has a role for some patients with acute leukemias, particularly for patients with relapsed disease. For patients with high-risk disease, allogeneic stem cell transplantation may be recommended once they are in remission. Allogeneic stem cell transplantation provides the potential benefit of a "graft-versus-leukemia" effect, which may reduce the chances of disease recurrence over chemotherapy alone. For individuals who achieve a remission but later relapse, treatment with reinduction, or salvage, chemotherapy is utilized to achieve a second remission. Allogeneic SCT is often recommended for such high-risk patients. The presence of CNS disease at diagnosis, or upon relapse, is considered a highly adverse risk factor and is frequently used to support a recommendation for allogeneic SCT.

The following outline summarizes the subtypes of leukemia that will be reviewed in detail.

- Myelodysplastic Syndromes (MDS)
- Myeloid Leukemias
  - Acute Myelogenous Leukemia (AML)
  - Chronic Myelogenous Leukemia (CML)

Lymphoid Leukemias
- Acute Lymphoblastic Leukemia (ALL)
  - B-cell subtype
    - Precursor B-cell
    - Mature B-cell
  - T-cell subtype
    - Precursor T-cell
    - Mature T-cell
- Chronic Lymphoblastic Leukemia (CLL)/Small Lymphocytic Lymphoma (SLL)

Myelodysplastic Syndromes (MDS)

Epidemiology and Etiology of MDS

Myelodysplastic syndromes (MDS) represent clonal malignant neoplasms of the bone marrow that result in cytopenias and, in some patients, heightened risk of developing AML. The median age of diagnosis is 68 years; there are approximately 15,000 cases of MDS in the United States each year, and the estimated prevalence is 50,000–100,000 cases. The disease is slightly more common in men compared to women with a ratio of 1.2:1, except for a rare variant of MDS known as the 5q-syndrome, which is more common in women at a ratio of 2:1.

Most patients with MDS have *de novo* disease – that is, disease which arises spontaneously. However, approximately 10% of patients have secondary disease, arising after an antecedent hematologic disorder, or after a period of exposure to chemotherapy or radiation. Individuals with secondary, or therapy-related, MDS have higher risk disease and require more aggressive treatment than those with *de novo* disease.

Clinical Presentation, Evaluation, and Staging of MDS

Cytopenias represent the most common manifestation of MDS and, because of the indolent clinical nature of MDS, the disease may be suspected upon routine blood testing. Anemia represents the most common cytopenia, experienced in 85% of patients. Approximately 50% of patients develop leukopenia and 25% thrombocytopenia. Symptoms are caused by the cytopenias. Patients with anemia develop dyspnea, fatigue, and depression, while those with leukopenia have increased risk of sinopulmonary and other infections. Individuals with thrombocytopenia may develop epistaxis, easy bruising, hematuria, hematochezia, and have an increased risk of intracranial hemorrhage after falls.

Diagnosis involves careful examination of the peripheral blood counts and exclusion of alternative causes of cytopenias. Thus, the CBC with differential, and measurements of serum B12, folate, iron, ferritin, and the transferrin saturation are useful. The erythropoietin level and reticulocyte count are also considered.

A bone marrow biopsy with cytogenetic analysis is required for the diagnosis of MDS. A hallmark of diagnosis is the presence of dysplasia within 10% or more of cells in at least one lineage. Dysplasia represents the morphologic abnormality, resulting from impaired cellular maturation due to the diseased hematopoietic stem cell clone responsible for MDS. Any of the three blood lineages may demonstrate dysplasia, though it is most commonly observed within the erythroid lineage. Red blood cells may demonstrate nuclear irregularities, frequent mitotic figures, and nuclear:cytoplasmic asynchrony. Myeloid cells may display nuclear atypia, hypogranulation, and the pseudo-Pelger-Huet nuclear abnormality. Lastly, dysplastic megakaryocytes may demonstrate nuclear hypolobation and clustering.

The bone marrow in MDS is hypercellular for age and may have increased myeloblasts as demonstrated on the bone marrow aspirate. The blasts may be normal in quantity, < 5% of the bone marrow cellularity, or may be increased in the range of 5–19%. If the blasts reach or exceed 20%, a diagnosis of AML is made.

Cytogenetic studies are important in the diagnosis and treatment of MDS. Cytogenetics are normal in 50% of individuals with MDS. However, when abnormal, the cytogenetics may suggest either low-, intermediate-, or high-risk disease based on the specific aberration(s) found. Cytogenetics are abnormal in > 80% of persons with secondary MDS. Chromosome 5q represents the most common chromosomal alteration in MDS, observed in 20% of individuals.

Individuals with an interstitial deletion within the long arm of chromosome 5q between bands 31 and 33 may have a 5q-syndrome. This syndrome is more commonly observed in women, is associated with anemia, thromobocytosis, excellent prognosis, and excellent clinical response to the class of medications known as immunomodulators, or IMiDs (ex. thalidomide, lenalidomide).

Natural History, Prognosis, and Treatment of MDS

Left untreated, MDS is associated with progressive cytopenias. Eventually, colony-stimulating factors, such as epoetin alfa to stimulate RBC production, and filgrastim to stimulate WBC production, are required. Individuals may develop transfusion dependence. Approximately 30% of patients with *de novo* disease, and most patients with secondary MDS, transform to AML. Thus, the goals of treatment are to improve quality of life, delay progression to AML, decrease transfusion dependence, and prolong overall survival.

The appropriate treatment for MDS is complex and is based on multiple factors, such as *de novo* versus secondary disease, cytogenetic status, patient age and wishes, and the presence of comorbid factors. The international prognostic scoring system (IPSS) takes into account the percentage of bone marrow blasts, cytogenetic status, and number and degree of cytopenias. The IPSS score correlates with median survival and time to development of AML, and may help guide treatment decision-making.

Allogeneic SCT represents the only possible cure for MDS, though it is a possible therapy for fewer than 20% of patients due to advanced age at diagnosis and lack of suitable donors. Supportive care consists of colony stimulating factors, blood product transfusions, and antibiotics. Hypomethylating agents, such as azacitidine and decitabine, have clinical benefit in reducing transfusion requirements and delaying development of AML. The primary cause of death is infection.

Acute Myelogenous Leukemia (AML)

Epidemiology and Etiology of AML

In the United States, there are roughly 10,000 new cases of AML diagnosed annually with a slight male predominance and a median age of onset of approximately 70 years. AML results from the improper maturation of myeloid cells, giving rise to a clonal population of myeloblasts. Excessive myeloblasts dominate the bone marrow and prevent normal hematopoiesis. No cause can be identified in most cases of AML; however, there are certain syndromes and exposures which can increase the risk of developing AML. Secondary AML, like secondary MDS, arises after a history of an antecedent hematologic disease or exposure to genotoxic agents, such as chemotherapy or radiation. A history of MDS is the most common risk factor for developing AML; other hematologic disorders, such as polycythemia vera and myelofibrosis, can also progress to AML. Individuals with trisomy 21, or Down's syndrome, have a 20-fold higher risk of leukemia than the general population. Smoking, exposure to benzene, and radiation exposure have also been associated with a higher risk of developing AML. A personal history of exposure to chemotherapy or radiation presents a risk for developing MDS and AML, and approximately 0.5% of patients receiving chemotherapy for a solid tumor will develop a myeloid malignancy. The agents most commonly associated with secondary AML include topoisomerase II inhibitors, which can predispose to AML within 1–3 years, and are frequently associated with abnormalities at chromosome11q23, the mixed-lineage leukemia (MLL) gene. Alkylating agents, such as melphalan, chlorambucil, cyclophosphamide, and ifosfamide increase the risk of MDS and AML, with peak incidence 3–7 years after exposure, and is often associated with aberrancies of chromosomes 5 and 7. A history of radiation therapy can also increase the risk of AML.

Clinical Presentation, Diagnosis, and Classification of AML

Presenting symptoms of AML include fatigue, dyspnea, bleeding (e.g. gastrointestinal, pulmonary, gingival), and/or infection, reflecting the patient's underlying anemia, thrombocytopenia, or neutropenia. Other individuals can present with abdominal fullness or pain from splenomegaly, gum swelling, or symptoms of leukostasis, like dyspnea or confusion, when the white blood cell count approaches > 100,000 cells/microliter. Symptoms and signs can include pallor, dyspnea, petechiae, ecchymoses, splenomegaly, or altered mental status.

Laboratory Findings

Common abnormal laboratory findings are anemia, thrombocytopenia, and leukopenia or leukocytosis. Coagulation studies may also be abnormal, especially in cases of acute promyelocytic leukemia (APML), which often presents with disseminated intravascular coagulopathy (DIC). The original French-American-British (FAB) system classified subtypes of AML based on the morphologic appearance of the myeloblasts. Under the FAB system, AML was defined by the presence of > 30% blast cells in the bone marrow. The more recent World Health Organization (WHO) system defines AML by the presence of at least 20% blasts in the peripheral blood or bone marrow; however, certain cytogenetic rearrangements are diagnostic of AML, regardless of the blast percentage. Classification is based on a combination of microscopy, histo- and cytochemical stains, cytogenetics, flow cytometry, and molecular analysis of peripheral blood and bone marrow.

Microscopy and Histochemistry

Blast cells often have prominent nucleoli and little cytoplasm. Auer rods, azurophilic granules within lysosomes, can sometimes be seen in myeloblasts on routine microscopy and are a characteristic of myeloid blasts, but not lymphoid blasts. AML cells stain positively with Sudan Black and myeloperoxidase, while ALL cells stain with periodic acid Schiff (PAS). Staining for nonspecific esterase, for example, can distinguish acute monocytic leukemia from other subtypes of AML.

Cytogenetics

Karyotyping and fluorescence in situ hybridization (FISH) often reveal characteristic cytogenetic abnormalities in AML and have become an integral part in the diagnosis, treatment, and prognosis of this disease. The t(15;17)(q22;q12) translocation is frequently seen in APML and creates a fusion product between the PML gene on chromosome 17 and the retinoic acid receptor alpha (RARα) gene on chromosome 15. This specific translocation is the basis for the excellent response and overall survival of APML to treatment with chemotherapy combined with all trans-retinoic acid (ATRA), which induces cellular differentiation. Other recurrent cytogenetic abnormalities in AML are summarized in Table 2.1. About 40% of individuals with AML have normal cytogenetics.

Table 2.1 Cytogenetic findings in AML

Cytogenetics	Prognosis	Distinguishing features
t(8;21)(q22;q22)	Good	AML1-ETO; myeloblastic with differentiation
t(15;17)(q22;q12)	Good	PML-RARα; (APML) excellent response to all trans-retinoic acid
Inversion 16(p13;q22)	Good	CBFb-MYH11; myelomonocytic with eosinophilia
Normal	Intermediate	Normal cytogenetics are observed in ~40% of AML
t(9;11)(p22;q23)	Intermediate	MLL3-MLL, monocytic, more common in children
Deletion 5q	Poor	Associated with prior treatment with alkylating agents
Deletion 7q	Poor	Associated with prior treatment with alkylating agents
11q23	Poor	MLL gene
>3 abnormalities	Poor	

Flow Cytometry and Molecular Analysis

Immunophenotyping (flow cytometry) is used to detect cell markers that help identify the lineage of leukemic cells. For example, myeloid cells often display markers such as CD13, CD33, and CD11c, whereas lymphoid cells more commonly demonstrate expression of the CD3, CD4, CD10, CD19 and CD20 markers. Other molecular studies provide additional diagnostic and prognostic information in patients with AML and are especially important in determining prognosis in patients with normal cytogenetics. The *FLT*3 gene (Fms-like tyrosine kinase 3) is commonly mutated, duplicated, or overexpressed in patients with AML and is associated with worse outcomes. Mutations in the *NPM*1 gene (nucleophosmin) are present in approximately 30% of AML cases; when found in the absence of other genetic abnormalities, *NPM*1 mutations confer a better prognosis. Similarly, *CEBPA* mutations, found in about 15% of AML patients, are associated with more favorable outcomes.

Natural History, Prognosis, and Treatment of AML

Approximately one-third of AML patients less than age 60 will survive longer than 5 years after diagnosis; the outcome in older patients is worse, with only about 10% surviving 5 years. As noted above, certain chromosomal rearrangements and genetic abnormalities correlate with patient outcome. Treatment regimens differ based on the subtype of AML, the age of the patient, and the presence of other co-morbidities. With the exception of APML (discussed below), most patients are treated initially with "7+3" induction therapy, which consists of 7 days of arabinosylcytosine (ara-C) and 3 days of an anthracycline (e.g. daunorubicin or idarubicin). Approximately

50–80% of patients achieve a remission with this combination; those with evidence of residual leukemia after a single induction can sometimes undergo reinduction with a second round of chemotherapy. After induction, AML patients with a favorable prognosis, such as those with the t(8;21) translocation, are often treated with consolidation therapy with several cycles of high-dose ara-C.

In patients with high-risk cytogenetic and molecular features, however, this strategy has a low probability of achieving cure. For these individuals, and for those who relapse after consolidation therapy, consideration is given to SCT. While allogeneic SCT offers the best chance of cure for AML, it is also associated with a high rate of treatment-related mortality, especially in older patients. Early life-threatening complications of SCT include infection, major bleeding, and organ failure. If engraftment of donor stem cells successfully occurs, transplant recipients can go on to develop graft-versus-host disease (GVDH), which itself carries a risk of morbidity and mortality.

In addition to induction, consolidation, and SCT, a number of novel therapeutic agents for AML are undergoing evaluation in clinical trials. These include demethylating agents (e.g. decitabine, azacitidine), Flt3 inhibitors (e.g. PKC 412), purine analogues (e.g. clofarabine), and monoclonal antibodies that target the CD33 cell surface marker present on many AML cells (e.g. lintuzumab, gemtuzumab).

Acute promyelocytic leukemia (APML) is a rare condition, but has a relatively high early mortality if it is not recognized and treated early. Induction therapy begins with oral all trans-retinoic acid (ATRA) followed by chemotherapy with an anthracycline and ara-C; this regimen can achieve complete remission in > 90% of APML cases. After remission, patients undergo multiple rounds of consolidation chemotherapy, often including arsenic trioxide (AsO3) and maintenance therapy with ATRA.

Diligent supportive care during treatment of AML is essential in avoiding adverse outcomes. This includes transfusion of red blood cells and platelets. Patients with APML are especially prone to disseminated intravascular coagulation (DIC) and its consequences, including intracranial hemorrhage, and thus should be supported with transfusions of fresh frozen plasma or cryoprecipitate and platelets. Prophylactic antibacterial, antifungal, and antiviral agents are usually administered once therapy is initiated. In neutropenic patients with fever, early treatment with broad-spectrum intravenous antibiotics is crucial.

Chronic Myelogenous Leukemia (CML)

Epidemiology and Etiology of CML

CML comprises roughly 20% of all adult leukemias, with a median age at diagnosis of approximately 50 years. CML is characterized by the translocation t(9;22), the so-called Philadelphia chromosome, which creates a fusion product between the *BCR* and *ABL* genes, and creates a fusion product with constitutive tyrosine kinase activity. The cause of this chromosomal rearrangement is unknown, but it may be observed at increased frequency in individuals previously exposed to radiation.

Clinical Presentation and Diagnosis of CML

Most patients with CML present in the stable phase of the disease (<5% of blasts in the bone marrow) and are asymptomatic at diagnosis. In these patients, diagnosis is often suspected when splenomegaly or leukocytosis is discovered on routine evaluations. Patients in the accelerated phase of CML (5–20% blasts) can sometimes present with weight loss, night sweats, and lymphadenopathy. Those in blast crisis (>20% blasts) present similarly to patients with acute leukemia, with symptoms of anemia, thrombocytopenia, or infection.

The CBC, peripheral blood smear, and bone marrow all usually reveal increased numbers of precursor and mature myeloid cells (blasts, myelocytes, metamyelocytes, granulocytes). These cells often have low enzyme activity, as reflected by the low leukocyte alkaline phosphatase (LAP) score. Definitive diagnosis is made by detection of the BCR-ABL translocation by cytogenetics or FISH. The translocation may also be detected by polymerase chain reaction (PCR) analysis of the blood and bone marrow.

Natural History, Prognosis, and Treatment of CML

The natural history and prognosis for patients with CML has improved dramatically in recent years since the development of molecular therapies that target the BCR-ABL fusion product. Prior to the development of tyrosine kinase inhibitors, most patients with CML would progress to blast crisis within 3–5 years, with generally a poor outcome at that point. These patients were formerly managed with medications such as hydroxyurea, busulfan, and interferon and, where possible, allogeneic stem cell transplantation. Imatinib mesylate, an oral tyrosine kinase inhibitor, revolutionized the treatment of CML. Among patients in the stable phase of disease, treatment with imatinib can achieve a 95% hematologic remission (normal WBC count), a 75% cytogenetic response (no detected Philadelphia chromosomes), and a 40% molecular remission (no BCR-ABL transcripts amplified by RT-PCR). Mutations in *BCR-ABL* or amplification of the gene can generate resistance to imatinib, as can activation of BCR-ABL-independent pathways. Second-generation tyrosine kinase inhibitors, such as dasatinib and nilotinib, are being used for treatment of imatinib-resistant CML.

SCT, once the only curative therapy for CML, is currently considered only for very young patients with CML or for those who do not respond to tyrosine kinase inhibitors. While SCT carries attendant risks, cure rates for CML reach 70%. Patients who develop chronic graft-versus-host disease (GVHD) after transplant have improved outcomes, implicating a strong role of graft-versus-leukemia effect in this disease.

Acute Lymphoblastic Leukemia (ALL)

Epidemiology and Etiology of ALL

Acute lymphoblastic leukemia (ALL) is a cancer of white blood cells of the lymphoid lineage (B- and T-cells). Approximately two-thirds of ALL cases occur in children under the age of 15, with a peak incidence in children ages 2–5. The incidence of ALL is higher among Caucasians and male children. Although ALL is the most common leukemia among children, it is relatively uncommon in adults. Specific causative factors have not been clearly linked to ALL, but it can occur in association with various genetic syndromes, such as Down syndrome, Klinefelter syndrome, neurofibromatosis, and ataxia telangectasia. A higher concordance rate is observed for ALL in monozygotic twins with a monochorionic placenta over dizygotic twins. The presence of leukemic translocations in neonatal blood spots from individuals who later developed ALL suggests that the initial leukemogenic mutations are prenatal in onset, at least in the pediatric form of this leukemia [12].

Clinical Presentation, Diagnosis, and Classification of ALL

Like other leukemias, ALL can present with anemia, neutropenia, and thrombocytopenia, as well as hepatosplenomegaly, lymphadenopathy, and bone pain. The CNS and testes form sanctuary sites for this leukemia and are potential sites for relapse, albeit less so in recent years. CNS involvement is more common in ALL than in myeloid leukemias; individuals with concurrent CNS and systemic ALL may present with headache, nausea, vomiting, and cranial nerve palsies.

Laboratory Findings

The diagnostic evaluation for ALL is similar to that for AML and includes CBC with differential, flow cytometry, cytogenetics, molecular studies, and analysis of the peripheral smear and bone marrow. The blood count and smear may demonstrate an elevated number of WBCs, with a lymphoblast predominance, often with anemia and thrombocytopenia. Other serum tests may reflect the rapid cell turnover that often accompanies ALL, such as high uric acid, phosphate, and lactate dehydrogenase (LDH), as well as low calcium. For diagnosis, bone marrow must demonstrate at least 25% lymphoblasts, although most patients present with an even greater percentage of blasts. Although other cell lines may be reduced in number, the general appearance and function of myeloid cells, erythroid cells, and megakaryocytes are preserved. Less than 5% of ALL patients have clinical manifestations of CNS leukemia; in this subset, LP and analysis of the CSF can reveal high opening pressure, low glucose, high protein, and pleocytosis with lymphoblasts. An LP is performed in all patients with ALL to detect CNS disease and concomitantly deliver prophylactic intrathecal chemotherapy. Imaging may demonstrate hepatosplenomegaly or lymphadenopathy; 5–15% of patients have an anterior mediastinal mass, which is more typical of T-cell ALL.

Flow Cytometry

Analysis of cell markers with flow cytometry is essential in the classification of ALL. Expression of terminal deoxynucleotidyltransferase (TdT), by IHC or flow cytometry, distinguishes precursor B- and T-cell leukemia/lymphomas from more mature non-Hodgkin lymphomas. Precursor B-cell ALL accounts for about 80% of ALL cases; these cells usually express the markers CD19 and CD10 (also called the common ALL antigen, cALLa), as well as other B-cell markers, such as CD20, CD24, CD22, CD21, or CD79. Mature B-cell ALL accounts for only 2–3% of ALL cases and represents disseminated Burkitt's lymphoma; these cells express CD19 and CD20.

The markers expressed by T-cell leukemias vary depending on their stage of maturation. Precursor T-cells usually express CD7, TdT, cytoplasmic CD3, and CD1a, whereas more differentiated cells express CD2, CD5, and then CD4 or CD8. Mature T-cells express T-cell receptor (TCR) and surface CD3.

Cytogenetics

As in AML, certain cytogenetic abnormalities are common in ALL and correlate with subtype, prognosis, and response to therapy, especially in precursor B-cell subtypes. In children, favorable cytogenetic findings include the t(12;21) translocation (*ETV*-6), hyperdiploidy (i.e. > 50 chromosomes per cell), and trisomies 4, 10, and 17. Unfavorable rearrangements in precursor B-cell ALL include the translocations t(4;11) (*MLL-AF*4), t(9;22) (Philadelphia chromosome, *BCR-ABL*), and t(1;19) (*E2A-PBX*1). Chromosomal and genetic abnormalities in T-cell ALL are not as well correlated with prognosis. About half of T-cell leukemias have activating mutations in the *NOTCH*1 gene and translocations involving the TCR are also common.

Natural History, Prognosis, and Treatment of ALL

For children with ALL, the rate of remission exceeds 95%, with four-fifths of patients surviving for 5 or more years after diagnosis. While 85% of adults achieve complete remission, only 25–40% survive 5 years. Unfavorable prognostic factors for children (summarized in Table 2.2) include age less than 1 year or over 10 years, high WBC count at presentation, poor response to initial therapy, mature B-cell or precursor T-cell ALL subtypes, certain cytogenetic rearrangements, and involvement of CNS.

Table 2.2 Prognostic factors for children with ALL

Characteristic	Favorable	Unfavorable
Age	1–9 years	<1 or >10 years
Subtype	Precursor B-cell	Mature B-cell Precursor T-cell
Location/distribution	No extramedullary disease	Involvement of mediastinum, and CNS
WBC count at presentation	<50,000/microliter	>50,000/microliter
Cytogenetics	t(12;21)ETV6-RUNX1 or TEL-AML1 Hyperdiploidy >50 Trisomies 4, 10, 17	t(9;22) BCR-ABL t(4;11) AF4/MLL t(1;19) E2A/PBX Hypodiploidy
Response to therapy	Clearance of peripheral blasts in 1 week; <5% marrow blasts at day 8 or 15; MRD < 0.1% at day 29	>5% marrow blasts on day 15 or > 0.1% MRD at day 29, failure to achieve CR by day 29

High-risk prognostic factors for adults have not been as clearly identified. Age > 30 is associated with a lower likelihood of achieving complete remission, earlier relapse, and worse overall survival. As with children, higher WBC count is unfavorable, as is the presence of a mediastinal mass.

For precursor-ALL subtypes, treatment involves a stepwise series of regimens: remission induction, intensification, maintenance, and CNS prophylaxis. The goal of remission induction is to normalize cell counts in the blood and marrow, reduce the blast burden to less than 5%, and eliminate extramedullary disease, including the CNS. This stage of treatment employs a steroid (e.g. prednisone), vincristine, L-asparaginase, and often, an anthracycline. In children, the presence of residual disease in a bone marrow aspirate 8 or 15 days after the start of induction predicts a higher risk of relapse [13]. For higher-risk patients and adults, additional agents are used. Intensification or consolidation aims to further reduce minimal residual disease (MRD) and prevent both relapse, as well as the selection of drug-resistant leukemic cells. In children, this phase may include courses of cyclophosphamide and cytarabine or high-dose methotrexate and is often followed by a reinduction regimen; for adults, a 5-drug regimen is typically used [14]. Maintenance therapy for children involves 2–3 years of weekly methotrexate and daily mercaptopurine with pulses of vincristine and steroid, along with intermittent intrathecal chemotherapy, in an effort to reduce relapse.

For mature B-cell ALL, Burkitt leukemia, the treatment regimen is similar to that of precursor ALL, with an emphasis on short intervals of time between cycles.

CNS Disease

Although clinically evident CNS leukemia is rarely seen and less than 10% of patients have blasts in the CSF at diagnosis, if the CNS is not treated prophylactically, leptomeningeal leukemic relapse is highly likely, despite a systemic remission. The initial diagnostic LP should be performed by a skilled clinician to avoid contamination of the CSF, with circulating leukemic lymphoblasts. At the time of the LP concomitant, intrathecal chemotherapy (methotrexate or cytarabine) should be given. Particularly in children, the LP may be performed under sedation to minimize the risk of trauma, especially given evidence that an initially traumatic LP in patients, with evidence of CNS disease at presentation is associated with inferior survival [15]. In adults, the LP is sometimes delayed until the peripheral blasts are cleared to minimize the theoretical risk of introducing blasts during the procedure.

In most children, CNS prophylaxis is accomplished using intrathecal chemotherapy, whereas cranial irradiation is reserved for patients who are at high-risk of CNS relapse (T cell ALL) or who have evidence for CNS disease at diagnosis or relapse [16]. Cranial irradiation is reserved for high-risk situations due to the concerns for long-term neurotoxicity. In adults, prophylactic intrathecal therapy and cranial irradiation are commonly utilized in combination, and are repeated at the time of CNS relapse. Intrathecal therapies commonly utilized include methotrexate and cytarabine, alone or in combination, and hydrocortisone is added when there is evidence for CNS disease. Liposomal cytarabine with systemic corticosteroids represents another therapeutic option. An Ommaya reservoir may be placed for patients who are receiving frequent intrathecal injections to enhance convenience and accuracy of drug administration, or where the LP is technically difficult due to anatomic considerations. However, hydrocortisone is often eliminated if administering chemotherapy through an Ommaya reservoir, as it may induce severe vomiting.

Stem Cell Transplantation

Autologous SCT is rarely utilized for adults with ALL, however, allogeneic SCT is considered for young adults with a matched sibling donor [17]. For individuals with relapsed disease, including within the CNS, allogeneic SCT is considered.

Chronic Lymphocytic Leukemia (CLL)

CLL, the appearance of mature, malignant lymphocytes within the blood may coexist with or occur independently of SLL when these cells involve lymph nodes. This is discussed in Chapter 1.

References

1. Dick JE (2003) Stem cells: self-renewal writ in blood. Nature 423(6937):231–233
2. Schofield R (1978) The relationship between the spleen colony-forming cell and the haemopoietic stem cell. Blood Cells 4(1–2):7–25

3. Hannum C, Culpepper J, Campbell D et al (1994) Ligand for FLT3/FLK2 receptor tyrosine kinase regulates growth of haematopoietic stem cells and is encoded by variant RNAs. Nature 368(6472):643–648
4. Uemura N, Ozawa K, Takahashi K et al (1993) Binding of membrane-anchored macrophage colony-stimulating factor (M-CSF) to its receptor mediates specific adhesion between stromal cells and M-CSF receptor-bearing hematopoietic cells. Blood 82(9):2634–2640
5. Chan JY, Watt SM (2001) Adhesion receptors on haematopoietic progenitor cells. Br J Haematol 112(3):541–557
6. Gong JK (1978) Endosteal marrow: a rich source of hematopoietic stem cells. Science 199(4336):1443–1445
7. Visnjic D, Kalajzic Z, Rowe DW et al (2004) Hematopoiesis is severely altered in mice with an induced osteoblast deficiency. Blood 103(9):3258–3264
8. Pittenger MF, Mackay AM, Beck SC et al (1999) Multilineage potential of adult human mesenchymal stem cells. Science 284(5411):143–147
9. Maitra B, Szekely E, Gjini K et al (2004) Human mesenchymal stem cells support unrelated donor hematopoietic stem cells and suppress T-cell activation. Bone Marrow Transplant 33(6):597–604
10. Wang L, Zhao RC (2009) Mesenchymal stem cells targeting the GVHD. Sci China C Life Sci 52(7):603–609
11. Dick JE, Lapidot T (2005) Biology of normal and acute myeloid leukemia stem cells. Int J Hematol 82(5):389–396
12. Greaves MF, Maia AT, Wiemels JL, Ford AM (2003) Leukemia in twins: lessons in natural history. Blood 102(7):2321–2333
13. Basso G, Veltroni M, Valsecchi MG et al (2009) Risk of relapse of childhood acute lymphoblastic leukemia is predicted by flow cytometric measurement of residual disease on day 15 bone marrow. J Clin Oncol 27(31):5168–5174
14. Larson RA, Dodge RK, Linker CA et al (1998) A randomized controlled trial of filgrastim during remission induction and consolidation chemotherapy for adults with acute lymphoblastic leukemia: CALGB study 9111. Blood 92(5):1556–1564
15. te Loo DM, Kamps WA, van der Does-van den Berg A et al (2006) Prognostic significance of blasts in the cerebrospinal fluid without pleiocytosis or a traumatic lumbar puncture in children with acute lymphoblastic leukemia: experience of the Dutch Childhood Oncology Group. J Clin Oncol 24(15):2332–2336
16. Pui CH, Campana D, Pei D et al (2009) Treating childhood acute lymphoblastic leukemia without cranial irradiation. N Engl J Med 360(26):2730–2741
17. Goldstone AH, Richards SM, Lazarus HM et al (2008) In adults with standard-risk acute lymphoblastic leukemia, the greatest benefit is achieved from a matched sibling allogeneic transplantation in first complete remission, and an autologous transplantation is less effective than conventional consolidation/maintenance chemotherapy in all patients: final results of the International ALL Trial (MRC UKALL XII/ECOG E2993). Blood 111(4):1827–1833

Part II
Central Nervous System Lymphomas

Chapter 3
Pathology of Primary Central Nervous System Lymphoma and Related Conditions

Judith A. Ferry, Rolf Pfannl, and Nancy L. Harris

Introduction

Primary Central Nervous System Lymphoma (PCNSL) is defined as lymphoma confined to the brain, eye, spinal cord, or leptomeninges without evidence of prior or concurrent lymphoma outside of the nervous system. Other types of lymphoma that involve the nervous system include lymphoma of peripheral nerves and nerve roots, lymphomatoid granulomatosis, and intravascular lymphoma; these lymphomas, as well as lymphoma of the dura mater are reviewed in the sections that follow.

Primary Central Nervous System Lymphoma

Background

PCNSL may develop in both immunocompetent patients and immunosuppressed patients. Among immunocompetent patients, PCNSL is rare, making up 4–5% of all primary central nervous system tumors and 1–2% of all non-Hodgkin's lymphomas [1–4]. Immunocompetent patients with PCNSL are predominantly older adults, with men affected slightly more often than women [1, 3–11]. PCNSL rarely occurs in immunocompetent individuals less than 21 years of age [5, 12, 13]. Immunodeficient patients who develop PCNSL are predominantly infected with the human immunodeficiency virus (HIV), with a risk of approximately 1,000 times that of immunocompetent individuals [14]. These patients are younger with a more striking male preponderance than immunocompetent patients [15]. In HIV+ individuals, PCNSL usually occurs late in the course of AIDS when the CD4 T-cell count is very low [15]. The use of highly active antiretroviral therapy (HAART) has been associated with a dramatic decrease in the incidence of PCNSL in HIV+ patients [16]. There is also an increased incidence of PCNSL in those with congenital and

J.A. Ferry (✉)
Department of Pathology, Massachusetts General Hospital, Boston, MA 02114, USA
e-mail: jferry@partners.org

T. Batchelor, L.M. DeAngelis (eds.), *Lymphoma and Leukemia of the Nervous System*, DOI 10.1007/978-1-4419-7668-0_3,

iatrogenic immunodeficiency, including transplant recipients. Other suggested but less well established predisposing factors include autoimmune disease and prior malignancy [1, 10, 17, 18]. Thus, immunologic abnormalities are important in the pathogenesis of a subset of PCNSL. The cause is unknown for those cases occurring sporadically. A detailed description of the epidemiology of PCNSL can be found in Chapter 4.

Establishing the Diagnosis

The diagnosis of PCNSL may be established by biopsy of the tumor, lumbar puncture for cerebrospinal fluid (CSF) cytology or, in patients with ocular involvement, vitreous aspirate or vitrectomy. However, CSF is often negative in patients with PCNSL. Because the lesions are often deep within the brain, involving vital structures, stereotactic biopsy is preferred. Tissue from biopsies performed in patients with suspected lymphoma should always be sent fresh to the pathologist for intraoperative examination and appropriate triage for permanent sections and special studies. Intraoperative diagnosis of brain biopsy specimens requires careful sampling to represent the tissue adequately. A very small amount of tissue from both tips of a stereotactic core needle biopsy can be smeared to prepare a "squash prep," or touch preps can be prepared, for microscopic examination. Intraoperative frozen section examination is usually performed to determine the adequacy of the specimen. Only a portion of the tissue should be frozen, and if it contains tumor or a lymphoid infiltrate, it should be retained frozen at –70° for molecular diagnostic studies in case these are necessary to establish the diagnosis. Preparing touch preps or squash preps is useful in evaluating cytologic features, and can complement evaluation of a frozen section. If a large amount of tissue is available, a portion may be sent for flow cytometry, as this may be a useful adjunct to histologic examination [1, 5, 8, 17, 19]. The CSF contains tumor cells in only a minority of cases, so while lumbar puncture is associated with little morbidity, it is relatively insensitive. Multicolor flow cytometry is a rapid and sensitive technique that can enhance the detection of lymphoma in paucicellular CSF samples [20]. CSF can also be evaluated using the polymerase chain reaction to investigate the presence of a B-cell population with clonally rearranged immunoglobulin heavy chain genes (*IGH*). PCR confirms the presence of a clonal B-cell population in some cases, in which CSF cytology is suspicious or positive, and also detects a clonal population in some cases in which cytology is negative. However, spurious clonality may be detected in CSF with only a few B cells. Thus, morphologic evaluation by cytopathology and molecular genetic evaluation using PCR are complementary techniques in detecting involvement of CSF by lymphoma [11]. Cytopathology, flow cytometry, and PCR can also be performed on vitreous fluid in those cases suspected to have ocular involvement by lymphoma.

For immunosuppressed patients whose lymphomas are almost always positive for the Epstein Barr virus (EBV), the presence of EBV DNA in the CSF detected by PCR is reported by some authorities to be a sensitive and specific technique for diagnosing PCNSL, which may be used as an alternative to routine diagnostic methods in selected cases [3, 10, 21, 22]. The presence of EBV DNA in CSF has been reported in HIV+ patients in disorders other than PCNSL, so that careful clinical and radiographic correlation is required. Absence of EBV DNA is reported to be a strong negative predictor for a diagnosis of PCNSL among HIV+ patients [23].

Primary CNS Diffuse Large B-Cell Lymphoma (PCNS DLBCL)

The great majority of PCNSL cases, including both primary intracerebral and intraocular lymphomas, are primary CNS diffuse large B-cell lymphoma (PCNS DLBCL). PCNS DLBCL has recently been recognized as a distinct subtype of DLBCL in the WHO Classification (Table 3.1) [11, 24]. It is defined as all primary intracerebral or intraocular diffuse large B-cell lymphomas [24]. Among immunocompromised patients, PCNSL are almost always PCNS DLBCL [15]; although considered separately from PCNS DLBCL in immunocompetent hosts in the WHO Classification, their pathologic features and the diagnostic problems they raise are similar, and so they are discussed together in the sections that follow. Intraocular lymphoma (IOL) is considered separately below [5, 17, 24, 25]. Other types of PCNSL are very uncommon among immunocompetent patients, and rare among immunosuppressed patients. These are discussed separately below.

Anatomic Distribution and Gross Pathology

The presentation of PCNS DLBCL is variable and can be deceiving to the untrained eye. It may mimic the appearance of tumors, such as glioblastomas or infectious diseases, such as toxoplasmosis. Not infrequently, it may present with periventricular changes resembling demyelination. Rarely, it may present only with subtle enhancement of cranial or radicular nerves, or with a focus of mild meningeal enhancement. PCNS DLBCL in immunocompetent patients usually presents as single or occasionally multiple lesions within the brain in the form of deep-seated masses in the periventricular white matter [3, 26]. Lesions are more often multiple in immunocompromised patients [15, 27]. Supratentorial disease is more common than infratentorial involvement among both immunocompetent and immunodeficient patients. Involvement of the spinal cord is uncommon, and lymphoma confined to the spinal cord at presentation is rare [2, 10, 15]. Although secondary leptomeningeal involvement in cases of PCNS DLBCL is not uncommon, lymphoma confined to the leptomeninges and cerebrospinal fluid at presentation, designated primary leptomeningeal lymphoma, is very rare. Autopsy examination typically reveals a poorly circumscribed mass lesion(s) with replacement or displacement of normal structures. The lesions are usually poorly circumscribed due to diffuse tumor infiltration of the surrounding tissue (Fig. 3.1). The adjacent gray matter nuclei and cortex may be involved to variable degrees [12]. PCNS DLBCL tumor masses usually contain varying degrees of tumor necrosis and hemorrhage. The extent of tumor

Table 3.1 Lymphoid neoplasms primary in the central nervous system and meninges

Type of lymphoma	PCNSL	Comments
Precursor neoplasms		
B lymphoblastic lymphoma/leukemia	Very rare	
Mature B-cell neoplasms		
Chronic lymphocytic leukemia/small lymphocytic lymphoma	Very rare, not well documented	
Lymphoplasmacytic lymphoma	Not well documented	
MALT lymphoma	Very rare	Mainly dural
Follicular lymphoma	Very rare, not well documented	
CNS Diffuse large B-cell lymphoma (DLBCL)	Approximately 95% of PCNSL	Most EBV–; EBV+ in immunodeficient patients
Lymphomatoid granulomatosis	May involve CNS, usually not in isolation	Neoplastic B cells EBV+
Intravascular large B-cell lymphoma	Presentation with CNS involvement is common; disease is often widespread	
Plasmablastic lymphoma	Very rare	Associated with HIV infection
Burkitt lymphoma	Rare	Associated with HIV infection
Mature T and NK-cell neoplasms		
Extranodal NK/T-cell lymphoma	Very rare	
Peripheral T-cell lymphoma, NOS	Rare	
ALCL, ALK+	Very rare	
ALCL, ALK–	Very rare	
Hodgkin lymphoma		
Classical Hodgkin lymphoma	Very rare	

Abbreviations: ALCL, anaplastic large cell lymphoma; EBV, Epstein–Barr virus.

necrosis may be significant, especially in previously treated tumors, highlighting the importance of acquiring tissue for diagnosis prior to the initiation or therapy. The mass effect of the tumor may be enhanced by tissue edema, causing expansion of the white matter and overlying gyri and narrowing of intervening sulci. Rare cases show extensive infiltration of the brain, and sometimes the spinal cord, without forming a recognizable tumor mass. Such a growth pattern is referred to as lymphomatosis cerebri [28, 29]. On occasion, the gross appearance of PCNS DLBCL can be deceiving and the widespread extent of the disease may be apparent on microscopy only.

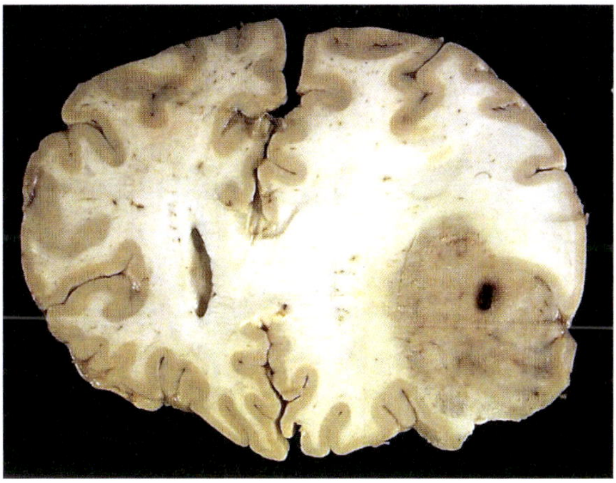

Fig. 3.1 PCNSL. Single ill-defined mass in the right frontal lobe with a small hemorrhagic area at the site of previous biopsy. The tumor borders and overlying cortical-white matter junction are effaced due to diffuse infiltration by tumor cells. Of note is the marked expansion of the white matter due to tissue edema

If leptomeningeal infiltration is present, the arachnoid is dull and gray, although in some cases the changes are subtle.

Microscopic Features

If solid tumor is sampled, the picture is that of sheets of fairly monotonous, atypical, discohesive mononuclear cells (Fig. 3.2). Tumor necrosis may be prominent and scattered foamy histiocytes may be present, and may be especially prominent if the patient has received steroids prior to biopsy [24]. When the edge of the tumor is sampled, the tumor cells are preferentially arranged around small blood vessels in otherwise normal brain parenchyma, or accompanied by a few reactive astrocytes (Fig. 3.3). Scattered to numerous mitotic figures can be seen. Endothelial cells are usually plump. Small blood vessel walls typically show infiltration by tumor cells with expansion of the reticulin framework. Scattered tumor cells can be seen invading the adjacent brain parenchyma. If corticosteroids have been administered prior to biopsy, the tumor may temporarily shrink or even disappear, and neoplastic cells may undergo apoptosis, making diagnosis difficult. In some cases, there is an associated perivascular loss of myelin, best demonstrated with the Luxol-fast blue stain. Demyelination has been described in association with PCNSL, but it may be due in some cases to myelin degeneration in the course of tumor regression related to therapy, rather than as a direct effect of the lymphoma alone [30, 31].

DLBCL are composed of centroblasts, immunoblasts, or a mixture of the two. Centroblasts are large lymphoid cells (typically three times the size of normal resting lymphocytes) with round to oval, vesicular nuclei, one or more small nucleoli usually present along the nuclear membrane, and scant cytoplasm. Immunoblasts are similar sized large cells with abundant cytoplasm, oval or irregular nuclei, and usually a single prominent nucleolus, sometimes with eccentric cytoplasm, indicating plasmacytic differentiation. The centroblastic variant of DLBCL is defined as

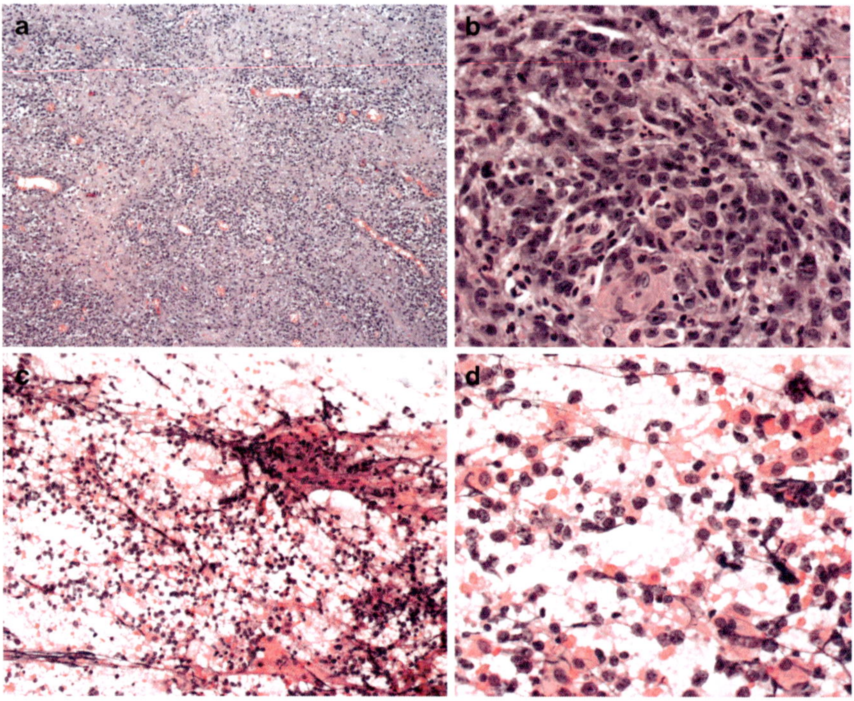

Fig. 3.2 Primary CNS diffuse large B-cell lymphoma. **a** Low power shows a patchy, but overall dense infiltrate of lymphoid cells with preferential distribution in broad perivascular cuffs. **b** High power shows large lymphoid cells, the majority of which are immunoblasts. **c** Low power examination of a squash prep shows scattered discohesive lymphoid cells in a background of strands of tissue. **d** High power of the squash prep shows large lymphoid cells with round to oval nuclei, small nucleoli and scant cytoplasm with scattered red blood cells and debris

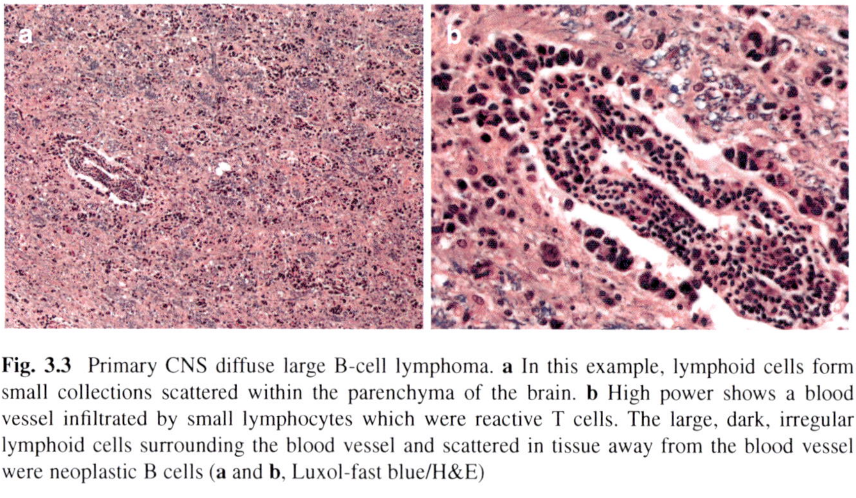

Fig. 3.3 Primary CNS diffuse large B-cell lymphoma. **a** In this example, lymphoid cells form small collections scattered within the parenchyma of the brain. **b** High power shows a blood vessel infiltrated by small lymphocytes which were reactive T cells. The large, dark, irregular lymphoid cells surrounding the blood vessel and scattered in tissue away from the blood vessel were neoplastic B cells (**a** and **b**, Luxol-fast blue/H&E)

being composed of centroblasts with or without admixed immunoblasts (up to 90% of the cells). The immunoblastic variant of DLBCL is composed entirely or almost entirely of immunoblasts (90% or more of all neoplastic cells) [32]. Compared to cases in immunocompetent patients, DLBCL in immunodeficient patients is more likely to be composed entirely of immunoblasts, to show plasmacytic differentiation or to be composed of more pleomorphic cells [1, 5, 6, 12, 15, 19, 33–35]. Post-transplantation lymphoproliferative disorders can be of a variety of polymorphic and monomorphic types (Table 3.2) [36], but those that are primary in the CNS are nearly all monomorphic, composed of large B cells [27, 28, 37]. A varying degree of reactive T-cell infiltration in the form of small mature lymphocytes around small cerebral blood vessels may be seen. On occasion, the T-cell population may be prominent and create diagnostic problems by raising the possibility of a reactive, rather than a neoplastic process. The reactive T-cell population may remain after the disappearance of the tumor after therapy.

Table 3.2 Categories of post-transplant lymphoproliferative disorders (PTLD)

1. Early lesions
   - Reactive plasmacytic hyperplasia
   - Infectious mononucleosis-like
2. Polymorphic PTLD
3. Monomorphic PTLD (classify according to lymphoma classification)
   - B-cell neoplasms
     Diffuse large B-cell lymphoma
     Burkitt lymphoma
     Plasma cell myeloma
     Plasmacytoma-like lesions
     Other
   - T-cell neoplasms
     Peripheral T-cell lymphoma, NOS
     Hepatosplenic T-cell lymphoma
     Other
4. Classical Hodgkin lymphoma-type PTLD

Cytological examination of the CSF can be useful in a subset of patients with PCNS DLBCL if tumor cells are adjacent to the CSF pathways [38]. The atypical lymphoid population most commonly consists of immunoblastic and centroblastic cells with large, sometimes irregular and convoluted nuclei, granular chromatin, prominent nucleoli and minimal cytoplasm. Mitotic figures may be identified [38].

Immunophenotype

PCNS DLBCL expresses pan-B cell antigens (CD20, CD79a). Monotypic expression of immunoglobulin (usually IgM) can often be detected when frozen tissue is available for immunohistochemistry or with flow cytometry, and occasionally on paraffin sections with immunohistochemistry or in situ hybridization

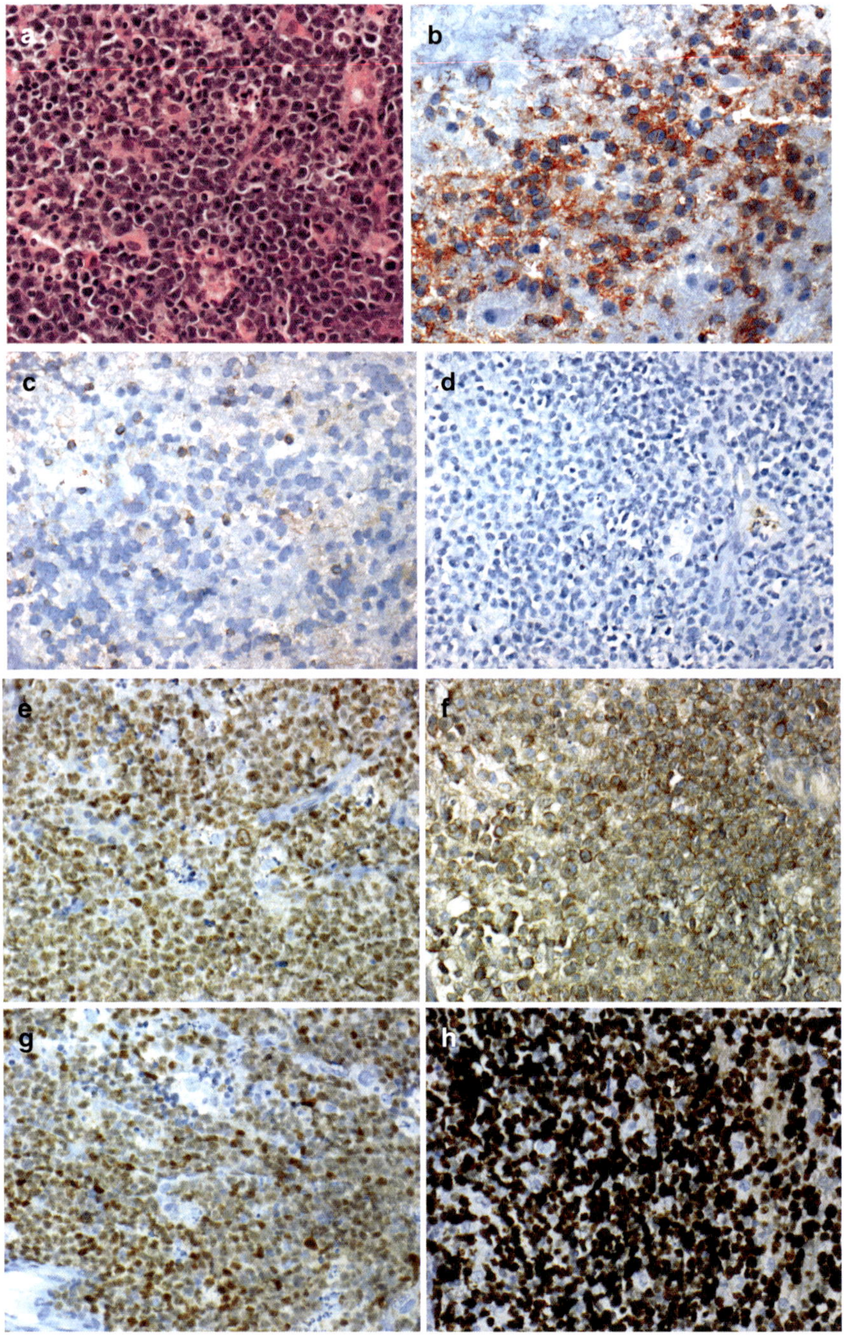

Fig. 3.4 Primary CNS diffuse large B-cell lymphoma, immunophenotype. **a** This lymphoma is composed of large atypical lymphoid cells with irregular nuclei. **b** and **c** Large atypical cells are CD20+ B cells (**b**) with few scattered small T cells (CD3+) (immunoperoxidase technique

[1, 35, 39, 40]. In one report, most HIV-associated PCNS DLBCL had undergone heavy chain class switch and expressed IgG or IgA [15], in contrast to the IgM expression found in immunocompetent patients. Nearly all HIV-associated and post-transplant cases of PCNSL contain EBV, readily detected with in situ hybridization for EBER. Many of them are positive for the EBV latent membrane protein (EBV-LMP) or the Epstein Barr nuclear antigen (EBNA) [12, 15, 21, 27, 39]. PCNSL in immunocompetent patients is typically negative for EBV [4, 6, 14].

A number of reports have described the immunophenotype of PCNS DLBCL of immunocompetent patients in more detail, using the findings to determine the stage of B-cell differentiation of the neoplastic cells. Results have varied among series, but CD10 is expressed in only a small minority of cases [13, 41–44], bcl6 is often expressed (46% or more of cases positive), bcl2 is variably expressed [6, 41, 43] and MUM1/IRF4 is nearly always positive [13, 41–43]. CD138, a marker most strongly associated with plasma cells, is uniformly negative [42–44]. Thus, only a minority of PCNSLs have a germinal center B-cell immunophenotype (CD10+, bcl6+ or CD10–, bcl6+, MUM1/IRF4) according to the criteria of Hans [45], while the great majority have a post-germinal center or non-germinal center immunophenotype (CD10–, bcl6– or CD10–, bcl6+, MUM1/IRF4+) (Fig. 3.4) [41]. A germinal center B-cell immunophenotype is less common among PCNSL compared to systemic diffuse large B-cell lymphoma [46]. We have seen the case of a patient with PCNSL (illustrated in Fig. 3.2) who achieved a complete remission and was well for 8 years, until he developed a cutaneous diffuse large B-cell lymphoma with histologic features similar to those of the PCNSL, and with an immunophenotype of the type most often seen in PCNS DLBCL (CD10–, bcl6+, MUM1/IRF4+) (Fig. 3.5). Although a clonal relationship between the two lymphomas was not formally demonstrated, the cutaneous lymphoma was considered most likely to be a relapse of the prior PCNS DLBCL. Primary CNS diffuse large B-cell lymphomas also, more often, have loss of HLA class I and/or HLA class II expression than primary nodal diffuse large B-cell lymphoma. The failure to express HLA antigens could result in neoplastic B cells escaping from immune surveillance by T cells [47], potentially contributing to the poor prognosis associated with PCNS DLBCL.

In one study, PCNS DLBCL was divided into two distinct groups based on morphology and immunophenotype: (1) lymphomas composed of centroblasts that are BCL-6+, LMP1–, BCL-2±, found both in HIV+ and HIV– patients, and (2) immunoblastic lymphomas that are BCL-6–, LMP1+, BCL-2+, found only in HIV+ patients [14]. Table 3.3 lists a panel of markers that should be done in the diagnostic evaluation of a biopsy specimen from a patient with suspected PCNSL.

Fig. 3.4 (continued) on frozen sections). **d–h**. The large neoplastic B cells are negative for CD10 (**d**), and positive for bcl6 (**e**), bcl2 (**f**) and MUM1/IRF4 (**g**); the vast majority of cells are Ki67+ (proliferation, **h**) (immunoperoxidase technique on paraffin sections)

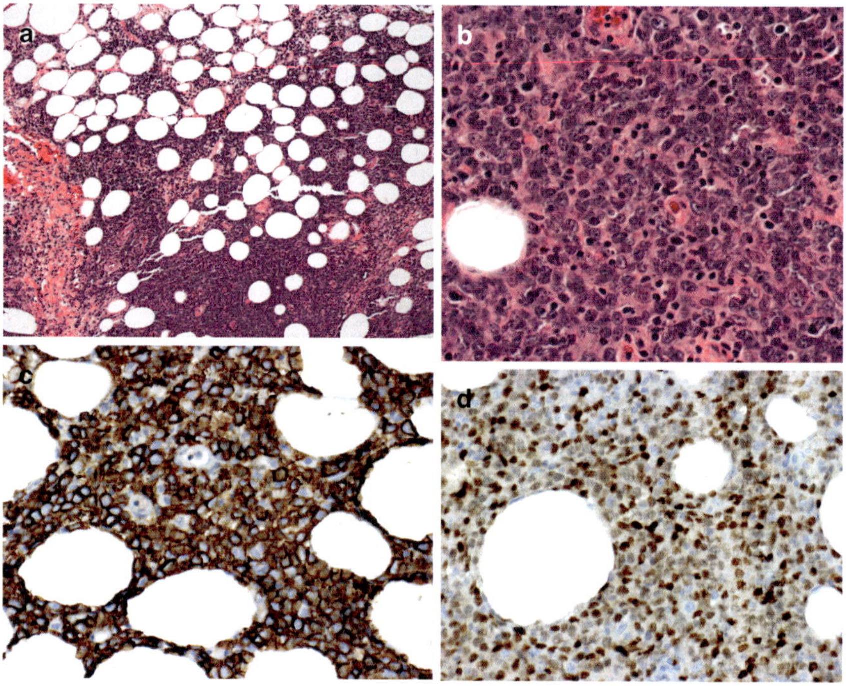

Fig. 3.5 Diffuse large B-cell lymphoma involving the skin, probably a relapse of the PCNSL illustrated in Fig. 3.2. **a** Low power shows a cellular lesion involving subcutaneous fat. **b** High power shows large atypical lymphoid cells with oval nuclei and scant cytoplasm; the appearance is similar to that of the lymphoma in Fig. 3.2b. **c** and **d** The lymphoid cells are CD20+ (**c**) and MUM1/IRF4+ (**d**) (immunoperoxidase technique on paraffin sections)

Table 3.3 Recommended evaluation of a specimen suspected to be PCNSL

Marker	Rationale
Leukocyte common antigen (CD45)	Confirms hematopoietic neoplasm
Cytokeratin; S100, HMB-45, MART1	Excludes metastatic carcinoma and melanoma
B-cell antigen (CD20)	Distinction of B cell from T cell lymphoma
T-cell antigen (CD3)	Distinction of B cell from T cell lymphoma; marker of T-cell infiltration
BCL-6	Follicle center origin; May have prognostic importance
CD10 (optional)	Follicle center origin; may have prognostic importance
BCL-2 (optional)	May have prognostic importance
MUM1/IRF4	May have prognostic importance
Ki-67 (optional)	Labels proliferating cells; may have prognostic significance
In situ hybridization for EBER	Positive in PCNSL in immunocompromised patients

Genetic Features

Molecular genetic analysis shows clonal immunoglobulin gene rearrangement in diffuse large B-cell lymphomas [9, 14]. *TP*53 and *CDKN2A/p*16 alterations may play a role in the pathogenesis of some cases of PCNSL [1]. In one study, 19/31 (61%) tumor specimens had either homozygous (13) or heterozygous (6) deletions of the *CDKN2A/p*16 gene. In this same study, 6/33 (18%) of the PCNSL tumor specimens were found to have *TP*53 alterations [43]. Neither of these genetic alterations was associated with prognosis in this study.

Approximately half of all PCNS DLBCL (more often in HIV– than HIV+ cases) have mutations of the *BCL*6 gene consistent with transition through the germinal center (GC) [14]. Aberrant somatic mutation of other genes, including *PAX*5 and *MYC*, is also reported [48]. *BCL*2 rearrangement is absent [14]. There appears to be preferential use of certain immunoglobulin VH families, as well as a very high load of somatic mutations, in some cases accompanied by intraclonal diversity. This pattern suggests that the neoplastic cells of PCNS DLBCL are derived from antigen-selected B cells of the GC. The extent of somatic hypermutation is greater than that encountered in diffuse large B-cell lymphomas arising outside the CNS [9, 35, 40, 49, 50]. Evaluation of PCNS DLBCL also shows evidence of activation of the NFκB pathway, in the form of expression of both MALT1 and BCL10, and increased transcript levels of genes of the NFκB complex and their target genes, suggesting that NFκB activation may play an important role in the pathogenesis of PCNS DLBCL [51].

A high load of somatic mutations is less common in HIV-associated PCNS DLBCL than in PCNS DLBCL in immunocompetent patients. Primary CNS diffuse large B-cell lymphoma in HIV+ patients also shows preferential use of certain IGV_H families, but the IGV_H family usage differs from that found in immunocompetent patients [33]. The failure to express HLA class I and II antigens noted above is related to deletions and genetic alterations of portions of the genes coding for the HLA class I and II molecules [47].

Intraocular Lymphoma

Intraocular lymphoma (IOL), i.e., lymphoma involving the eye itself, is uncommon but its frequency has increased in recent years [25, 52–55]. IOL may occur in isolation, or may be the presenting symptom of more widespread CNS disease. The eyes may also be secondarily involved by spread from PCNSL, initially presenting in the brain or from systemic lymphoma arising in nodal or extranodal primary sites [52, 56–58].

IOL predominantly affects older adults [53–55, 59, 60], less commonly young adults [55, 61, 62], and rarely, children [54, 61, 63]. Among patients with IOL, there is a female preponderance [52–55, 60, 62, 64–68]. The majority of IOL apparently arise sporadically, but a few cases have arisen in the setting of HIV infection [25, 69] or in association with iatrogenic immunosuppression in allograft recipients [61, 70, 71].

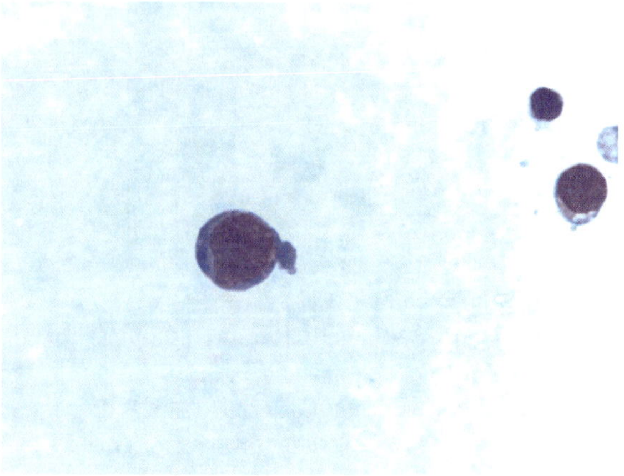

Fig. 3.6 Intraocular lymphoma, aspirate of vitreous fluid. The image shows a large atypical lymphoid cell with prominent nucleoli and deep blue cytoplasm that is much larger then the small lymphocyte also present. Flow cytometric analysis detected a population of CD45+, CD19+, CD20+, CD5–, CD10– B cells expressing monotypic kappa light chain involving the vitreous of both eyes

A variety of techniques may be used to establish the diagnosis of IOL, including vitreous aspirate, vitrectomy, biopsy, or in patients with a blind, painful eye, ocular enucleation. The technique most commonly used is microscopic examination of aspirated vitreous fluid, but the sensitivity of this procedure may be limited by admixed inflammatory cells, which may obscure the neoplastic population, or by prior corticosteroid therapy, which may eliminate many of the tumor cells [54, 55, 72, 73]. An elevated IL-10 level in the vitreous is strongly associated with IOL, and could prompt repeat biopsy if the initial specimen is non-diagnostic [52]. In contrast, elevated levels of IL-6, likely derived from reactive cells, tend to support a diagnosis of uveitis. Although not completely specific, an IL-10:IL-6 ratio > 1 is suspicious for lymphoma, while a ratio < 1 is more supportive of uveitis [69].

Nearly all cases of IOL are diffuse large B-cell tumors [25, 54, 55, 70, 71, 73]. The histologic and immunophenotypic features are essentially identical to diffuse large B-cell lymphoma presenting in the brain (Fig. 3.6), and intraocular DLBCL falls within the WHO category of PCNS DLBCL, as noted above [24]. EBV is present in intraocular diffuse large B-cell lymphoma in immunodeficient patients, but not in immunocompetent patients. Rare cases of peripheral T-cell lymphoma presenting with ocular involvement have also been described [56, 69, 74–77].

Postulated Normal Counterpart of PCNS DLBCL

The immunophenotypic features suggest derivation of most cases of PCNS DLBCL from a post-GC B cell. The prominent somatic hypermutation of immunoglobulin genes and the frequent aberrant somatic hypermutation of other genes strongly suggest prolonged exposure to the GC microenvironment. The neoplastic cells thus share features corresponding to GC and post-GC stages of B-cell differentiation. Since the CNS is devoid of GCs, the implication of these observations is that PCNSL may represent a tumor that arises outside the CNS. Subsequent localization to the CNS might involve the development of a "neurotropic" cellular phenotype, or failure of the host immune system to eliminate malignant lymphoid cells that have reached the immunologically privileged CNS [43].

Primary Central Nervous System Lymphomas: Rare Types

A small subset of DLBCL presenting with CNS involvement (1–2%) are intravascular large B-cell lymphoma [1, 12]. Lymphomatoid granulomatosis may also affect the CNS. Intravascular large B-cell lymphoma and lymphomatoid granulomatosis are discussed below. Rare low-grade B-cell lymphomas primary in the CNS have been described; they have been classified as small lymphocytic, small lymphocytic plasmacytoid or follicular lymphoma [78, 79]. Rare peripheral T-cell lymphomas [78, 79], including cases of ALK+ and ALK– anaplastic large cell lymphoma are also described [80–82]. Burkitt's lymphoma is occasionally encountered, particularly in immunocompromised patients [15, 83]. A case of plasmablastic lymphoma, apparently primary in the CNS, has been described in an HIV+ male [84]. Plasmablastic lymphoma is an uncommon type of DLBCL, strongly associated with immunosuppression, characterized by a tendency to present in extranodal sites, especially the oral cavity, to have a plasma cell immunophenotype with expression of markers associated with a late stage in B-cell differentiation with lack of CD20, with EBV present in neoplastic cells in most cases, and with an unfavorable prognosis [85]. Rare cases of extranodal marginal zone lymphoma (MALT lymphoma) arising in the brain are reported [86]. We have seen the case of a well-documented B lymphoblastic lymphoma/leukemia confined to the CNS in a young woman; this patient eventually succumbed to her disease, and even at autopsy, no lymphoma was identified outside the CNS. Isolated cases of extranodal NK/T-cell lymphoma, nasal-type, primary in the brain, including one case in an allograft recipient, are described [87, 88]. Classical Hodgkin lymphoma primary in the CNS is very rare [89, 90].

Intravascular Large B-Cell Lymphoma

In the WHO Classification, intravascular large B-cell lymphoma is defined as an extranodal large B-cell lymphoma characterized by selective growth within the lumens of blood vessels, particularly capillaries [91]. Prior to its recognition as a type of lymphoma, this neoplasm was known as malignant angioendotheliomatosis, and was thought most likely to be derived from endothelial cells [92]. Modern immunohistochemical techniques have permitted the recognition of this malignancy as a lymphoma. In nearly all cases, the neoplastic cells are large B cells [91].

Subsequently within the entity of intravascular large B-cell lymphoma several distinct clinicopathologic variants have been recognized: the classical, visceral form of the disease (also referred to as the Western form of intravascular large B-cell lymphoma) [91], a cutaneous variant [93, 94] and an Asian variant. Patients with the cutaneous variant of intravascular large B-cell lymphoma, with disease confined to the skin, have a relatively favorable prognosis. Patients with the Asian variant of intravascular lymphoma commonly have fever, peripheral blood cytopenias, hepatosplenomegaly, respiratory insufficiency, hemophagocytosis, and evidence of disseminated intravascular coagulation, usually without conspicuous involvement of skin or CNS [95, 96]. Involvement of the CNS is common in the classic, or Western form of this lymphoma; the discussion below thus focuses on that variant of intravascular large B-cell lymphoma.

Middle-aged and older adults are affected. Patients present with symptoms related to vascular obstruction in a wide variety of extranodal sites, among which the most common is the CNS. The brain is affected most often, but the spinal cord may also be involved. Other commonly involved sites include kidneys, adrenal glands, lungs, heart and skin, but intravascular lymphoma may involve almost any anatomical site. Involvement of lymph nodes and spleen is rare. The mortality is high, but prognosis appears to be better when therapy appropriate for lymphoma is given [91, 95, 97–99].

On gross examination, involved tissues may appear normal or may show hemorrhage and necrosis. The characteristic microscopic finding in this disorder is the presence of blood vessels that are filled and distended by large transformed lymphoid cells generally with the appearance of centroblasts or immunoblasts. This infiltrate may be associated with thrombosis (Fig. 3.7). Extravascular lymphoma can be found in some cases. Immunophenotyping shows that these cells express pan-B cell antigens, such as CD19, CD20, and CD79a, usually with co-expression of MUM1/IRF4. In a number of cases, CD5 co-expression by the neoplastic B cells has been observed; CD10 is expressed in a few cases [91, 98, 100]. Rare cases of intravascular lymphoma are of T-lineage [95]. The pathogenesis of this unusual lymphoma is uncertain, but it has been postulated that lack of certain adhesion molecules or a homing receptor defect could contribute to the widespread anatomic distribution and the intravascular localization characteristic of this lymphoma [98, 100–102].

Lymphomatoid Granulomatosis

Lymphomatoid granulomatosis (LyG) is defined as an angiocentric, angiodestructive EBV+ B-cell lymphoproliferative disorder involving extranodal sites; there is a variable admixture of reactive T cells with the neoplastic B cells [103]. Lymphomatoid granulomatosis tends to affect individuals with immunologic abnormalities. LyG has a strong tendency to involve extranodal sites; the CNS is among the more common of these, although LyG confined to the CNS is uncommon. LyG in the CNS is usually accompanied by involvement of other sites, especially the lungs, which are involved in more than 90% of cases. Biopsy reveals the presence

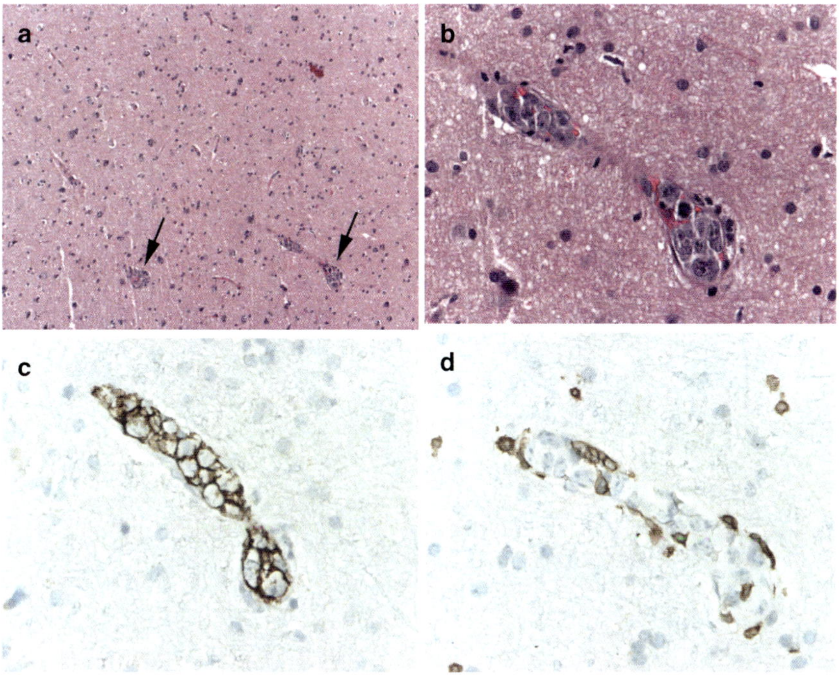

Fig. 3.7 Intravascular large B-cell lymphoma, involving the right frontal lobe. **a** Isolated blood vessels within the parenchyma are filled with cells (*arrow*). **b** Higher power view of the blood vessel shows that its lumen is filled by large, atypical cells with irregular nuclei, one or more distinct nucleoli and scant cytoplasm. **c** The large atypical cells are CD20+ B cells; B cells are confined to the lumen of the blood vessel. **d** A few small, non-neoplastic T cells (CD3+) are present around and within the blood vessel (immunoperoxidase technique on paraffin sections)

of a variable number of large, atypical, EBV+ B cells in a background of small T cells and histiocytes [103].

Peripheral T-Cell Lymphomas

Primary T-cell lymphomas are rare in the CNS, but they appear to account for a higher proportion of PCNSL in Asian series compared to Western series [104]. Most have been peripheral T-cell lymphoma, not otherwise specified. Some authors suggest that peripheral T-cell lymphomas are more likely to arise in the posterior fossa, or the leptomeninges than B-cell lymphomas [30, 105], but others have reported them to be predominantly supratentorial, similar to B-cell lymphomas [104, 106]. Histologic and immunophenotypic features are variable. They may be composed predominantly of small cells or of a mixed population of small, medium, and large cells with cleaved nuclei and pale cytoplasm, or of pleomorphic large cells. ALK+ anaplastic large cell lymphomas have been reported. In contrast to

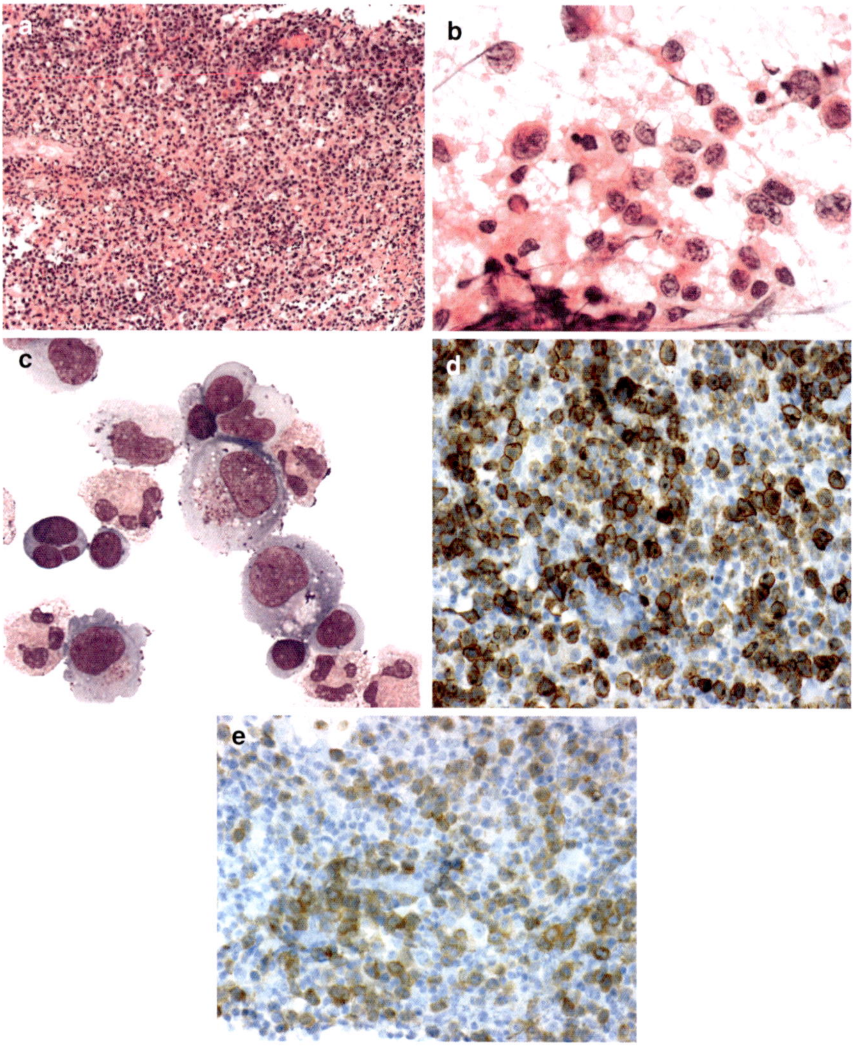

Fig. 3.8 ALK+ anaplastic large cell lymphoma, involving the right frontal lobe of a young man. **a** The lymphoma forms a dense, destructive infiltrate replacing normal tissue. **b** The squash prep shows large, atypical, discohesive cells with oval, irregular, occasionally slightly indented nuclei and scant to moderate quantity of pink cytoplasm. **c** The cerebrospinal fluid contains several large atypical lymphoid cells with oval to slightly flattened nuclei, abundant basophilic cytoplasm and collections of azurophilic granules, consistent with cytotoxic granules, in a paranuclear location. Also present are a few non-neoplastic granulocytes, small lymphocytes and monocytes (Wright stain). **d** and **e** The large atypical cells are diffusely strongly positive for CD30 (**d**) and for ALK (**e**). ALK is present in a cytoplasmic distribution, but not in the nucleus, consistent with a variant *ALK* translocation with a partner other than the common *NPM*, which yields staining for ALK in a nuclear and cytoplasmic distribution (immunoperoxidase technique on paraffin sections)

most other PCNSL, these mainly affect children and young adults. ALK+ anaplastic large cell lymphoma has a tendency to invade the leptomeninges and dura, and may even invade the skull. Their histologic and immunophenotypic features are similar to those in other sites more commonly involved by this type of lymphoma: they are composed of large mononuclear or multinucleated cells, often with horseshoe-shaped or doughnut-shaped nuclei, and abundant cytoplasm, expressing CD30, ALK (typically in a nuclear and cytoplasmic pattern), and sometimes, T-cell associated antigens (Fig. 3.8) [80–82]. The outcome of ALK+ anaplastic large cell lymphoma primary in the CNS does not appear to be as favorable as that in other sites. A few cases of primary CNS ALK– anaplastic large cell lymphoma have been reported; this type of lymphoma affects adults. Its pathologic features are similar to those of ALK– anaplastic large cell lymphoma in other sites. Its prognosis appears to be poor, and seems to be worse than that of ALK+ anaplastic large cell lymphoma [80].

Differential Diagnosis

Sampling artifact or prior corticosteroid therapy can result in a biopsy showing a predominance of small reactive T cells, mimicking a chronic inflammatory process, including a demyelinating disorder [1, 46]. Avoiding corticosteroids prior to biopsy and obtaining intraoperative frozen sections to be certain that tissue is representative in any case of suspected PCNSL are helpful in establishing a diagnosis. There can be a surrounding glial reaction that may mimic astrocytoma. Other neoplasms, including primitive neuroectodermal tumors, oligodendroglioma and metastases from undifferentiated carcinoma or melanoma can grow in sheets and mimic lymphoma [12]. Areas of lymphoma with perivascular growth can suggest arteritis [12, 46]. Among HIV+ patients, the clinical and radiographic features can mimic toxoplasma encephalitis [10, 39, 46].

In the rare cases of low-grade B-cell and T-cell lymphomas, the neoplastic cells may resemble small mature lymphocytes and thus, may mimic a reactive condition. In such cases, detailed immunophenotyping by immunohistochemistry or flow cytometry, and possibly also molecular studies to investigate the presence of a clonal population, are often required for definitive diagnosis.

Lymphoma of Peripheral Nerves and Nerve Roots

Lymphoma can affect the peripheral nervous system in several ways. The most common is in the form of a paraneoplastic syndrome related to a serum paraprotein, most often in association with Waldenström's macroglobulinemia. Less often, there is direct extension into nerves or compression of nerves by lymphoma in adjacent tissues [107]. Preferential infiltration of the nerves themselves is quite uncommon. In such cases, patients may present with symptoms of polyradiculoneuropathy, but

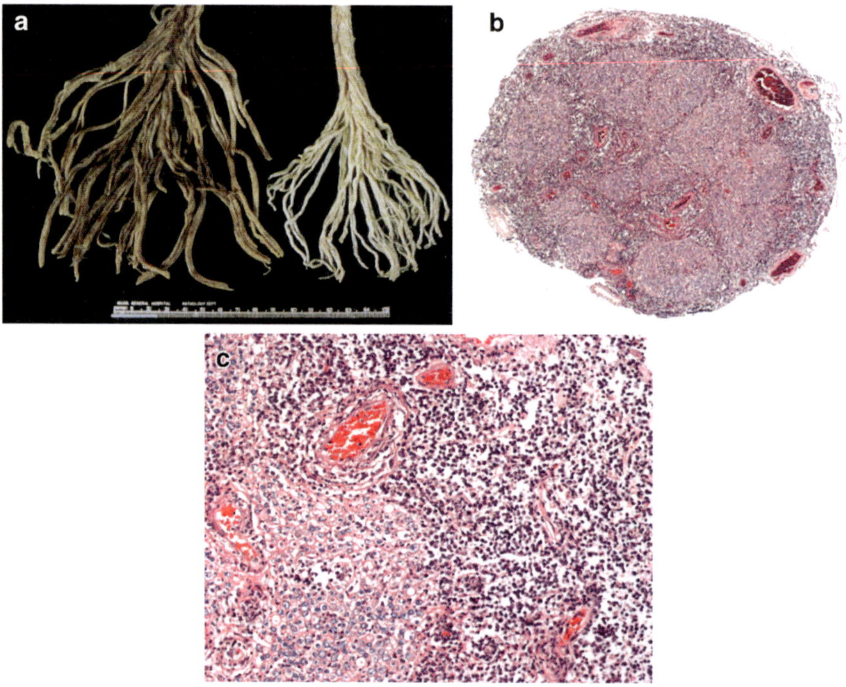

Fig. 3.9 Neurolymphomatosis. **a** The nerve roots of the cauda equina are diffusely expanded (*left*); compare to normal cauda equina (*right*). **b** This nerve root is diffusely infiltrated by neoplastic lymphoid cells. **c** Higher magnification reveals large atypical lymphoid cells shown to be B cells on immunohistochemical evaluation. Reproduced from Case records of the Massachusetts General Hospital, Case 39-1997. N Engl J Med 1997;337:1829–1837, with permission

staging usually reveals more widespread disease, involving the CNS or sites outside the nervous system. Lymphoma arising in other sites can relapse in peripheral nerves after successful initial treatment [108, 109]. Primary lymphoma confined to peripheral nerves is rare. Involvement of multiple nerves with or without involvement of spinal nerve roots, dorsal root ganglia, and meninges (neurolymphomatosis) is more common than involvement of a single nerve (Fig. 3.9) [107, 109, 110].

Patients with peripheral nerve lymphoma are usually adults; men and women are equally affected. These patients typically present with subacute onset of neuropathic pain, often accompanied by motor and sensory deficits. Gross examination or MRI reveals a tumor associated with or expanding involved nerves, sometimes imparting a fusiform contour [107, 108, 111]. When a single nerve is involved, it is usually the sciatic nerve [107, 112]. Lymphoma infiltrates the nerve and results in segmental demyelination and axonal degeneration [109, 110]. These lymphomas are most often diffuse large B-cell lymphomas, but low grade B-cell lymphomas and T-cell lymphomas have been described [107, 111–113].

Lymphomas of the Dura Mater

Lymphoma arising in the dura mater is quite uncommon, but a number of cases have been described. Patients are mostly middle-aged and older adults, with women more often affected than men. There is no apparent association with immunosuppression. These patients usually present with seizures, headache, cranial nerve abnormalities, radicular pain, syncope, or a combination of these findings [3, 114–121]. Radiologic evaluation usually reveals a localized, expansile mass or plaque-like thickening of the dura [3, 116, 121] that may be mistaken for a meningioma, a nerve sheath tumor or a subdural hematoma [116, 120, 121].

Extranodal marginal zone lymphoma of mucosa-associated lymphoid tissue (MALT lymphoma) is the most common type of lymphoma to arise in this site [116, 120]. Rare cases of dural lymphoma are diffuse large B-cell lymphoma [114]. The marginal zone lymphomas have histologic and immunohistochemical features similar to their counterparts that occur in other sites more commonly involved by marginal zone lymphoma although in the dura, these lymphomas may be associated with prominent sclerosis. These tumors are composed of small lymphocytes and/or marginal zone cells with oval to slightly irregular nuclei and a small amount of clear cytoplasm, often with plasmacytic differentiation (Fig. 3.10). Reactive follicles may be seen; if they are not recognizable on routinely stained sections, they can be highlighted with antibodies to follicular dendritic cells, such as CD21 and CD23. Entrapped meningothelial cells may be identified. Amyloid deposition has been described in one case [117]. The neoplastic cells are B cells (CD20+), sometimes with co-expression of CD43, but without CD5, CD10 or CD23 expression. Most cases have a prominent component of plasma cells (CD138+), expressing monotypic cytoplasmic immunoglobulin. There are usually scattered, admixed reactive T cells (CD3+) [117, 120]. A clonal population of B cells can generally be demonstrated by molecular genetic analysis without *BCL*1 or *BCL*2 rearrangement [120, 122]. In one case, a MALT lymphoma-associated translocation, t(14;18)(q32;q21), involving *MALT*1 and *IGH*, was identified by FISH [122]. It has been suggested that dural marginal zone lymphomas arise in association with the meningothelium, just as marginal zone lymphomas usually arise in association with epithelium in other sites [116, 120]. Dural lymphomas are usually localized (stage IE) tumors. Therapy has varied from case to case, but almost all patients fare well [116, 117, 120, 121].

Other low grade B-cell lymphomas, such as lymphoplasmacytic lymphoma and chronic lymphocytic leukemia may have histologic features mimicking those of marginal zone lymphoma, but the immunophenotype and the typically localized nature of marginal zone lymphoma can be used to exclude other low grade lymphomas. Some cases previously interpreted as dural plasmacytoma may actually represent marginal zone lymphoma with marked plasmacytic differentiation [116, 120]. Some cases thought to represent lymphoplasmacyte-rich meningiomas may actually be marginal zone lymphomas. Some marginal zone lymphomas resemble inflammatory pseudotumor or a chronic inflammatory process, but immunophenotyping and/or genotyping can help establish a diagnosis [121].

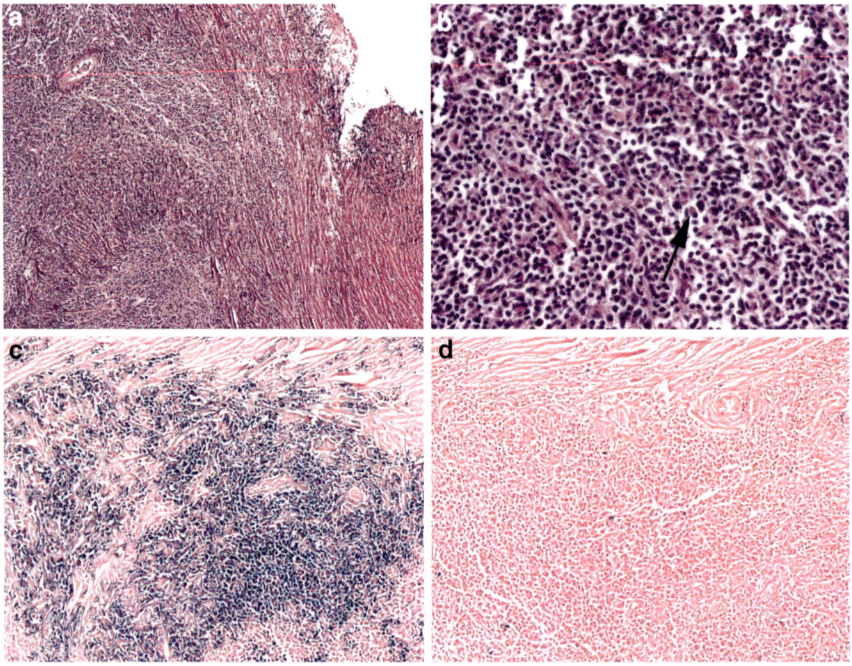

Fig. 3.10 Extranodal marginal zone lymphoma (MALT lymphoma) of the dura mater. **a** Low power shows a dense lymphoid infiltrate involving the dense collagenous tissue of the dura. **b** Higher power shows lymphocytes as well as many plasma cells with abundant cytoplasm and eccentrically placed nuclei (*arrows*). **c** and **d** In situ hybridization on paraffin sections shows kappa light chain expression by numerous plasma cells (**c**) while there is staining of very rare cells for lambda (**d**), consistent with a monotypic kappa+ population

References

1. van der Valk P (1996) Central nervous system lymphomas. Curr Diagn Pathol 3:45–52
2. Iwamoto FM, DeAngelis LM (2006) An update on primary central nervous system lymphoma. Hematol Oncol Clin North Am 20:1267–1285
3. Rubenstein J, Ferreri AJ, Pittaluga S (2008) Primary lymphoma of the central nervous system: epidemiology, pathology and current approaches to diagnosis, prognosis and treatment. Leuk Lymphoma 49(Suppl 1):43–51
4. Cady FM, O'Neill BP, Law ME et al (2008) Del(6)(q22) and BCL6 rearrangements in primary CNS lymphoma are indicators of an aggressive clinical course. J Clin Oncol 26:4814–4819
5. Nuckols J, Liu K, Burchette J et al (1999) Primary central nervous system lymphomas: a 30-year exprerience at a single institution. Mod Pathol 12:1167–1173
6. Camilleri-Broet S, Martin A, Moreau A et al (1998) Primary central nervous system lymphomas in 72 immunocompetent patients: pathologic findings and clinical correlations. Am J Clin Pathol 110:607–612
7. Eby N, Grufferman S, Flannelly C et al (1988) Increasing incidence of primary brain lymphoma in the US. Cancer 62:2461–2465

8. McAllister LD, Doolittle ND, Guastadisegni PE et al (2000) Congnitive outcomes and long-term follow-up results after enhanced chemotherapy delivery for primary central nervous system lymphoma. Neurosurgery 46:51–61
9. Sekita T, Tamaru J, Kaito K et al (2001) Primary central nervous system lymphomas express Vh genes with intermediate to high somatic mutations. Leuk Lymphoma 41:377–385
10. Eichler AF, Batchelor TT (2006) Primary central nervous system lymphoma: presentation, diagnosis and staging. Neurosurg Focus 21:E15
11. Fischer L, Martus P, Weller M et al (2008) Meningeal dissemination in primary CNS lymphoma: prospective evaluation of 282 patients. Neurology 71:1102–1108
12. Miller D, Hochberg F, Harris N et al (1994) Pathology with clinical correlations of primary central nervous system non-Hodgkin's lymphoma. The Massachusetts General Hospital experience 1958–1989. Cancer 74:1383–1397
13. Lin CH, Kuo KT, Chuang SS et al (2006) Comparison of the expression and prognostic significance of differentiation markers between diffuse large B-cell lymphoma of central nervous system origin and peripheral nodal origin. Clin Cancer Res 12:1152–1156
14. Larocca L, Capello D, Rinelli A et al (1998) The molecular and phenotypic profile of primary central nervous system lymphoma identifies distinct categories of the disease and is consistent with histogenetic derivation from germinal center related B cells. Blood 92:1011–1019
15. Camilleri-Broet S, Davi F, Feuillard J et al (1997) AIDS-related primary brain lymphomas: histopathologic and immunohistochemical study of 51 cases. The French Study Group for HIV-Associated Tumors. Hum Pathol 28:367–374
16. Kirk O, Pedersen C, Cozz-Lepri A et al (2001) Non-Hodgkin's lymphoma in HIV-infected patients in the era of highly active antiretroviral therapy. Blood 98:3406–3412
17. Herrlinger U, Schabet M, Brugger W et al (2001) Primary central nervous system lymphoma 1991–1997: outcome and late adverse effects after combined modality treatment. Cancer 91:130–135
18. DeAngelis L (1991) Primary central nervous system lymphoma as a secondary malignancy. Cancer 67:1431–1435
19. DeAngelis L (1999) Primary central nervous system lymphoma. J Neurol Neurosurg Psychiatry 66:699–701
20. Finn WG, Peterson LC, James C, Goolsby CL (1998) Enhanced detection of malignant lymphoma in cerebrospinal fluid by multiparameter flow cytometry. Am J Clin Pathol 110:341–346
21. Antinori A, Larocca L, Fassone L et al (1999) HHV-8/KSHV is not associated with AIDS-related primary central nervous system lymphoma. Brain Pathol 9:199–208
22. DeLuca A, Antinori A, Cingolani A et al (1995) Evaluation of cerebrospinal fluid EBV-DNA and IL-10 as markers for in vivo diagnosis of AIDS-related primary central nervous system lymphoma. Brit J Haematol 90:844–849
23. Corcoran C, Rebe K, van der Plas H et al (2008) The predictive value of cerebrospinal fluid Epstein–Barr viral load as a marker of primary central nervous system lymphoma in HIV-infected persons. J Clin Virol 42:433–436
24. Kluin P, Deckert M, Ferry J (2008) Primary diffuse large B-cell lymphoma of the CNS. In: Swerdlow S, Campo E, Harris N et al(eds) WHO classification tumours of haematopoietic and lymphoid tissues, 4th edn. IARC Press, Lyon, 240–241
25. Rivero M, Kuppermann B, Wiley C et al (1999) Acquired immunodeficiency syndrome-related intraocular B-cell lymphoma. Arch Ophthalmol 117:616–622
26. Porter AB, Giannini C, Kaufmann T et al (2008) Primary central nervous system lymphoma can be histologically diagnosed after previous corticosteroid use: a pilot study to determine whether corticosteroids prevent the diagnosis of primary central nervous system lymphoma. Ann Neurol 63:662–667

27. Castellano-Sanchez AA, Li S, Qian J et al (2004) Primary central nervous system posttransplant lymphoproliferative disorders. Am J Clin Pathol 121:246–253
28. Commins DL (2006) Pathology of primary central nervous system lymphoma. Neurosurg Focus 21:E2
29. Rollins KE, Kleinschmidt-DeMasters BK et al (2005) Lymphomatosis cerebri as a cause of white matter dementia. Hum Pathol 36:282–290
30. Grove A, Vyberg M (1993) Primary leptomeningeal T-cell lymphoma: a case and a review of primary T-cell lymphoma of the central nervous system. Clin Neuropathol 12:7–12
31. Alderson L, Fetell MR, Sisti M et al (1996) Sentinel lesions of primary CNS lymphoma. J Neurol Neurosurg Psychiatry 60:102–105
32. Stein H, Warnke R, Chan W et al (2008) Diffuse large B-cell lymphoma, not otherwise specified. In: Swerdlow S, Campo E, Harris N et al(eds) WHO classification tumours of haematopoietic and lymphoid tissues, 4th edn. IARC Press, Lyon, 233–237
33. Capello D, Martini M, Gloghini A et al (2008) Molecular analysis of immunoglobulin variable genes in human immunodeficiency virus-related non-Hodgkin's lymphoma reveals implications for disease pathogenesis and histogenesis. Haematologica 93: 1178–1185
34. Herrlinger U, Schabet M, Clemens M et al (1998) Clinical presentation and therapeutic outcome in 26 patients with primary CNS lymphoma. Acta Neurol Scand 97:257–264
35. Thompsett A, Ellison D, Stevenson F, Zhu D (1999) VH gene sequences from primary central nervous system lymphomas indicate derivation from highly mutated germinal center B cells with ongoing mutational activity. Blood 94:1738–1746
36. Swerdlow S, Webber S, Chadburn A, Ferry J (2008) Post-transplant lymphoproliferative disorders. In: Swerdlow S, Campo E, Harris N et al(eds) WHO classification tumours of haematopoietic and lymphoid tissues, 4th edn. IARC Press, Lyon, 343–349
37. Cavaliere R, Petroni G, Lopes MB, Schiff D (2010) Primary central nervous system post-transplantation lymphoproliferative disorder: an International Primary Central Nervous System Lymphoma Collaborative Group report. Cancer 116(4):863–870
38. Bigner SH (1992) Cerebrospinal fluid (CSF) cytology: current status and diagnostic applications. J Neuropathol Exp Neurol 51:235–245
39. Haldorsen IS, Krakenes J, Goplen AK et al (2008) AIDS-related primary central nervous system lymphoma: a Norwegian national survey 1989–2003. BMC Cancer 8:225
40. Montesinos-Rongen M, Schmitz R, Courts C et al (2005) Absence of immunoglobulin class switch in primary lymphomas of the central nervous system. Am J Pathol 166:1773–1779
41. Levy O, Deangelis LM, Filippa DA et al (2008) Bcl-6 predicts improved prognosis in primary central nervous system lymphoma. Cancer 112:151–156
42. Camilleri-Broet S, Criniere E, Broet P et al (2006) A uniform activated B-cell-like immunophenotype might explain the poor prognosis of primary central nervous system lymphomas: analysis of 83 cases. Blood 107:190–196
43. Braaten KM, Betensky RA, de Leval L et al (2003) BCL-6 expression predicts improved survival in patients with primary central nervous system lymphoma. Clin Cancer Res 9:1063–1069
44. Sugita Y, Tokunaga O, Nakashima A, Shigemori M (2004) SHP-1 expression in primary central nervous system B-cell lymphomas in immunocompetent patients reflects maturation stage of normal B cell counterparts. Pathol Int 54:659–666
45. Hans CP, Weisenburger DD, Greiner TC et al (2004) Confirmation of the molecular classification of diffuse large B-cell lymphoma by immunohistochemistry using a tissue microarray. Blood 103:275–282
46. Bhagavathi S, Wilson JD (2008) Primary central nervous system lymphoma. Arch Pathol Lab Med 132:1830–1834
47. Riemersma SA, Jordanova ES, Schop RF et al (2000) Extensive genetic alterations of the HLA region, including homozygous deletions of HLA class II genes in B-cell lymphomas arising in immune-privileged sites. Blood 96:3569–3577

48. Montesinos-Rongen M, Van Roost D, Schaller C et al (2004) Primary diffuse large B-cell lymphomas of the central nervous system are targeted by aberrant somatic hypermutation. Blood 103:1869–1875
49. Schwindt H, Akasaka T, Zuhlke-Jenisch R et al (2006) Chromosomal translocations fusing the BCL6 gene to different partner loci are recurrent in primary central nervous system lymphoma and may be associated with aberrant somatic hypermutation or defective class switch recombination. J Neuropathol Exp Neurol 65:776–782
50. McCann KJ, Ashton-Key M, Smith K et al (2009) Primary central nervous system lymphoma: tumor-related clones exist in the blood and bone marrow with evidence for separate development. Blood 113:4677–4680
51. Montesinos-Rongen M, Siebert R, Deckert M (2009) Primary lymphoma of the central nervous system: just DLBCL or not? Blood 113:7–10
52. Cassoux N, Merle-Beral H, Leblond V et al (2000) Ocular and central nervous system lymphoma: clinical features and diagnosis. Ocul Immunol Inflamm 8:243–250
53. Freeman L, Schachat A, Knox D (1987) Clinical features, laboratory investigations, and survival in ocular reticulum cell sarcoma. Ophthalmology 94:1631–1639
54. Peterson K, Gordon K, Heinemann M-H, DeAngelis L (1993) The clinical spectrum of ocular lymphoma. Cancer 72:843–849
55. Whitcup S, de Smet M, Rubin B et al (1993) Intraocular lymphoma. Clinical and histopathologic diagnosis. Ophthalmology 100:1399–1406
56. Ridley M, McDonald H, Sternberg P Jr. et al (1992) Retinal manifestations of ocular lymphoma (reticulum cell sarcoma). Ophthalmology 99:1153–1161
57. Hochberg F, Miller D (1988) Primary central nervous system lymphoma (Review). J Neurosurg 68:835–853
58. Stephenson P, Duffey R, Ferguson J Jr. (1989) Intraocular histiocytic lymphoma: a pediatric case presentation. J Pediatr Ophthalmol Strabismus 26:296–298
59. Buggage R, Chan C, Nussenblatt R (2001) Ocular manifestations of central nervous system. Curr Opin Oncol 13:137–142
60. Grimm SA, McCannel CA, Omuro AM et al (2008) Primary CNS lymphoma with intraocular involvement: International PCNSL Collaborative Group report. Neurology 71:1355–1360
61. Maier W, Laubert A, Weinel P (1994) Acute bilateral blindness in childhood caused by rhabdomyosarcoma and malignant lymphoma. J Laryngol Otol 108:873–877
62. Baehring JM, Androudi S, Longtine JJ et al (2005) Analysis of clonal immunoglobulin heavy chain rearrangements in ocular lymphoma. Cancer 104:591–597
63. Clark W, Scott I, Murray T et al (1998) Primary intraocular posttransplantation lymphoproliferative disorder. Arch Ophthalmol 116:1667–1669
64. Karma A, von Willebrand EO, Tommila PV et al (2007) Primary intraocular lymphoma: improving the diagnostic procedure. Ophthalmology 114:1372–1377
65. Merle-Beral H, Davi F, Cassoux N et al (2004) Biological diagnosis of primary intraocular lymphoma. Br J Haematol 124:469–473
66. Frenkel S, Hendler K, Siegal T et al (2008) Intravitreal methotrexate for treating vitreoretinal lymphoma: 10 years of experience. Br J Ophthalmol 92:383–388
67. Maiuri F (1990) Visual involvement in primary non-Hodgkin's lymphomas. Clin Neurol Neurosurg 92:119–124
68. Dean JM, Novak MA, Chan CC, Green WR (1996) Tumor detachments of the retinal pigment epithelium in ocular/central nervous system lymphoma. Retina 16:47–56
69. Chan CC (2003) Molecular pathology of primary intraocular lymphoma. Trans Am Ophthalmol Soc 101:275–292
70. Ziemianski M, Godfrey W, Lee K, Sabates F (1980) Lymphoma of the vitreous associated with renal transplantation and immunosuppressive therapy. Ophthalmology 87:596–601
71. Schanzer MC, Font RL, O'Malley RE (1991) Primary ocular malignant lymphoma associated with the acquired immune deficiency syndrome. Ophthalmology 98:88–91

72. Char D, Ljung B-M, Miller T, Phillips T (1988) Primary intraocular lymphoma (ocular reticulum cell sarcoma) diagnosis and management. Ophthalmology 95:625–630
73. Buettner H, Bolling J (1993) Intravitreal large-cell lymphoma. Mayo Clin Proc 68:1011–1015
74. Brown S, Jampol L, Cantrill H (1994) Intraocular lymphoma presenting as retinal vasculitis. Surv Ophthalmol 39:133–140
75. Kohno T, Uchida H, Inomata H et al (1993) Ocular manifestations of adult T-cell leukemia/lymphoma. A clinicopathologic study. Ophthalmology 100:1794–1799
76. Coupland SE, Hummel M, Muller HH, Stein H (2005) Molecular analysis of immunoglobulin genes in primary intraocular lymphoma. Invest Ophthalmol Vis Sci 46:3507–3514
77. Gunduz K, Pulido JS, McCannel CA, O'Neill BP (2006) Ocular manifestations and treatment of central nervous system lymphomas. Neurosurg Focus 21:E9
78. Jahnke K, Korfel A, O'Neill BP et al (2006) International study on low-grade primary central nervous system lymphoma. Ann Neurol 59:755–762
79. Jahnke K, Thiel E, Schilling A et al (2005) Low-grade primary central nervous system lymphoma in immunocompetent patients. Br J Haematol 128:616–624
80. George DH, Scheithauer BW, Aker FV et al (2003) Primary anaplastic large cell lymphoma of the central nervous system: prognostic effect of ALK-1 expression. Am J Surg Pathol 27:487–493
81. Merlin E, Chabrier S, Verkarre V et al (2008) Primary leptomeningeal ALK+ lymphoma in a 13-year-old child. J Pediatr Hematol Oncol 30:963–967
82. Rupani A, Modi C, Desai S, Rege J (2005) Primary anaplastic large cell lymphoma of central nervous system – a case report. J Postgrad Med 51:326–327
83. Paulus W (1999) Classification, pathogenesis and molecular pathology of primary CNS lymphomas. J Neurooncol 43:203–208
84. Shuangshoti S, Assanasen T, Lerdlum S et al (2008) Primary central nervous system plasmablastic lymphoma in AIDS. Neuropathol Appl Neurobiol 34:245–247
85. Stein H, Harris N, Campo E (2008) Plasmablastic lymphoma. In: Swerdlow S, Campo E, Harris N et al(eds) WHO classification tumours of haematopoietic and lymphoid tissues, 4th edn. IARC Press, Lyon, 256–257
86. Park I, Huh J, Kim JH et al (2008) Primary central nervous system marginal zone B-cell lymphoma of the basal ganglia mimicking low-grade glioma: a case report and review of the literature. Clin Lymphoma Myeloma 8:305–308
87. Omori N, Narai H, Tanaka T et al (2008) Epstein–Barr virus-associated T/NK cell-type central nervous system lymphoma which manifested as a post-transplantation lymphoproliferative disorder in a renal transplant recipient. J Neurooncol 87:189–191
88. Kaluza V, Rao DS, Said JW, de Vos S (2006) Primary extranodal nasal-type natural killer/T-cell lymphoma of the brain: a case report. Hum Pathol 37:769–772
89. Klein R, Mullges W, Bendszus M et al (1999) Primary intracerebral Hodgkin's disease: report of a case with Epstein–Barr virus association and review of the literature. Am J Surg Pathol 23:477–481
90. Gerstner ER, Abrey LE, Schiff D et al (2008) CNS Hodgkin lymphoma. Blood 112:1658–1661
91. Nakamura S, Ponzoni M, Campo E (2008) Intravascular large B-cell lymphoma. In: Swerdlow S, Campo E, Harris N et al(eds) WHO classification tumours of haematopoietic and lymphoid tissues. IARC Press, Lyon, 252–253
92. Pfleger L, Zur TJ (1959) Kenntnis der systemisierten Endotheliomatose der cutanen Blutgefässe (Reticuloendotheliose?). Hautarzt 10:359–363
93. Ferreri AJ, Campo E, Seymour JF et al (2004) Intravascular lymphoma: clinical presentation, natural history, management and prognostic factors in a series of 38 cases, with special emphasis on the 'cutaneous variant'. Br J Haematol 127:173–183
94. Roglin J, Boer A (2007) Skin manifestations of intravascular lymphoma mimic inflammatory diseases of the skin. Br J Dermatol 157:16–25

95. Ferreri AJ, Dognini GP, Campo E et al (2007) Variations in clinical presentation, frequency of hemophagocytosis and clinical behavior of intravascular lymphoma diagnosed in different geographical regions. Haematologica 92:486–492
96. Murase T, Nakamura S, Kawauchi K et al (2000) An Asian variant of intravascular large B-cell lymphoma: clinical, pathological and cytogenetic approaches to diffuse large B-cell lymphoma associated with haemophagocytic syndrome. Br J Haematol 111:826–834
97. DiGiuseppe JA, Nelson WG, Seifter EJ et al (1994) Intravascular lymphomatosis: a clinicopathologic study of 10 cases and assessment of response to chemotherapy. J Clin Oncol 12:2573–2579
98. Ferry JA, Harris NL, Picker LJ et al (1988) Intravascular lymphomatosis (malignant angioendotheliomatosis). A B-cell neoplasm expressing surface homing receptors. Mod Pathol 1:444–452
99. Zuckerman D, Seliem R, Hochberg E (2006) Intravascular lymphoma: the oncologist's 'great imitator'. Oncologist 11:496–502
100. Ponzoni M, Arrigoni G, Gould VE et al (2000) Lack of CD 29 (beta1 integrin) and CD 54 (ICAM-1) adhesion molecules in intravascular lymphomatosis. Hum Pathol 31:220–226
101. Kutzner H, Jaffe E (2006) Intravascular large B-cell lymphoma. In: LeBoit P, Burg G, Weedon D, Sarasin A, (eds) Pathology and genetics: skin tumours. IARC Press, Lyon, 200–201
102. Gatter K, Warnke R (2001) Intravascular large B-cell lymphoma. In: Jaffe E, Harris N, Stein H, Vardiman J, (eds) Pathology and genetics of tumours of haematopoietic and lymphoid tissues. IARC Press, Lyon, 177–178
103. Pittaluga S, Wilson W, Jaffe E (2008) Lymphomatoid granulomatosis. In: Swerdlow S, Campo E, Harris N et al(eds) WHO classification tumours of haematopoietic and lymphoid tissues, 4th edn. IARC Press, Lyon, 247–249
104. Choi JS, Nam DH, Ko YH et al (2003) Primary central nervous system lymphoma in Korea: comparison of B- and T-cell lymphomas. Am J Surg Pathol 27:919–928
105. Villegas E, Villa S, Lopez-Guillermo A et al (1997) Primary central nervous system lymphoma of T-cell origin: description of two cases and review of the literature. J Neurooncol 34:157–161
106. Shenkier TN, Voss N, Chhanabhai M et al (2005) The treatment of primary central nervous system lymphoma in 122 immunocompetent patients: a population-based study of successively treated cohorts from the British Colombia Cancer Agency. Cancer 103:1008–1017
107. Misdraji J, Ino Y, Louis D et al (2000) Primary lymphoma of peripheral nerve. Am J Surg Pathol 24:1257–1265
108. Quinones-Hinojosa A, Friedlander R, Boyer P et al (2000) Solitary sciatic nerve lymphoma as an initial manifestation of diffuse neurolymphomatosis. J Neurosurg 92:165–169
109. Abad S, Zagdanski A, Sabine B et al (1999) Neurolymphomatosis in Waldenstrom's macroglobulinaemia. Br J Haematol 106:100–103
110. Diaz-Arrastia R, Younger D, Hair L et al (1992) Neurolymphomatosis: a clinicopathologic syndrome re-emerges. Neurology 42:1136–1141
111. Baehring JM, Damek D, Martin EC et al (2003) Neurolymphomatosis. Neurooncol 5: 104–115
112. Descamps MJ, Barrett L, Groves M et al (2006) Primary sciatic nerve lymphoma: a case report and review of the literature. J Neurol Neurosurg Psychiatry 77:1087–1089
113. Ghobrial IM, Buadi F, Spinner RJ et al (2004) High-dose intravenous methotrexate followed by autologous stem cell transplantation as a potentially effective therapy for neurolymphomatosis. Cancer 100:2403–2407
114. Yamada SM, Ikawa N, Toyonaga S et al (2006) Primary malignant B-cell-type dural lymphoma: case report. Surg Neurol 66:539–543; discussion 43
115. Iwamoto FM, DeAngelis LM, Abrey LE (2006) Primary dural lymphomas: a clinicopathologic study of treatment and outcome in eight patients. Neurology 66:1763–1765
116. Kumar S, Kumar D, Kaldjian E et al (1997) Primary low-grade B-cell lymphoma of the dura: a mucosa associated lymphoid tissue-type lymphoma. Am J Surg Pathol 21:81–87

117. Lehman N, Horoupian D, Warnke R et al (2002) Dural marginal zone lymphoma with massive amyloid deposition: rare low-grade primary central nervous system B-cell lymphoma. J Neurosurg 96:368–372
118. Altundag M, Ozisik Y, Yalcin S et al (2000) Primary low grade B-cell lymphoma of the dura in an immunocompetent patient. J Exp Clin Cancer Res 19:249–251
119. Freudenstein D, Bornemann A, Ernemann U et al (2000) Intracranial malignant B-cell lymphoma of the dura. Clin Neuropathol 19:34–37
120. Kambham N, Chang Y, Matsushima A (1998) Primary low-grade B-cell lymphoma of mucosa-associated lymphoma tissue (MALT) arising in dura. Clin Neuropathol 17:311–317
121. Miranda R, Glantz L, Myint M et al (1996) Stage IE non-Hodgkin's lymphoma involving the dura: A clinicopathologic study of five cases. Arch Pathol Lab Med 120:254–260
122. Bhagavathi S, Greiner T, Kazmi S et al (2008) Extranodal marginal zone lymphoma of the dura mater with IgH/MALT1 translocation and review of the literature. J Hematopathol 1:131–137

Part III
Primary CNS Lymphoma

Chapter 4
Epidemiology of Primary Central Nervous System Lymphoma

Ingfrid Salvesen Haldorsen and Brian Patrick O'Neill

Introduction

Primary central nervous system lymphoma (PCNSL) is commonly lethal, affects vulnerable immunosuppressed populations, and continues to increase in incidence among immunocompetent individuals in several countries. During the last decades, epidemiological studies from different parts of the world have demonstrated varying incidence rates of PCNSL, as well as discrepant findings concerning whether the incidence of PCNSL is increasing or stable. These findings suggest that there may be some factor or factors other than immunodeficiency that either causes or increases the susceptibility of an individual to PCNSL.

Recent advances in the molecular characterization of PCNSL have resulted in increased understanding of how PCNSLs differ from systemic lymphoma [1], identified a potential chromosomal location for a tumor suppressor gene or genes [2], and have characterized the signature of a poor prognosis tumor [3]. Because of unique biological, clinical, and therapeutic features a PCNSL "signature" is emerging [1].

There are several important reasons to study this rare tumor. First, important discoveries of new tumorigenic agents and mechanisms have been made from studies of rare tumors; e.g. asbestos and mesothelioma. Second, the information we learn about the cause of a rare, but well-defined subgroup of lymphomas may also provide insight into the causes of other extranodal lymphomas, e.g. testicular lymphoma. Third, PCNSL, like other brain tumors, may have a disproportionate effect on quality of life because of their disabling impact on cognition, memory, language, mobility, and adaptive skills. This morbidity is further amplified because of the advanced age of the average patient and the well documented neurotoxicity of standard therapy [4]. Fourth, although long-term survival may be achieved in PCNSL, the tumor most often recurs eventually leading to death. Fifth, the incidence rate continues to increase among immunocompetent individuals in most (but not all) populations.

B.P. O'Neill (✉)
Department of Neurology, Mayo Medical School, Mayo Clinic Cancer Center, Rochester, MN 55905, USA
e-mail: boneill@mayo.edu

T. Batchelor, L.M. DeAngelis (eds.), *Lymphoma and Leukemia of the Nervous System*, DOI 10.1007/978-1-4419-7668-0_4,

It is in this context that this chapter reviews epidemiologic studies to date, speculates on reasons for the apparent increased frequency among immunocompetent patients, and projects a view of where etiologic research in PCNSL is headed.

Studies on Incidence Rates

PCNSL is a relatively rare type of primary brain tumor. Prior to the 1980s, PCNSL reportedly comprised approximately 1% of all brain tumors [5, 6] and 1% of all non-Hodgkin lymphomas [7]. From the early 1980s, increasing incidence rates of PCNSL were reported both among acquired immunodeficiency syndrome (AIDS)-patients [8, 9] and in the non-AIDS population [8–11] (Fig. 4.1).

However, increasing incidence has not been reported from all parts of the world. While increasing incidence rates were observed in the United States [5, 8–11] (from the time periods 1973–1984, 1981–1990, 1973–1992, 1958–1989, and 1973–1997, respectively), the United Kingdom [12] (1973–1990), the Netherlands [13] (1989–1994), Japan [14] (1989–2004), and Norway [15] (1989–2003), stable incidence rates have been found in Canada [16] (1975–1996), Denmark [17] (1983–1992), Scotland [18] (1991–1995), Hong Kong [19] (1982–1997), and India [20] (1985–1999). Most of these studies are based on recordings in registries without a review of the medical records [5, 8, 9, 11], potentially reducing the validity of their data. Only three studies [15–17] (two reporting stable incidence rates and one an increasing incidence rate) are based on review of medical records of the patients recorded in cancer registries; these studies reported exclusion rates of approximately 50% after review of medical records [15–17]. Furthermore, some studies [12, 13] (reporting increasing incidence rates) have not been able to discriminate between AIDS-related PCNSL and non-AIDS PCNSL, as the HIV-status of all included patients was not available. Thus, the discrepant findings from different parts of the world may be partly explained by methodological factors. Nevertheless, it seems reasonable to assume that true regional differences in the incidence of PCNSL may exist. So far, etiological factors explaining these differences remain to be identified.

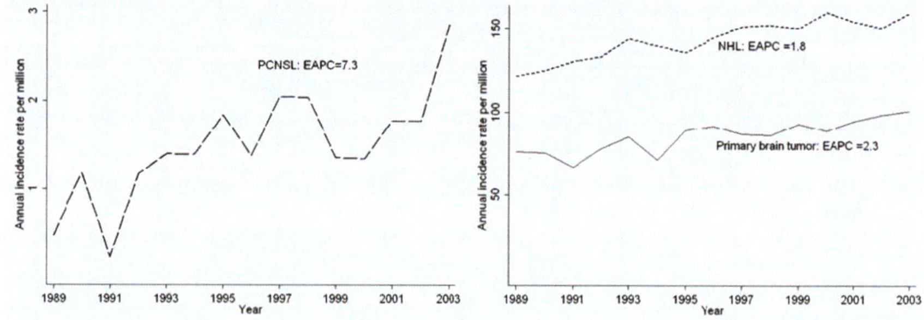

Fig. 4.1 Incidence rates of non-AIDS PCNSL, NHL and primary brain tumors in Norway 1989–2003. EAPC, estimated annual percent change; NHL, non-Hodgkin lymphoma; PCNSL, primary central nervous system lymphoma

There have also been discrepant reports during the last decades regarding the relative frequency of PCNSL, compared to primary brain tumors in general. Of all primary brain tumors, PCNSL accounted for 1.2% at a hospital in India in 1985–1999 [20], 1.6% in a region of Denmark in 1983–1992 [17], 1.7% in Norway in 1989–2003 [15], 5.1% in Southeast Netherlands in 1989–1994 [13], and 6.6% at Massachusetts General Hospital in the US in 1978–1989 [10]. Since these reports came from the modern neuroimaging era, the change in incidence is unlikely due to technology advances. Many of these discrepancies, however, may be related to ascertainment bias; reports from institutions, such as the Mayo Clinic [21] and the Massachusetts General Hospital [10] have a distinct referral bias.

Non-AIDS PCNSL

The reported average annual incidence rate of non-AIDS-related PCNSL ranges from 1.0 to 4.8 per million in different studies, during the last two decades. In a region of Denmark, it was 1.6 per million in 1983–1992 [17], in Hong Kong, 1.0 per million in 1982–1997 [19], in Norway, 1.5 per million in 1989–2003 [15], and in Canada (Alberta), 1.1 per million in 1975–1996 [16]. In the US, increasing incidence rates have been reported; 0.8 per million in 1982–1984 (Surveillance, Epidemiology and End Results program; covering approximately 10% of the US population) [1], 2.0 per million in 1986–1989 (California, Florida, New Jersey and metropolitan Atlanta) [8], and 4.8 per million in 1985–1997 (Surveillance, Epidemiology and End Results program; excluding patients with Kaposi's sarcoma, never-married men, and those with unknown marital status to avoid possible HIV-infection) [11]. In Southeast England, the average annual incidence rate of PCNSL was 2.1 per million in 1985–1990 [12], and in Southeast Netherlands, 2.7 per million in 1989–1994 [13]. These two studies from England and Netherlands included some HIV-positive patients; 21% of the patients with available HIV status were HIV-positive in the study from England [8], whereas <15% were HIV-positive (estimated indirectly) in the study from the Netherlands [13]. As many studies are based on recordings in registries only [5, 8, 9, 11, 12], and some materials may have included patients with HIV-infection [8, 9], the estimates on incidence rates may be inaccurate.

AIDS-Related PCNSL

PCNSL is an AIDS-defining disease, and it represents approximately 20% of all AIDS-related non-Hodgkin lymphomas (NHL) [22]. During the last decade, in the era of highly active antiretroviral therapy (HAART; introduced in 1996), the incidence of PCNSL among HIV infected patients has declined [23–28]. The absolute incidence rate of PCNSL per 1,000 person-years, among AIDS patients in the US, was 4.7 in 1981–1990 [8] and declined from 8.4 to 1.1 from 1988–1995 to 1996–2000, respectively [23]. In Norway, the absolute incidence rate of PCNSL among AIDS patients per 1,000 person-years in 1989–2003 was 1.7 (95%CI: 1.1–2.4), and decreased from 3.6, to 2.5, to 0.4 in the consecutive 5-year periods [28].

Incidence rates of PCNSL per 1,000 person-years among HIV-infected individuals in Europe were 0.3–5.3 in 1983–2002 [25], 0.4–8.3 in 1994–2000 [24], and 2.8 and 1.0 in 1993–1994 and 1997–1998 [27], respectively. PCNSL is diagnosed in approximately 2% of individuals infected with HIV [22, 29], and in 9–14% of AIDS–autopsies [30]. In Norway, up to 5.5% (28/508) of AIDS patients who died in 1989–2003 had PCNSL, explained by the relatively high autopsy rate (>25%) among AIDS deaths [28]. The diagnosis of PCNSL was first established by autopsy in 93% (27/29) of the patients [28]; in 15% (4/27) of these patients, imaging of the brain before death did not reveal focal lesions, so PCNSL was unexpected. Furthermore, based on imaging and clinical course, PCNSL was considered a likely differential diagnosis prior to death in only 35% (8/23) of those with focal brain lesions, whereas cerebral toxoplasmosis was considered likely in 91% (21/23) [28]. Thus, autopsy, in all AIDS patients, seems to be needed to estimate the incidence of AIDS-related PCNSL accurately.

Etiology, Pathogenesis, and Risk Factors

Cancer epidemiology has typically sought relationships that would inform etiologic hypotheses. Newer biologic tools have spawned scientifically robust cancer epidemiology domains, such as molecular epidemiology, which often requires paired blood and frozen tumor specimens from each patient. Because PCNSL tends to involve deep structures of the brain, most PCNSL patients are diagnosed by stereotactic biopsy [31]. The tissue cores removed in the biopsy technique are often exhausted during the diagnostic workup. Even if some residual tumor remains, it is usually formalin-fixed and paraffin embedded, and newer techniques of analysis, such as DNA and RNA microarray analyses require substantial frozen specimens. (As an example, a recent study from the Mayo Clinic reported the gene expression profiling of PCNSL and systemic lymphoma patients. Within a list of approximately 11,500 genes, 50 PCNSL genes were expressed at a twofold or greater differential expression compared to nodal and extranodal systemic lymphoma [2].)

Immunocompromised patients have an increased risk for developing PCNSL. In this setting, PCNSL occurs in the setting of congenital immunodeficiency or is secondary to AIDS, to iatrogenic immunosuppression for transplantation or arises in the context of autoimmune diseases, such as rheumatoid arthritis [32, 33]. Patients with congenital immune deficiency have an approximate 4% life time risk for developing PCNSL [33]. The life time risk for developing PCNSL is reported to be 1–5% for all transplant patients, with incidence figures varying from 1–2% for renal transplants recipients, to 2–7% for cardiac, lung, or liver transplant recipients [33]. Time trends in post-transplant PCNSL suggest a relationship with T-cell specific immunosuppression by agents, such as mycophenolate mofetil (MM) [34]. More recently, use of MM for treatment of autoimmune disorders has been associated with the form of PCNSL seen post-organ transplant [35, 36]. A causal relationship is suggested by the clear improvement in outcome associated with withdrawal of MM [35].

The etiology of PCNSL differs based on whether the affected patients are immunocompromised or immunocompetent. In the context of an immunocompromised patient, PCNSL arises from B-cells latently infected with Epstein–Barr virus (EBV) [32, 37]. Affected B-cells proliferate unchecked by the immune system and have a propensity to form tumors in the immuno-privileged environment of the central nervous system. The pathogenesis is unclear, but may involve cellular transformation by EBV gene products, resulting in over-expression of bcl-2, a protein that inhibits apoptosis [38]. The association between AIDS-related PCNSL and EBV is almost 100%, whereas the association between AIDS-related systemic NHL and EBV is less pronounced (20–75%, depending on histological subtype) [29]. In AIDS patients, advanced disease with severe immunodeficiency and a very low CD4 cell count (less than 50/μL) is the most important predisposing factor for PCNSL [27]. Among HIV-infected individuals in the French Hospital Database on HIV (for the time periods 1993–1994 and 1997–1998), the incidence rate of PCNSL was 9.7 and 0.15/1,000 person years at risk (PYAR) in patients with CD4 count <50/μL and >350/μL, respectively [27].

In contrast to immunocompromised patients, immunocompetent patients have no well-established cause of PCNSL. EBV and the human herpes viruses have been investigated, but no convincing association with PCNSL has been discovered [32]. As B-cells have no known role in the brain, it is puzzling how these neoplasms may develop. Some have proposed that PCNSL arises secondary to a systemic malignancy that is eliminated by the immune system, suggesting that neoplastic tumor cells have a propensity for the CNS since the CNS potentially offers immune protection for these cells [32, 39]. Others have hypothesized that trauma or infectious processes may attract lymphoid cells that proliferate locally to a monoclonal neoplastic state [39, 40]. Alternatively, it has been proposed that lymphomatous cells generated in other tissues might develop adhesion molecules and acquire selective homing receptors for cerebral endothelia [39, 40]. Lastly, in the early part of the last century, PCNSL was thought to arise by dedifferentiation of pluripotential perivascular cells. This led to the now outdated term, *perithelial sarcoma*. Very recent data derived from studies of Kaposi's sarcoma (KS) have reoriented research back towards a pluripotential precursor cell, such as a pericyte transformed via infection by human herpesvirus 8 (HHV-8) [41]. The transformation appears to correlate with neoplastic development *and* response to therapy. No candidate infectious agent in immunocompetent PCNSL has emerged. So far, no convincing data to support or refute any of these mechanisms have been published.

Different from other lymphomas, there has been no direct evidence to suggest a hereditary component in the pathogenesis of PCNSL [37]. A dual case control study (neurologic disease controls and cancer controls) from the Mayo Clinic failed to confirm an association with a family history of cancer [42]. PCNSL, developing as a second neoplasm, is reported to occur in 8–13% of PCNSL patients [43, 44]. This may represent an inherent individual predisposition to cancer, or it may be a consequence of the carcinogenic effect of the antineoplastic therapy administered for the first malignancy [37]. PCNSLs among immunocompetent patients have a slight propensity for men [33] and the elderly [32]. A recent study using the expanded SEER Registry demonstrated that there were differences in PCNSL incidence between races. United States (US) Black patients had twice the incidence of PCNSL in the ages between 20 and 49 years compared to White patients. However, in those 50 years of age or older, the PCNSL incidence in Whites was twofold higher than the incidence in Blacks [45]. The study instrument (SEER) was not structured to determine the HIV status of patients or their socio-economic class. It is tempting to think of race as a surrogate for "genetic," but the complex intersection of race, socio-economic class, and HIV risk precluded any definite conclusion in this study.

Tumor Biomarkers and Histogenetic Origin

The expression of different tumor biomarkers and its impact on survival in PCNSL have been increasingly explored during the last decade. The histogenetic origin of PCNSL, with respect to stage of B-cell differentiation, has been elucidated, using panels of immunohistochemical markers. CD10 and Bcl-6 are expressed in germinal center B-cells, whereas MUM1 (multiple myeloma-1) and CD138 are expressed in activated B-cells [46]. High expression of Bcl-6 has been linked to a likely germinal center B-cell origin [46, 47], and in most studies, confers a survival advantage [48]. Genetic studies have also suggested PCNSL is derived from a late germinal center B-cell [49]. The majority of PCNSLs express MUM1 and Bcl-6 [46]. Based on these findings characteristic of late germinal center and early post germinal center B-cells, a histogenetic origin of PCNSL in a "time-slot" overlapping late germinal center and early post germinal center has been postulated [34].

In the NCI Dictionary of Cancer Terms (http://www.cancer.gov/dictionary/db), a "biomarker" is defined as "A biological molecule found in blood, other body fluids, or tissues that is a sign of a normal or abnormal process, or of a condition or disease". It is often used as a surrogate for how well the body responds to a treatment for a disease or condition (prognostic); whether a person has or will get the disease or condition (predictive), or the presence of the disease or condition in a population. A number of biologic discoveries have been reported in PCNSL over the past five years, but only a few studies have matched these with population analyses to determine if the putative marker has prognostic or predictive value. The reader is referred to several excellent, recent reviews of this subject with an emphasis on biologic data that may lead to epidemiologic studies [50, 51].

A common aberration in hematologic malignancies is deletion of the long arm of chromosome 6. Deletions may have prognostic value as markers of poor outcome. In addition, these deletions may have a pathogenetic role since they occur as the sole cytogenetic abnormality in some cases of systemic diffuse large cell B-cell lymphoma [52]. Nakamura et al. were the first to suggest that a 140-kb deletion, located at 6q22–23, may contain the putative tumor suppressor, PTPRK [53]. In that study, loss of heterozygosity (LOH) on 6q in 29 samples of surgically resected PCNSL was found at 1 or more loci at 6q22–23 in 19 samples (66%); 18 of these samples shared a deletion in a ~140 kb region, in which the human *R-PTP-κ* gene (*PTPRK*) is said to be located. Furthermore, LOH on 6q22–q23 significantly correlated with shorter patient survival (12.8 ± 4.3 *versus* 23.4 ± 3.5 months; $P < 0.0001$). This work was confirmed and expanded by Cady et al. [2]. The latter investigators found that the presence of del(6)(q22) or a BCL6 translocation was associated with inferior overall survival (OS; P =.0097). Univariate results held after adjusting for age, deep structure involvement, and use of high-dose intravenous methotrexate in a multivariate model. Lastly, a report by Rubenstein et al. [54] used microarray analysis to identify more than 100 genes upregulated in PCNSL, compared to systemic lymphoma. Of these, expression of IL-4 and STAT6, a mediator of IL-4 signaling, predicted early progression and short survival independent of methotrexate treatment.

References

1. Mrugala MM, Rubenstein JL, Ponzoni M, Batchelor TT (2009 Jan) Insights into the biology of primary central nervous system lymphoma. Curr Oncol Rep 11(1).73–80; review
2. Cady FM, O'Neill BP, Law ME et al (2008) Del(6)(q22) and BCL6 rearrangements in primary CNS lymphoma are indicators of an aggressive clinical course. J Clin Oncol 26:4814–4819
3. Tun HW, Personett D, Baskerville KA et al (2008 Mar 15) Pathway analysis of primary central nervous system lymphoma. Blood 111(6):3200–3210
4. Blay JY, Conroy T, Chevreau C et al (1998 Mar) High-dose methotrexate for the treatment of primary cerebral lymphomas: analysis of survival and late neurologic toxicity in a retrospective series. J Clin Oncol 16(3):864–871
5. Eby NL, Grufferman S, Flannelly CM et al (1988) Increasing incidence of primary brain lymphoma in the US. Cancer 62:2461–2465
6. Hochberg FH, Miller DC (1988) Primary central nervous system lymphoma. J Neurosurg 68:835–853
7. Levitt LJ, Dawson DM, Rosenthal DS, Moloney WC (1980) CNS involvement in the non-Hodgkin's lymphomas. Cancer 45:545–552
8. Cote TR, Manns A, Hardy CR et al (1996) Epidemiology of brain lymphoma among people with or without acquired immunodeficiency syndrome. AIDS/Cancer Study Group. J Natl Cancer Inst 88:675–679
9. Corn BW, Marcus SM, Topham A et al (1997) Will primary central nervous system lymphoma be the most frequent brain tumor diagnosed in the year 2000? Cancer 79:2409–2413
10. Miller DC, Hochberg FH, Harris NL et al (1994) Pathology with clinical correlations of primary central nervous system non-Hodgkin's lymphoma. The Massachusetts General Hospital experience 1958–1989. Cancer 74:1383–1397
11. Olson JE, Janney CA, Rao RD et al (2002) The continuing increase in the incidence of primary central nervous system non-Hodgkin lymphoma: a surveillance, epidemiology, and end results analysis. Cancer 95:1504–1510
12. Lutz JM, Coleman MP (1994) Trends in primary cerebral lymphoma. Br J Cancer 70:716–718
13. van der Sanden GA, Schouten LJ, van Dijck JA et al (2002) Primary central nervous system lymphomas: incidence and survival in the Southern and Eastern Netherlands. Cancer 94:1548–1556
14. Makino K, Nakamura H, Kino T et al (2006) Rising incidence of primary central nervous system lymphoma in Kumamoto, Japan. Surg Neurol 66:503–506
15. Haldorsen IS, Krossnes BK, Aarseth JH et al (2007) Increasing incidence and continued dismal outcome of primary central nervous system lymphoma in Norway 1989–2003: time trends in a 15-year national survey. Cancer 110:1803–1814

16. Hao D, DiFrancesco LM, Brasher PM et al (1999) Is primary CNS lymphoma really becoming more common? A population-based study of incidence, clinicopathological features and outcomes in Alberta from 1975 to 1996. Ann Oncol 10:65–70
17. Krogh-Jensen M, D'Amore F, Jensen MK et al (1994) Incidence clinicopathological features and outcome of primary central nervous system lymphomas. Population-based data from a Danish lymphoma registry. Danish Lymphoma Study Group, LYFO. Ann Oncol 5:349–354
18. Yau YH, O'Sullivan MG, Signorini D et al (1996) Primary lymphoma of central nervous system in immunocompetent patients in south-east Scotland. Lancet 348:890
19. Au WY, Chan AC, Srivastava G et al (2000) Incidence and pathology of primary brain lymphoma in Hong Kong Chinese patients. Leuk Lymphoma 37:175–179
20. Powari M, Radotra B, Das A, Banerjee AK (2002) A study of primary central nervous system lymphoma in northern India. Surg Neurol 57:113–116
21. Tomlinson FH, Kurtin PJ, Suman VJ et al (1995) Primary intracerebral malignant lymphoma: a clinicopathological study of 89 patients. J Neurosurg 82:558–566
22. Chamberlain MC, Kormanik PA (1999) AIDS-related central nervous system lymphomas. J Neurooncol 43:269–276
23. Diamond C, Taylor TH, Aboumrad T, Anton-Culver H (2006) Changes in acquired immunodeficiency syndrome-related non-Hodgkin lymphoma in the era of highly active antiretroviral therapy: incidence, presentation, treatment, and survival. Cancer 106: 128–135
24. Kirk O, Pedersen C, Cozzi-Lepri A et al (2001) Non-Hodgkin lymphoma in HIV-infected patients in the era of highly active antiretroviral therapy. Blood 98:3406–3412
25. Wolf T, Brodt HR, Fichtlscherer S et al (2005) Changing incidence and prognostic factors of survival in AIDS-related non-Hodgkin's lymphoma in the era of highly active antiretroviral therapy (HAART). Leuk Lymphoma 46:207–215
26. Ammassari A, Cingolani A, Pezzotti P et al (2000) AIDS-related focal brain lesions in the era of highly active antiretroviral therapy. Neurology 55:1194–1200
27. Besson C, Goubar A, Gabarre J et al (2001) Changes in AIDS-related lymphoma since the era of highly active antiretroviral therapy. Blood 98:2339–2344
28. Haldorsen IS, Krakenes J, Goplen AK et al (2008) AIDS-related primary central nervous system lymphoma: a Norwegian national survey 1989–2003. BMC Cancer 8:225
29. Kasamon YL, Ambinder RF (2005) AIDS-related primary central nervous system lymphoma. Hematol Oncol Clin North Am 19:665–687
30. Cingolani A, Fratino L, Scoppettuolo G, Antinori A (2005) Changing pattern of primary cerebral lymphoma in the highly active antiretroviral therapy era. J Neurovirol 11 Suppl 3:38–44
31. O'Neill BP, Kelly PJ, Earle JD et al (1987) Computer-assisted sterotactic biopsy for the diagnosis of primary central nervous system lymphoma. Neurology 37:1160–1164
32. Mohile NA, Abrey LE (2007) Primary central nervous system lymphoma. Semin Radiat Oncol 17:223–229
33. Schabet M (1999) Epidemiology of primary CNS lymphoma. J Neurooncol 43:199–201
34. Snannoudj R, Durrbach A, Leblond V et al (2003) Primary brain lymphomas after kidney transplantation presentation and outcome. Transplantation 76:930–937
35. O'Neill BP, Vernino S, Dogan A et al (2007) EBV-associated lymphoproliferative disorder of CNS associated with the use of mycophenolate mofetil. Neurooncol 9:364–369
36. Kleinschmidt-DeMasters BK, Damek DM, Lillehe KO et al (2008) Epstein Barr virus-associated primary CNS lymphomas in elderly patients on immunosuppressive medications. J Neuropathol Exp Neurol 67(11):1103–1111
37. Ferreri AJ, Reni M (2007) Primary central nervous system lymphoma. Crit Rev Oncol Hematol 63:257–268
38. Gates AE, Kaplan LD (2002) AIDS malignancies in the era of highly active antiretroviral therapy. Oncology 16:657–665

39. Nakamura M, Shimada K, Ishida E, Konishi N (2004) Histopathology pathogenesis and molecular genetics in primary central nervous system lymphomas. Histol Histopathol 19: 211–219
40. Paulus W (1999) Classification, pathogenesis and molecular pathology of primary CNS lymphomas. J Neurooncol 43:203–208
41. Nicholas J (2007) Human herpesvirus 8 encoded proteins with potential roles in virus-associated neoplasia. Front Biosci 12:265–281
42. Schiff D, Suman VJ, Yang P et al (1998) Risk factors for primary central nervous system non-Hodgkin's lymphoma (PCNSL). Cancer 82:975–992
43. DeAngelis LM (1991) Primary central nervous system lymphoma as a secondary malignancy. Cancer 67:1431–1435
44. Reni M, Ferreri AJ, Zoldan MC, Villa E (1997) Primary brain lymphomas in patients with a prior or concomitant malignancy. J Neurooncol 32:135–142
45. Pulido JS, Vierkant RA, Olson JE et al (2009 Jun) Racial differences in primary central nervous system lymphoma incidence and survival rates. Neurooncol 11(3):318–322
46. Camilleri-Broet S, Criniere E, Broet P et al (2006) A uniform activated B-cell-like immunophenotype might explain the poor prognosis of primary central nervous system lymphomas: analysis of 83 cases. Blood 107:190–196
47. Braaten KM, Betensky RA, de Leval L et al (2003) BCL-6 expression predicts improved survival in patients with primary central nervous system lymphoma. Clin Cancer Res 9: 1063–1069
48. Levy O, DeAngelis LM, Fillipa DA et al (2008) Bcl-6 predicts improved prognosis in primary central nervous system lymphoma. Cancer 112(1):151–156
49. Montesinos-Rongen M, Brunn A, Bentink S et al (2008) Gene expression profiling suggests primary central nervous system lymphomas to be derived from a late germinal center B cell. Leukemia 22:400–405
50. Algazi AP, Kadoch C, Rubenstein JL (2009) Biology and treatment of primary central nervous system lymphoma. Neurotherapeutics 6:587–597
51. Rubenstein J, Ferreri AJM, Pittaluga S (2008) Primary lymphoma of the central nervous system: epidemiology, pathology and current approaches to diagnosis, prognosis and treatment. Leuk Lymphoma 49:32–51
52. Thelander EF, Ichimura K, Corcoran M et al (2008) Characterization of 6q deletions in mature B-cell lymphomas and childhood acute lymphoblastic leukemia. Leuk Lymphoma 49(3): 477–487
53. Nakamura M, Kishi M, Sakaki T et al (2003) Novel tumor suppressor loci on 6q22-23 in primary central nervous system lymphomas. Cancer Res 63:737–741
54. Rubenstein JL, Fridlyand J, Shen A et al (2006) Gene expression and angiotropism in primary CNS lymphoma. Blood 107:3716–3723

Chapter 5
Biology of Primary Central Nervous System Lymphoma

James L. Rubenstein

Introduction

Insights into the biology of primary central nervous system lymphoma (PCNSL) are essential to facilitate the development of more effective treatment for this uncommon variant of extranodal non-Hodgkin lymphoma (NHL). An accumulating body of evidence suggests that the molecular pathogenesis of PCNSL is distinct from systemic lymphomas of the same histological type. First, 90% of NHL cases that present in the central nervous system (CNS) will, upon staging, prove to be confined to the brain, leptomeninges, optic nerves, and intraocular structures and thus be classified as PCNSL. Over the natural history of the disease, it is rare for PCNSL tumors to recur outside of the brain, underscoring this unique tropism for the CNS. Second, PCNSL tumors are associated with an inferior prognosis compared to other localized extranodal NHL tumors confined to a single extranodal site, such as bone. Third, CNS lymphomas tend to exhibit a heightened responsiveness to high-dose methotrexate-based therapy compared to systemic lymphomas with a concomitant diminished responsiveness to adriamycin-based chemotherapy regimens [1]. The molecular and cellular basis for this apparent increased sensitivity to methotrexate has not been discovered, but the impact of methotrexate is profound in that a subset of CNS lymphoma patients exhibit significant progression-free survival with methotrexate-based monotherapy [2]. This is particularly striking given that methotrexate has no role in the treatment of aggressive NHL outside of the brain. This chapter will highlight the molecular features of PCNSL, which may account for the unique phenotypic properties of this neoplasm.

J.L. Rubenstein (✉)
Division of Hematology/Oncology, Department of Medicine, University of California, San Francisco, CA 94143-1270, USA
e-mail: jamesr@medicine.ucsf.edu

T. Batchelor, L.M. DeAngelis (eds.), *Lymphoma and Leukemia of the Nervous System*, DOI 10.1007/978-1-4419-7668-0_5,

Potential CNS Homing Mechanisms

The CNS is an immunologically privileged site, normally devoid of B-cells, and the origin of the tumor cells in PCNSL has yet to be elucidated. One proposed mechanism postulates that a malignant clone of B-cells of systemic origin might evolve to express selective molecular properties such as specific adhesion molecule(s) that facilitate homing to the CNS, where the tumor cells proliferate and undergo secondary mutations in the absence of regulatory control by the immune system. Indeed, recent evidence suggests that subclinical tumor-related clones are detectable in the blood and bone marrow of PCNSL patients, suggesting that the CNS microenvironment might promote a more aggressive phenotype [3, 4]. However, to date, no differences in the expression of adhesion molecules have been definitively established between PCNSL and systemic lymphomas [5].

In immunosuppressed populations, such as AIDS patients or those receiving immunosuppression in the setting of organ transplantation, PCNSL is usually linked to latent infection of the neoplastic B-cells by Epstein–Barr virus (EBV) [6]. Infection of normal B-cells may result in their immortalization, however, proliferation of EBV-infected B-cells is usually suppressed by normal T-cell immunity. With diminished T-cell function, however, the EBV-infected clone may progress to malignant lymphoma [7]. Moreover, EBV infection correlates with CNS tropism of lymphoma. The risk of CNS tumor dissemination in EBV-positive systemic AIDS-related NHL is approximately tenfold higher than the risk for EBV-negative cases [8]. In addition, the concordance of EBV DNA in the cerebrospinal fluid (CSF), as quantified by polymerase chain reaction, with suggestive abnormalities on neuroimaging, including MRI and SPECT studies may permit the presumptive diagnosis of CNS lymphoma in patients with AIDS [9]. The precise molecular basis for EBV-driven CNS tropism in NHL remains to be defined.

Chemokines are an important class of molecules that regulate a number of properties of leukocytes including their trafficking, proliferation, and adhesion. Chemokine:chemokine receptor interactions contribute to the development of normal lymph node structure. Recently, a B-cell attracting chemokine, CXCL13 (BCA-1) was noted to be expressed at significant levels in PCNSL tumors [10]. CXCL13 is a lymphoid chemokine that promotes B-cell homing to secondary lymphoid organs [11]. Notably, CXCL13 is expressed in *Helicobacter pylori*-induced mucosa-associated lymphoid tissue (MALT), as well as in gastric lymphoma [12]. Binding of CXCL13 to its receptor CXCR5, also expressed by B-cells in PCNSL, may be involved in the extranodal localization of CNS lymphomas. While CXCL13 is known to be expressed by lymphoma cells, it does not appear to be produced by tumor endothelia in PCNSL, and therefore it may not directly contribute to the unique angiotropic pattern of growth seen in PCNSL. Similarly, expression of the chemokine stromal derived factor-1 (SDF-1) has also been demonstrated by malignant B-cells in PCNSL [13]. Elevated levels of CXCL13 were recently demonstrated in the CSF of PCNSL patients, further supporting a role for this chemokine in the pathogenesis of lymphoma within the CNS [14]. Notably, the expression of the B-cell chemokines CXCL13 and SDF-1 by the retinal pigment epithelium has also been demonstrated in primary intraocular lymphoma [15]. Ectopic expression of these chemokines within the intraocular compartment may contribute to lymphoma cell homing to the retinal pigment epithelium from the choroidal circulation [16].

Transcriptional Profiling of PCNSL

Recently, PCNSL tumors have been analyzed using large-scale genomic classification involving microarrays. Data from these studies demonstrated that while PCNSL may be classified among the three established molecular subclasses of large B-cell lymphoma, two independent reports identified molecular characteristics that distinguish CNS lymphomas from nodal and/or extranodal large B-cell lymphoma. Using a cDNA-microarray-based platform, Rubenstein et al. identified greater than 400 clones that distinguished 23 cases of PCNSL from nine cases of nodal large B-cell lymphoma [17]. Using an oligonucleotide-based platform, Tun et al. identified more than sixty genes which distinguished 13 cases of PCNSL from 11 nodal and 19 extranodal large B-cell lymphomas [18].

Genes whose expression was shown to be upregulated in PCNSL in the Rubenstein et al. study included X-box binding protein 1, a transcriptional mediator of the unfolded protein response pathway, which may facilitate tumor adaptation in conditions of glucose deprivation and hypoxia [19]. In addition, the proto-oncogenes c-myc and Pim-1 also were shown to be expressed at high levels in these brain tumors.

In addition, ectopic expression of the B-cell growth factor interleukin-4 (IL-4) was also demonstrated in PCNSL tumors. IL-4 is not only a potential autocrine growth factor for lymphoma cells, but may also function as a significant paracrine growth factor given its novel expression by tumor-associated endothelia in PCNSL. IL-4 was not detected in the vasculature of normal brain nor by the vasculature in malignant astrocytic neoplasms. These findings support the hypothesis that IL-4 may be important in the pathogenesis and progression of PCNSL, and may contribute to the angiotropic growth pattern demonstrated by lymphoma cells within the CNS. In addition, the activated form of the transcription factor, STAT-6, a mediator of IL-4-dependent gene expression, was also shown to be expressed by tumor cells and tumor endothelia in PCNSL, suggesting a significant functional role of IL-4 signaling in the pathogenesis of this type of lymphoma. Signaling through the IL-4 pathway might drive lymphomagenesis via a number of different mechanisms: First, given the established role of IL-4 as a B-cell survival factor [20, 21], IL-4 may promote lymphoma survival signaling as an autocrine growth factor. Second, IL-4 may regulate tumor angiogenesis and thus, may contribute to lymphomagenesis via promotion of tumor neovasculature [22, 23]. Third, IL-4 may subvert the function of macrophages within tumors via polarization from a classically-active phenotype which antagonizes cancer growth to an alternatively-activated or M2 phenotype, which supports angiogenesis and suppresses the anti-tumor immune response [24].

Indeed, Kadoch et al. recently provided evidence for the M2 polarization of tumor macrophages in diagnostic specimens of PCNSL [25]. Disruption of the IL-4 signaling pathway therefore represents a potential avenue for therapeutic intervention in this disease.

Rubenstein et al. noted that high-density PCNSL tumors in which lymphoma cells and tumor endothelia express activated STAT-6 exhibit a worse prognosis after treatment with standard methotrexate-based regimens than tumors of low cell density, independent of STAT-6 activation status [17]. Subsequently it was reported that the intratumoral expression of STAT-6 protein (an IL-4 induced gene) was associated with short survival in PCNSL patients treated with high-dose methotrexate [26]. In summary, these data support the hypothesis that the expression pattern of STAT-6 constitutes a novel biomarker for prognostic determination in newly diagnosed PCNSL.

The gene expression study of Tun et al. compared PCNSL and non-CNS lymphomas (both nodal and extranodal), and used pathway analysis software to highlight the differential expression of extracellular matrix molecules in PCNSL, in particular osteopontin and chitinase 3-like 1. Osteopontin may regulate B cell adhesion, activation, and proliferation. Notably, osteopontin is overexpressed in other CNS diseases including multiple sclerosis, and astrocytomas, suggesting an important role for this molecule in the adaptation of inflammatory and tumor cells for growth within the brain microenvironment [27, 28].

The significance of each of these two microarray studies is limited given that each analyzed a relatively small number of specimens and each lacked an independent validation set of tumor samples. Also, each study used distinct microarray platforms. It is therefore notable that a subset of overlapping genes, which are concordant in distinguishing CNS from non-CNS large B-cell lymphoma, in each study was elucidated [29] (Table 5.1)

The majority of genes that reproducibly distinguished PCNSL and systemic NHL are components of the extracellular matrix. For example, osteopontin and chitinase-3-like 1 were independently found to be expressed at higher levels in cases of PCNSL by Rubenstein et al. and Tun et al. In contrast, collagen type VI, laminin alpha-4 and lumican, a keratin sulfate proteoglycan, were consistently expressed at higher levels in systemic NHL in each study. In the Rubenstein et al. study, it was observed that other collagens, specifically types IV and V, were expressed at higher levels in nodal lymphomas. The differential expression of collagen subtypes between CNS versus systemic large B-cell NHL may impact the apoptotic threshold to specific types of genotoxic stress. For example, the expression of extracellular matrix proteins in the "lymph node signature" has been associated with outcomes in systemic large B-cell lymphoma [30]. Also, high expression of collagen type VI may modulate chemotherapy drug resistance in cancer [31].

Each analysis independently detected higher expression of genes involved in signaling and cell proliferation. For example, expression of regulator of G-protein signaling (RGS)-13 was twofold higher in PCNSL tumor specimens compared to systemic lymphomas. RGS proteins negatively regulate the signaling of G-proteins, including chemokine receptors [32]. This observation suggests

Table 5.1 Gene microarray studies in PCNSL

	Symbol	Fold-change Rubenstein study	*p*-value Rubenstein study	Fold-change Tun study	*p*-value Tun study
CNS to non-CNS: upregulated					
Osteopontin	SPP1	11.4	8.00E–06	9.73	3.03E–08
Complement component 1, q subcomponent	C1QB	2.8	8.29E–06	2	2.40E–02
Hemoglobin alpha 2	HBA2	2	6.26E–04	2.5	1.90E–02
Regulator of G-protein signaling 13	RGS13	2.3	3.34E–02	2.4	2.70E–02
Chitinase 3-like 1	CH13L1	2.8	5.02E–02	2.72	5.10E–05
T-cell leukemia/lymphoma 1A	TCL1A	2.8	1.07E–01	2.96	5.55E–05
CNS to non-CNS: downregulated					
Nicotinamide N-methyltransferase	NNMT	0.56	5.26E–03	0.43	8.99E–04
Vascular endothelial growth factor C	VEGFC	0.51	7.16E–03	0.4	1.00E–03
Collagen type VI, alpha 1	COL6A1	0.45	1.32E–02	0.45	3.25E–04
Latexin	LXN	0.76	1.99E–02	0.48	2.67E–02
Lumican	LUM	0.5	2.27E–02	0.28	8.45E–03
Laminin alpha 4	LAMA4	0.74	4.54E–02	0.37	8.00E–03

that RGS-13 may enhance the response to relevant chemokines in CNS lymphoma, for example, CXCL13, to selectively modulate lymphoma homing within the CNS.

Distinct from coding messenger RNA transcripts whose differential expression in lymphoma subtypes has been extensively evaluated using DNA microarrays, there is emerging evidence that non-coding short microRNAs (miRNAs) can act to promote or to suppress cell transformation, as well as regulate tumor invasion and metastasis [33]. The first survey of the differential expression of miRNA in nodal versus extranodal diffuse large B-cell lymphoma, including CNS and testicular NHL was conducted by Robertus et al. who demonstrated significantly higher expression of a miRNA miR-17-5p in CNS lymphomas compared to nodal and testicular DLBCL [34]. Data suggests that miR-17-5p microRNA may promote tumor growth via a variety of mechanisms, including the down-modulation of expression of negative regulators of mitogen activated protein kinase (MAPK) signaling cascade [35]. While this preliminary observation requires validation, it will be interesting to determine the functional significance of differential expression of miR-17-5p microRNA in terms of the organotropism and pathogenesis of lymphoma within the CNS microenvironment.

For a variety of reasons, the determination of the molecular features of CNS lymphoma is significantly more challenging than for systemic NHL. The architecture of CNS lymphoma is often heterogeneous, with variable cell density and neovascularization, and infiltration by immune effector cells [17, 36, 37]. The molecular profiling of individual small brain biopsy specimens using array platforms may therefore provide an incomplete analysis of the tumor and its microenvironment. Rubenstein et al. proposed that there are at least two major growth patterns of PCNSL, as evidenced by the histopathology of diagnostic tumor specimens; approximately half of cases of PCNSL are of low tumor cellularity, in which normal brain elements are evident within the neoplasm; the remainder of tumors are of high cellular density without intervening normal brain elements between the neoplastic cells [29] (Fig. 5.1). As above, there is evidence that high-density tumors that express activated STAT-6 are associated with a worse prognosis after treatment with standard, methotrexate-based regimens than tumors of low cell density, independent of STAT-6 activation status.

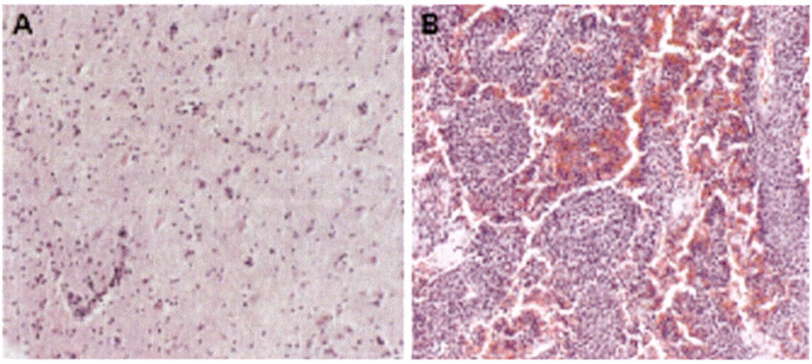

Fig. 5.1 Low density (**a**) and high density (**b**) PCNSL tumors, each of large B-cell histology, are distinguished by the presence (**a**), or absence (**b**), of intervening normal brain elements between the tumor cells in pathological specimens. Magnification X100 (hematoxylin and eosin). This research was originally published in Blood [29]. © The American Society of Hematology

Given that neurons and glia are a rich source of molecules involved in signal transduction, including proto-oncogenes, such as bcl-2 [38, 39] the molecular profiling of PCNSL specimens of low tumor density would be prone to sampling error, given the presence of interspersed normal brain elements. It follows, therefore, that microarray studies of this disease may tend to be biased toward the analysis of the most aggressive cases.

Genetics of PCNSL

Because aberrant somatic hypermutation has an established role in the pathogenesis of DLBCL, Montesinos-Rongen et al. pursued the potential contribution of this pathogenic mechanism to the development of PCNSL. These investigators detected a high relative mutation frequency for immunoglobulin H (*IgH*) genes in PCNSL. Moreover, these investigators also found that PCNSL tumors commonly displayed aberrant somatic hypermutation involving four proto-oncogenes – *PAX5*, *PIM1*, *c-MYC*, and *RhoH/TTF* genes, which have an established role in B cell development and differentiation, as well as in the regulation of proliferation and apoptosis [40].

The mean mutation frequencies were twofold to fivefold higher in PCNSL compared to extraneural DLBCL [40]. Such high mutation frequencies may arise during a prolonged interaction of the tumor cell (or its precursor) in the germinal center microenvironment [41].

The $p16^{INK4a}$ gene is frequently inactivated by either homozygous deletion (40–50%) or 5′-CpG hypermethylation (15–30%) in PCNSL patients [42]. Inactivation of $p14^{ARF}$ and $p16^{INK4a}$ genes by either homozygous deletion or promoter hypermethylation may represent an important step in the molecular pathogenesis of PCNSL. The $p14^{ARF}$ gene, for example, normally induces growth arrest and stabilizes p53 protein in the cell nucleus. Its deletion has been reported in glioblastoma and systemic NHL. Both $p14^{ARF}$ and $p16^{INK4a}$ genes are frequently co-deleted in human neoplasms; moreover, mice lacking the murine homologue of $p14^{ARF}$ develop a variety of tumors, including lymphomas, sarcomas, and gliomas [37, 43–45]. In contrast, mutations in the *TP*53 gene have been observed in only a small proportion of PCNSL specimens.

Comparative genomic hybridization has identified other potentially important genetic lesions in PCNSL. Gains have been detected on chromosome 12, as well as on the long arms of chromosomes 1, 7, and 18. Gain on chromosome 12 appears to be the most common chromosomal alteration, specifically in the 12q region harboring MDM2, CDK4, and GLI1 [37, 44, 46]. Reduced number of DNA copies was detected on chromosome 6 and the short arms of chromosomes 17 and 18. Chromosome 6q deletions, in particular 6q21–23, a locus containing the putative tumor suppressor gene *PTPRK*, may be most frequent and occur in between 40 and 60% of PCNSL tumors [47].

Cady and colleagues from the Mayo Clinic used interphase fluorescence in situ hybridization (FISH) to evaluate four candidate genomic loci which they hypothesized to have prognostic significance in PCNSL tumors: 6q22–23, as well as translocations involving BCL-6, MYC and IgH. PCNSL tumors isolated from 75 immunocompetent patients treated at a single institution were analyzed. Deletion of 6q22 was determined to be the most prevalent genomic aberration identified, occurring in 45% of tumors; BCL6 translocations were the next most common and were detected in 17% of tumors. The presence of del(6)(q22) and/or a BCL6 translocation was associated with inferior overall survival ($p=0.0097$). Notably, deletion of (6)(q22) is more common in PCNSL (45%) than in systemic DLBCL (25%) and IGH translocations are less common in PCNSL (13%) than in systemic DLBCL (45–51%) [48]. These observations support the body of evidence that PCNSL has a distinct molecular pathogenesis compared to systemic diffuse large B-cell lymphoma.

Proteomics of PCNSL

To test the hypothesis that the CSF proteome harbors biological information, which might provide insights into the pathogenesis of PCNSL as well as immediately practical information to facilitate diagnosis, prognosis and the detection of minimal residual disease, Roy et al. conducted an in-depth proteomic analysis of the CSF from CNS lymphoma patients using two-dimensional liquid chromatography followed by mass spectrometry (2D-LC/MS). As controls, CSF was obtained from patients with benign brain tumors, other non-malignant CNS conditions, or patients with systemic cancer who had no evidence of CNS disease. The analysis was repeated 1 year later with samples from different patients to test its reproducibility: a total of 30 CSF specimens were subjected to proteomic profiling to identify candidate CSF biomarkers. There was a high degree of concordance between the two sets of results (Spearman correlation 0.71) indicating the highly reproducible nature of this technology when applied to differential protein identification and quantification in the CSF. Approximately 80 differentially-expressed CSF proteins were identified, both upregulated in CSF from CNS lymphoma patients, as well as downregulated in CSF from CNS lymphoma patients relative to the CSF from control subjects [49] (Fig. 5.2). The majority of proteins that were upregulated in CNS lymphoma were serine proteases or protease inhibitors, complement mediators and

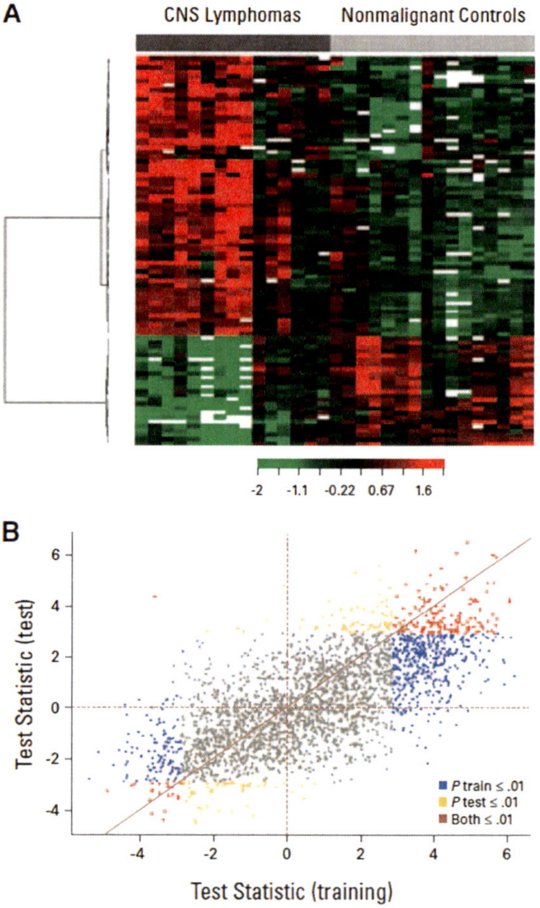

Fig. 5.2 **a** Differential expression of CSF proteins that distinguish CNS lymphoma from patients without CNS malignancy. Values are shown as a color scale with positive values represented by *red*, negative represented by *green*, and *black* corresponding to values close to zero. Missing values are shown in *white*. **b** The concordance between training and test sets was exceptional, as shown by comparing the test statistics from the two data sets. Reprinted with permission from [49]. © 2008. All rights reserved

inhibitors, serum glycoproteins and lipoproteins, well as components of the extracellular matrix, notably osteopontin and chitinase-3-like-1, as predicted by gene expression analyses [18, 29]. Most of the proteins whose expression was downregulated in CSF of CNS lymphoma patients were associated with normal neuronal function, such as neuropeptides or proteins involved in the regulation of neuronal signaling.

To further validate this approach and to illustrate the potential of protein biomarkers to facilitate decision-making in CNS lymphoma, the investigators defined the CSF expression of the serine protease inhibitor antithrombin III (ATIII), using a different technology, ELISA. ATIII was of particular interest because this molecule had been independently identified by gene expression studies as being expressed at the transcriptional level in CNS lymphoma, particularly in cases associated with short survival. Elevated CSF concentration of ATIII in CNS lymphoma patients was confirmed by ELISA in an independent validation set of 100 cases. Receiver operating characteristic curve analysis demonstrated that ATIII protein determination may have better diagnostic accuracy than CSF cytology in the diagnosis of CNS lymphoma. However, elevated CSF concentration of ATIII was also noted in cases of glioblastoma, as well as metastatic carcinomas, highlighting the need to identify protein biomarkers, which are specific to CNS lymphoma.

Biomarkers of Prognosis in PCNSL

In agreement with other studies which associate *BCL*-6 expression with a favorable prognosis in diffuse large B-cell lymphoma (DLBCL), Braaten et al. demonstrated that overexpression of *BCL*-6 in PCNSL patients was associated with improved survival (101 months) compared to patients whose tumors did not express *BCL*-6 (14.7 months) [50]. The prognostic significance of *BCL*-6 in CNS lymphoma was subsequently corroborated by Levy et al. [51] and Lin et al. [52]. Another potential prognostic marker in PCNSL is the presence of reactive perivascular T-cell infiltrates (RPVI). In a large, multicenter, retrospective series of 100 PCNSL cases, the presence of RPVI significantly correlated with a better outcome [53]. As noted previously, STAT6 expression and activation by tumor cells and tumor endothelia were implicated as a possible marker of poor prognosis in PCNSL patients receiving therapy with methotrexate [17, 36]. Finally, vascular expression of endoglin (CD105) was shown to be a marker of neoangiogenesis and strong expression of endoglin by tumor endothelia correlates with adverse prognosis in PCNSL [54].

Chromosomal imbalances determined by comparative genomic hybridization (CGH) demonstrate deletions on 6q in 60% of PCNSL patients [47]. As noted above, the incidence of chromosome 6q deletions as demonstrated either by CGH or FISH appears to be higher in PCNSL than in extraneural lymphomas and patients with del (6)(q22) may have shorter survival compared to PCNSL patients without LOH on 6q. While this locus is known to contain the *PTPRK* gene, precise identification of the candidate tumor suppressor gene responsible for the adverse

Table 5.2 Prognostic biomarkers in PCNSL

Gene	Biological effects	Possible clinical significance
CD105 (Endoglin)	Modulates TGF-beta signaling Marker of proliferating tumor endothelia	• Aggressive tumor growth • Poor prognosis
STAT6	Mediator of IL-4 Signaling Expressed by lymphoma cells and tumor endothelia	• Decreased survival in patients treated with methotrexate
Del 6*q*(22)	Possible locus of tumor suppressor gene *PTPRK* which may regulate cell contact and adhesion	• Shorter survival in patients with loss of expression
BCL-6	Transcriptional repressor, oncogene, malignant transformation of germinal center B cells	• Overexpression associated with favorable prognosis

phenotype associated with del 6q22 patients awaits further study (Table 5.2). It is also likely that with the development of high-resolution genomic sequencing, additional genomic aberrations will be identified that may also be significant in terms of prognosis.

References

1. Bokstein F, Lossos A, Lossos IS, Siegal T (2002) Central nervous system relapse of systemic non-Hodgkin's lymphoma: results of treatment based on high-dose methotrexate combination chemotherapy. Leuk Lymphoma 43:587–593
2. Batchelor T, Carson K, O'Neill A et al (2003) Treatment of primary CNS lymphoma with methotrexate and deferred radiotherapy: a report of NABTT 96-07. J Clin Oncol 21:1044–1049
3. McCann KJ, Ashton-Key M, Smith K et al (2009) Primary central nervous system lymphoma: tumor-related clones exist in the blood and bone marrow with evidence for separate development. Blood 113:4677–4680
4. Jahnke K, Hummel M, Korfel A et al (2006) Detection of subclinical systemic disease in primary CNS lymphoma by polymerase chain reaction of the rearranged immunoglobulin heavy-chain genes. J Clin Oncol 24:4754–4757
5. Paulus W, Jellinger K (1993) Comparison of integrin adhesion molecules expressed by primary brain lymphomas and nodal lymphomas. Acta Neuropathol 86:360–364
6. Forsyth PA, DeAngelis LM (1996) Biology and management of AIDS-associated primary CNS lymphomas. Hematol Oncol Clin North Am 10:1125–1134
7. Thomas JA, Crawford DH, Burke M (1995) Clinicopathologic implications of Epstein–Barr virus related B cell lymphoma in immunocompromised patients. J Clin Pathol 48:287–290
8. Cingolani A, Gastaldi R, Fassone L et al (2000) Epstein–Barr virus infection is predictive of CNS involvement in systemic AIDS-related non-Hodgkin's lymphomas. J Clin Oncol 18:3325–3330
9. Antinori A, De Rossi G, Ammassari A et al (1999) Value of combined approach with thallium-201 single-photon emission computed tomography and Epstein–Barr virus DNA polymerase

chain reaction in CSF for the diagnosis of AIDS-related primary CNS lymphoma. J Clin Oncol 17:554–560
10. Smith JR, Braziel RM, Paoletti S et al (2003) Expression of B-cell-attracting chemokine 1 (CXCL13) by malignant lymphocytes and vascular endothelium in primary central nervous system lymphoma. Blood 101:815–821
11. Ansel KM, Harris RB, Cyster JG (2002) CXCL13 is required for B1 cell homing, natural antibody production, and body cavity immunity. Immunity 16:67–76
12. Mazzucchelli L, Blaser A, Kappeler A et al (1999) BCA-1 is highly expressed in Helicobacter pylori-induced mucosa-associated lymphoid tissue and gastric lymphoma. J Clin Invest 104:R49–R54
13. Smith JR, Falkenhagen KM, Coupland SE et al (2007) Malignant B cells from patients with primary central nervous system lymphoma express stromal cell-derived factor-1. Am J Clin Pathol 127:633–641
14. Fischer L, Korfel A, Pfeiffer S et al (2009) CXCL13 and CXCL12 in central nervous system lymphoma patients. Clin Cancer Res 15:5968–5973
15. Chan CC, Shen D, Hackett JJ et al (2003) Expression of chemokine receptors, CXCR4 and CXCR5, and chemokines, BLC and SDF-1, in the eyes of patients with primary intraocular lymphoma. Ophthalmology 110:421–426
16. Falkenhagen KM, Braziel RM, Fraunfelder FW, Smith JR (2005) B-cells in ocular adnexal lymphoproliferative lesions express B-cell attracting chemokine 1 (CXCL13). Am J Ophthalmol 140:335–337
17. Rubenstein JL, Fridlyand J, Shen A et al (2006) Gene expression and angiotropism in primary CNS lymphoma. Blood 107:3716–3723
18. Tun HW, Personett D, Baskerville KA et al (2008) Pathway analysis of primary central nervous system lymphoma. Blood 111:3200–3210
19. Park HR, Tomida A, Sato S et al (2004) Effect on tumor cells of blocking survival response to glucose deprivation. J Natl Cancer Inst 96:1300–1310
20. Dancescu M, Rubio-Trujillo M, Biron G et al (1992) Interleukin 4 protects chronic lymphocytic leukemic B cells from death by apoptosis and upregulates Bcl-2 expression. J Exp Med 176:1319–1326
21. Conticello C, Pedini F, Zeuner A et al (2004) IL-4 protects tumor cells from anti-CD95 and chemotherapeutic agents via up-regulation of antiapoptotic proteins. J Immunol 172:5467–5477
22. Nelms K, Keegan AD, Zamorano J et al (1999) The IL-4 receptor: signaling mechanisms and biologic functions. Annu Rev Immunol 17:701–738
23. Fukushi J, Ono M, Morikawa W et al (2000) The activity of soluble VCAM-1 in angiogenesis stimulated by IL-4 and IL-13. J Immunol 165:2818–2823
24. Mantovani A, Sozzani S, Locati M et al (2002) Macrophage polarization: tumor-associated macrophages as a paradigm for polarized M2 mononuclear phagocytes. Trends Immunol 23:549–555
25. Kadoch C, Dinca EB, Voicu R et al (2009) Pathologic correlates of primary central nervous system lymphoma defined in an orthotopic xenograft model. Clin Cancer Res 15:1989–1997
26. Yang SH, Lee KS, Kim IS et al (2009) Long-term survival in primary CNS lymphoma treated by high-dose methotrexate monochemotherapy: role of STAT6 activation as prognostic determinant. J Neurooncol 92:65–71
27. Selkirk SM, Morrow J, Barone TA et al (2008) Elevation of osteopontin levels in brain tumor cells reduces burden and promotes survival through the inhibition of cell dispersal. J Neurooncol 86:285–296
28. Chabas D, Baranzini SE, Mitchell D et al (2001) The influence of the proinflammatory cytokine, osteopontin, on autoimmune demyelinating disease. Science 294:1731–1735
29. Rubenstein JL, Shen A, Batchelor TT et al (2009) Differential gene expression in central nervous system lymphoma. Blood 113:266–267; author reply 7–8

30. Rosenwald A, Wright G, Chan WC et al (2002) The use of molecular profiling to predict survival after chemotherapy for diffuse large-B-cell lymphoma. N Engl J Med 346:1937–1947
31. Sherman-Baust CA, Weeraratna AT, Rangel LB et al (2003) Remodeling of the extracellular matrix through overexpression of collagen VI contributes to cisplatin resistance in ovarian cancer cells. Cancer Cell 3:377–386
32. Shi GX, Harrison K, Wilson GL et al (2002) RGS13 regulates germinal center B lymphocytes responsiveness to CXC chemokine ligand (CXCL)12 and CXCL13. J Immunol 169:2507–2515
33. Ma L, Teruya-Feldstein J, Weinberg RA (2007) Tumour invasion and metastasis initiated by microRNA-10b in breast cancer. Nature 449:682–688
34. Robertus JL, Harms G, Blokzijl T et al (2009) Specific expression of miR-17-5p and miR-127 in testicular and central nervous system diffuse large B-cell lymphoma. Mod Pathol 22: 547–555
35. Cloonan N, Brown MK, Steptoe AL et al (2008) The miR-17-5p microRNA is a key regulator of the G1/S phase cell cycle transition. Genome Biol 9:R127
36. Kadoch C, Treseler P, Rubenstein JL (2006) Molecular pathogenesis of primary central nervous system lymphoma. Neurosurg Focus 21:E1
37. Rubenstein JL, Treseler P, O'Brien JM (2005) Pathology and genetics of primary central nervous system and intraocular lymphoma. Hematol Oncol Clin North Am 19:705–717
38. Merry DE, Korsmeyer SJ (1997) Bcl-2 gene family in the nervous system. Annu Rev Neurosci 20:245–267
39. Skene JH (1984) Growth-associated proteins and the curious dichotomies of nerve regeneration. Cell 37:697–700
40. Montesinos-Rongen M, Roost DV, Schaller C et al (2004) Primary diffuse large B-cell lymphomas of the central nervous system are targeted by aberrant somatic hypermutation. Blood 103:1869–1875
41. Montesinos-Rongen M, Kuppers R, Schluter D et al (1999) Primary central nervous system lymphomas are derived from germinal-center B cells and show a preferential usage of the V4-34 gene segment. Am J Pathol 155:2077–2086
42. Nakamura M, Sakaki T, Hashimoto H et al (2001) Frequent alterations of the p14(ARF) and p16(INK4a) genes in primary central nervous system lymphomas. Cancer Res 61:6335–6339
43. Kamijo T, Bodner S, van de Kamp E et al (1999) Tumor spectrum in ARF-deficient mice. Cancer Res 59:2217–2222
44. Nakamura M, Shimada K, Ishida E, Konishi N (2004) Histopathology pathogenesis and molecular genetics in primary central nervous system lymphomas. Histol Histopathol 19:211–219
45. Mrugala MM, Rubenstein JL, Ponzoni M, Batchelor TT (2009) Insights into the biology of primary central nervous system lymphoma. Curr Oncol Rep 11:73–80
46. Harada K, Nishizaki T, Kubota H et al (2001) Distinct primary central nervous system lymphoma defined by comparative genomic hybridization and laser scanning cytometry. Cancer Genet Cytogenet 125:147–150
47. Weber T, Weber RG, Kaulich K et al (2000) Characteristic chromosomal imbalances in primary central nervous system lymphomas of the diffuse large B-cell type. Brain Pathol 10:73–84
48. Cady FM, O'Neill BP, Law ME et al (2008) Del(6)(q22) and BCL6 rearrangements in primary CNS lymphoma are indicators of an aggressive clinical course. J Clin Oncol 26:4814–4819
49. Roy S, Josephson SA, Fridlyand J et al (2008) Protein biomarker identification in the CSF of patients with CNS lymphoma. J Clin Oncol 26:96–105
50. Braaten KM, Betensky RA, de Leval L et al (2003) BCL-6 expression predicts improved survival in patients with primary central nervous system lymphoma. Clin Cancer Res 9:1063–1069
51. Levy O, Deangelis LM, Filippa DA et al (2008) Bcl-6 predicts improved prognosis in primary central nervous system lymphoma. Cancer 112:151–156

52. Lin CH, Kuo KT, Chuang SS et al (2006) Comparison of the expression and prognostic significance of differentiation markers between diffuse large B-cell lymphoma of central nervous system origin and peripheral nodal origin. Clin Cancer Res 12:1152–1156
53. Ponzoni M, Berger F, Chassagne-Clement C et al (2007) Reactive perivascular T-cell infiltrate predicts survival in primary central nervous system B-cell lymphomas. Br J Haematol 138:316–323
54. Sugita Y, Takase Y, Mori D et al (2007) Endoglin (CD 105) is expressed on endothelial cells in the primary central nervous system lymphomas and correlates with survival. J Neurooncol 82:249–256

Chapter 6
Clinical and Diagnostic Considerations in Primary Central Nervous System Lymphoma

Tracy Batchelor, Edward Neuwelt, Daphne L. Wang, and R. Gilberto Gonzalez

Introduction

Primary central nervous system lymphoma (PCNSL) is characterized by unique clinical features and diagnostic requirements. The extent of disease evaluation differs from that recommended for other non-Hodgkin lymphoma (NHL) patients or for patients with other primary brain tumors. Diagnostic and therapeutic knowledge of PCNSL is rapidly advancing and the former will be reviewed in this chapter.

Clinical Presentation

In immunocompetent patients, the median age at diagnosis of PCNSL is 53–57 years, with a male:female ratio of 1.2–1.7:1 [1]. The highest risk group appears to be those $\geq$ 60 years, in whom the incidence has increased disproportionately since the mid 1990s [2]. The only characteristics shared by immunocompetent patients who develop PCNSL are advanced age and a slight propensity for the male sex.

Symptoms and Signs

The symptoms and signs of PCNSL at presentation usually reflect the neuroanatomical location of the lesion(s). PCNSL patients typically present with one of four distinct anatomical patterns: (1) Discrete intracranial mass lesions that are solitary or multiple, often in contact with ventricular or meningeal surfaces, (2) leptomeningeal lesions, (3) ocular lymphoma with or without other lesions, and (4) rare spinal cord lesions.

The average time between the onset of symptoms to the diagnosis of PCNSL is 3 months, reflecting the high proliferative capacity of this lymphoid malignancy [3].

T. Batchelor (✉)
Stephen E. and Catherine Pappas Center for Neuro-Oncology, Departments of Neurology and Radiation Oncology, Division of Hematology and Oncology, Massachusetts General Hospital, Harvard Medical School, 55 Fruit Street, Boston, MA 02114, USA
e-mail: tbatchelor@partners.org

T. Batchelor, L.M. DeAngelis (eds.), *Lymphoma and Leukemia of the Nervous System*, DOI 10.1007/978-1-4419-7668-0_6,

In a review of 64 patients with a history of rapid, progressive neurological deterioration undergoing brain biopsy, the most common etiology for the clinical syndrome was PCNSL (20%) [4]. Administration of corticosteroids can delay or confound the diagnosis, due to cytolysis of lymphoma cells [5]. Although corticosteroids should be avoided until a histopathological diagnosis is achieved, one study demonstrated that radiographic response to this class of drug was a positive prognostic marker [6].

As with all masses in the central nervous system (CNS), the location of PCNSL lesions determines the clinical presentation. Presenting symptoms and signs in a series of 248 immunocompetent patients with PCNSL included: focal neurological deficits in 70% of patients; neuropsychiatric symptoms in 43%; headache/nausea/vomiting suggestive of increased intracranial pressure (ICP) in 33%; seizures in 14%; and ocular symptoms in 4% [7]. Focal deficits included dysphasia, hemiparesis, and ataxia due to discrete intracerebral lesions, as well as less common cranial nerve palsies secondary to leptomeningeal deposits. Neuropsychiatric changes such as apathy, depression, slowed thinking, and confusion have been attributed to the infiltration of white matter tracts by PCNSL lesions that involve the periventricular regions or the corpus callosum. Seizures are the presenting symptom of PCNSL in only 10–15% of immunocompetent patients with PCNSL possibly due to the deeper, subcortical location typical of PCNSL [3].

The range of leptomeningeal dissemination in different series of PCNSL patients is 7–42% [8] and may depend on the method of ascertainment (lumbar puncture, autopsy) in each study. Dissemination of lymphoma cells to the leptomeninges is asymptomatic in the majority of patients. In one study, less than one-third of PCNSL patients with definite leptomeningeal involvement showed any symptoms or signs suggestive of leptomeningeal tumor [9]. Primary leptomeningeal lymphoma is a rare condition.

For the 15–25% of immunocompetent patients found at diagnosis of PCNSL to have ocular involvement, and for those with primary intraocular lymphoma (PIOL), both eyes are affected in the majority of cases. These patients typically report nonspecific ocular symptoms. In a study of 83 patients with PIOL, the most common symptoms were blurred vision (52%), decreased visual acuity (37%) and floaters (30%) [10].

The rare spinal cord lesions found in patients with PCNSL are primarily discrete intramedullary nodules. The symptoms and signs of intramedullary spinal cord lymphoma resemble those of other intramedullary spinal tumors and depend upon the location within the spinal cord. Presenting symptoms may include limb parasthesias and/or numbness, limb weakness (often asymmetric), impaired gait, and perineal numbness with bladder or bowel dysfunction.

Differential Diagnosis

For the immunocompetent patient population, a solitary lesion that infiltrates the corpus callosum or other periventricular location, enhances homogenously, and is associated with only a moderate amount of edema is highly suggestive of PCNSL.

However, in addition to PCNSL, the radiographic differential diagnosis of a single homogenously enhancing lesion surrounded by edema includes: glioma, metastatic brain tumor, abscess, and focal demyelinating lesion. Diffuse periventricular disease without any discrete mass is a less common presentation of PCNSL and may be misdiagnosed as multiple sclerosis [11].

Neuroimaging

The appearance of PCNSL on cranial computerized tomography (CT) and magnetic resonance imaging (MRI) studies has been well described [12–19]. In a study of the radiographic presentation of 100 immunocompetent PCNSL patients, lesions were solitary in 65% of cases and were located in a cerebral hemisphere (38%) (Fig. 6.1), thalamus/basal ganglia (16%), corpus callosum (14%) (Fig. 6.2), periventricular region (12%), and cerebellum (9%) [20]. Infiltration of the corpus callosum is commonly observed in only one other brain neoplasm, glioblastoma (Fig. 6.3 – see comments below). While the cerebral hemispheres and the deep gray matter are the most common locations for PCNSL masses, they can occur virtually anywhere within the brain including the cerebellum, brainstem, infundibulum, and within the ventricle [21]. In patients with PIOL, it is uncommon to visualize discrete lesions by CT and MRI.

Tumor contrast enhancement on CT and MRI is typical and is observed in over 90% of PCNSL patients. Absence of enhancement with contrast administration is

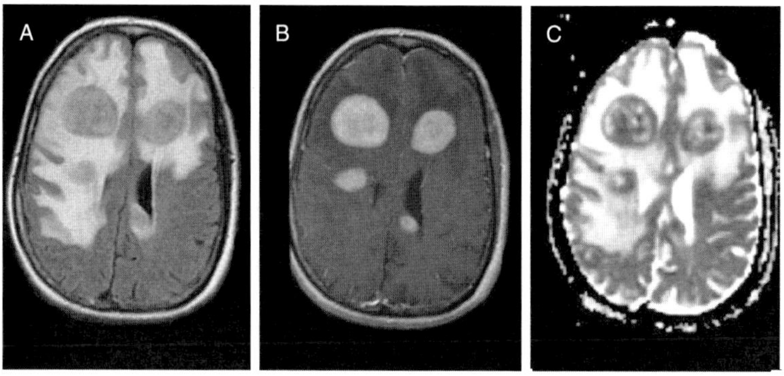

Fig. 6.1 PCNSL with multiple enhancing cerebral masses. **a** Axial FLAIR MRI. Four mass lesions that are isointense to brain are identified at this level. Two are in the right frontal lobe, one is in the left frontal lobe and one has an ependymal location in the left lateral ventricle. The isointense masses are surrounded by extensive areas of hyperintensity suggestive of edema. **b** Post-contrast, T1-weighted axial MRI image. There is intense enhancement of all four masses. **c** Apparent diffusion coefficient (ADC) axial MRI. The masses are slightly heterogeneous but they have predominantly low signal consistent with reduced diffusion, which is characteristic of PCNSL (source: R. Gilberto Gonzalez, M.D., Massachusetts General Hospital)

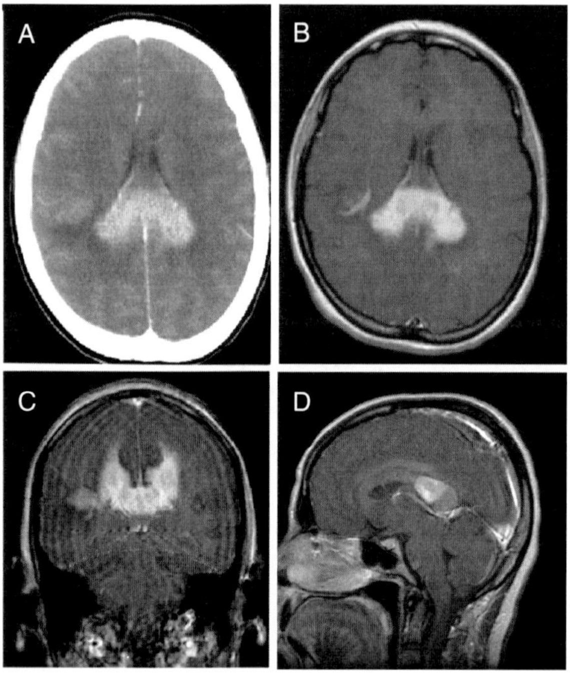

Fig. 6.2 PCNSL involving the corpus callosum. **a** A contrast-enhanced head CT at the level of the splenium of the corpus callosum demonstrates an intensely enhancing mass infiltrating the splenium of the corpus callosum and extending into both hemispheres. Hypodensity surrounding the enhancing mass suggests edema. **b** Contrast enhanced T1-weighted MRI. Intense enhancement of the mass is observed after contrast administration. Additionally, a satellite lesion is seen in the right hemisphere. **c** Coronal FLAIR MRI The mass lesion involving the splenium of the corpus callosum is hyperintense on this pulse sequence. In addition to the lesion that enhances, there is hyperintensity that extends beyond the enhancing component, which suggests edema although lymphomatous cellular infiltration is also possible. **d** Sagittal FLAIR MRI through the corpus callosum. The expansile mass in the splenium of the corpus callosum has variable signal characteristics. The most posterior aspect is isointense with brain, which can be seen with highly cellular tumors such as lymphoma. More anteriorly, the signal is hyperintense. Abnormal signal is also seen throughout the body and genu of the corpus callosum as well as in the cingulate gyrus (source: R. Gilberto Gonzalez, M.D., Massachusetts General Hospital)

observed typically after administration of anti-tumor therapy. However, absence of contrast enhancement has been reported in a small proportion of PCNSL patients who have not undergone treatment [13]. Typically, the enhancement is homogeneous and results in a sharply demarcated mass. On occasion, the enhancement pattern is heterogeneous. Ring-like enhancement is less common except in the immunocompromised patient population (Fig. 6.4).

Although most immunocompetent PCNSL patients present with a single brain lesion on CT or MRI, a minority (10–50%) of these patients will manifest multiple

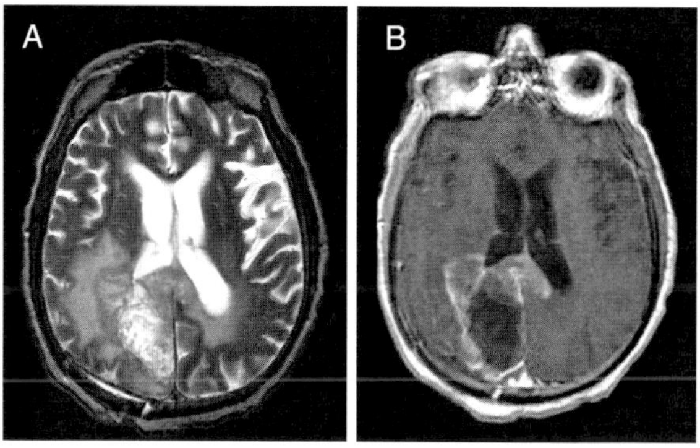

Fig. 6.3 Glioblastoma involving the corpus callosum. Differentiating glioblastoma from PCNSL is aided by the appearance of necrosis, which is common in glioblastoma as demonstrated in this figure, but rare in the patient with PCNSL unless immunocompromised. **a** Axial, T2-weighted MRI. The infiltrative mass lesion expands the splenium of the corpus callosum. The mass is isointense to brain. The mass extends posteriorly and to the right hemisphere where it is more heterogeneous with central areas of hyperintensity suggesting necrosis. There is substantial surrounding T2 hyperintensity suggesting edema. **b** Axial, post-contrast, T1-weighted MRI. The mass enhances intensely except for the posterior right hemisphere component, which has irregular ring enhancement confirming necrosis (source: R. Gilberto Gonzalez, M.D., Massachusetts General Hospital)

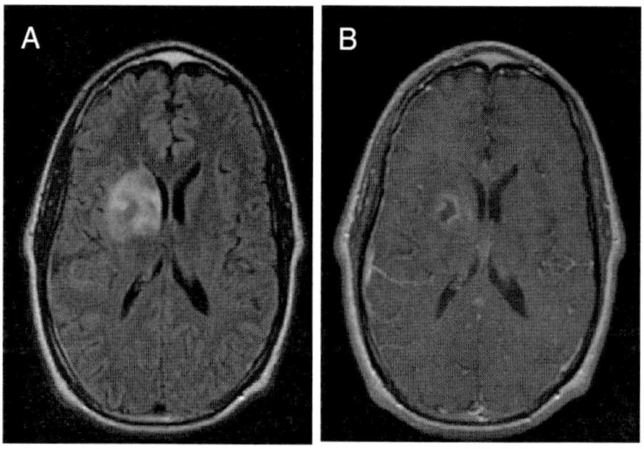

Fig. 6.4 Ring-enhancing PCNSL. **a** Axial FLAIR MRI. Well-circumscribed, predominantly hyperintense mass lesion is identified in the right basal ganglia region. **b** Axial, postcontrast, T1-weighted MRI. The mass in the right basal ganglia has a ring enhancing pattern. Ring enhancement is much less common than uniform enhancement in PCNSL, and is observed more often in immunocompromised patients (source: R. Gilberto Gonzalez, M.D., Massachusetts General Hospital)

brain lesions (Figs. 6.1, 6.2, 6.5, and 6.6). The reported rate of multiple lymphomatous masses is higher in immunocompromised PCNSL patients. The degree of mass effect exerted by PCNSL is largely dependent on the degree of associated edema.

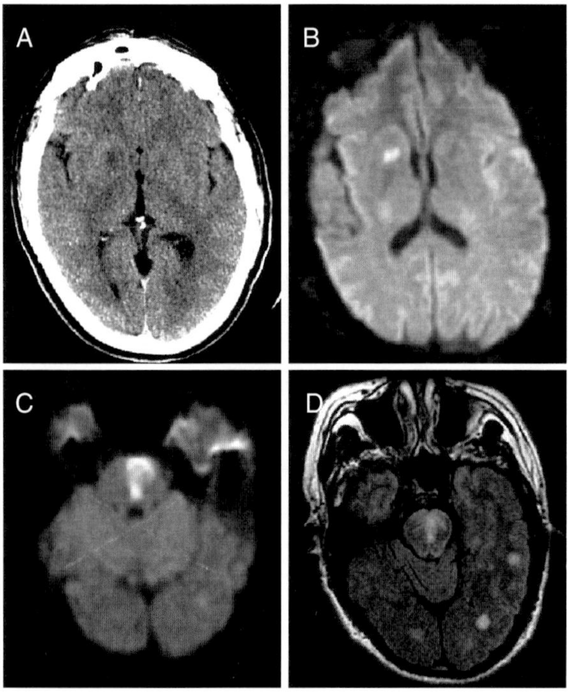

Fig. 6.5 Intravascular Lymphoma mimics multiple embolic strokes. **a** Axial, postcontrast head CT. There is a focal hypodensity in the head of the right caudate nucleus. **b** Axial diffusion-weighted MRI. There is a focus of hyperintense signal abnormality in the head of the right caudate nucleus that was confirmed to be due to reduced diffusion on the ADC images. This appearance is also commonly seen in acute ischemic stroke. **c** Axial diffusion-weighted MRI at the level of the pons. There is a large hyperintensity in the left hemi-pons in the distribution of the a pontine penetrating artery. **d** Axial FLAIR MRI at the level of the pons. There is a hyperintense signal abnormality in the left hemi-pons that corresponds to the DWI abnormality shown on figure **c**. In addition there are two FLAIR hyperintense lesions in the left temporal and occipital lobes that are not well seen on the DWI study. This appearance can be seen in ischemic strokes of multiple ages, but in this case the signal abnormalities are due to intravascular lymphoma (source: R. Gilberto Gonzalez, M.D., Massachusetts General Hospital)

Early reports suggested relatively minimal mass effect considering the size of the lesions, and this was attributed to the infiltrative nature of the tumor. However, extensive edema causing marked mass effect with brain distortion and even herniation is not uncommon (Fig. 6.1). Primary CNS lymphomas are commonly in locations near the subarachnoid space. In one report, all patients had at least one lesion adjacent to CSF pathways [12]. Dissemination along perivascular spaces and along ependymal surfaces (Fig. 6.6) has also been reported in PCNSL.

The signal intensity of PCNSL masses is variable on both CT and MRI. However, a large proportion of these masses appear iso- to hyper-dense on CT and iso- to hypo-intense on T2-weighted images on MRI. This appearance, uncommon

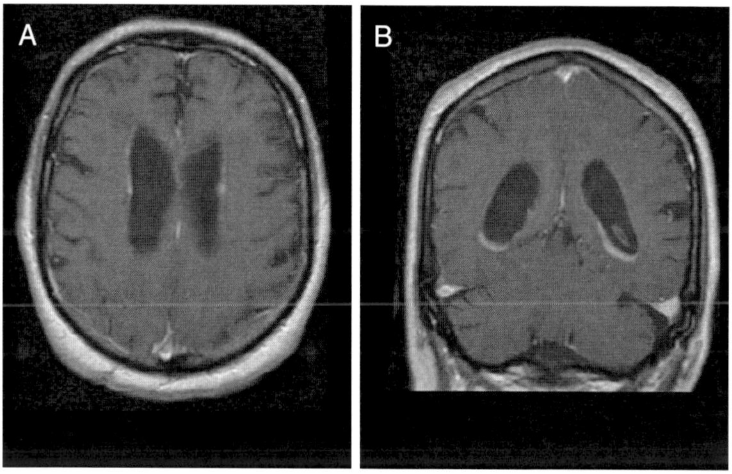

Fig. 6.6 Ependymal involvement by lymphoma. Axial and coronal post-contrast, T1-weighted MRI images. **a** Axial images reveal nodular enhancement involving the ependyma of the lateral ventricles. **b** Coronal images demonstrate a thick, rind like area of enhancement involving the ependyma of the inferior portions of the lateral ventricles (source: R. Gilberto Gonzalez, M.D., Massachusetts General Hospital)

in other brain neoplasms and infections, is thought to be due to a highly cellular tumor characterized by a high nuclear to cytoplasmic ratio. A reduction of the rate of water diffusion in many PCNSL masses results in hyperintense lesions on diffusion weighted images (DWI) and hypointense lesions on apparent diffusion coefficient (ADC) maps (Fig. 6.1). In a report of 18 immunocompetent PCNSL patients, ADC maps demonstrated an inverse correlation between cellular density and ADC measurements. Moreover, patients in the "low ADC group" were noted to have shorter, progression-free survival and overall survival, whereas patients who experienced a decrease in ADC measurements after methotrexate chemotherapy experienced improved clinical outcomes [22]. This preliminary report raises the possibility that ADC measurements by MRI may serve as a useful prognostic and predictive "imaging biomarker" in the PCNSL patient population.

The differential diagnosis of brain masses that have the appearance of PCNSL includes metastasis, other primary brain tumors, and infections. When multiple lesions are seen, metastasis becomes an important consideration. Certain metastases are often iso- to hypo-intense on T2-weighted MRI images and may have a similar appearance as PCNSL. These types of neoplasms include adenocarcinomas from the gastrointestinal tract, breast, or lung. An enhancing mass crossing the corpus callosum represents PCNSL, or glioblastoma in the large majority of cases. Differentiating these two tumors is aided by the appearance of necrosis, which is common in GBM, but is unusual in the patient with PCNSL, unless immunocompromised (Figs. 6.2 and 6.5). Ring-enhancing lesions raise the possibility of an abscess. As previously noted, ring-enhancement is unusual in immunocompetent PCNSL patients.

The capability of FDG-PET to accurately differentiate between PCNSL and non-malignant CNS lesions has been evaluated in several small studies. Two of these studies arrived at similar conclusions [23, 24]. Using both qualitative and quantitative criteria, PCNSL was distinguished from non-neoplastic brain lesions by a higher uptake of FDG by lymphoma. However, these studies cannot be considered definitive because of the small number of subjects involved. It is unclear whether FDG-PET is superior to thallium SPECT imaging for this purpose. Cranial FDG-PET may become an important imaging modality to monitor response to therapy in PCNSL patients. In a study of 28 PCNSL patients, residual hypermetabolic lesions were noted in 10/20 (50%) patients who responded to therapy, and had only nonspecific MRI findings at the time of response assessment. The authors concluded that cranial FDG-PET in these situations was useful in guiding further management in this subset of patients [25].

Other Diagnostic Studies

After structural neuroimaging of the brain suggests PCNSL, definitive histopathological diagnosis must be established via other diagnostic modalities prior to treatment. In one prospective study of 96 immunocompetent patients with PCNSL, 15% were diagnosed by CSF cytology alone, 5% by vitrectomy alone, and 78% by surgical methods [9].

Cerebrospinal Fluid

As in all cases of intracranial mass lesions, lumbar puncture for CSF examination should only be performed on PCNSL patients who are not at risk for herniation. Examination of CSF includes: (a) basic studies such as cell count, protein, glucose; (b) cytology and flow cytometry; and (c) PCR for clonal immunoglobulin gene rearrangements, or in AIDS patients, PCR for EBV-DNA. CSF cytology is the diagnostic test most commonly performed, with PCR used at specialized centers. In the largest study of this subject, 49/282 (17.4%) PCNSL patients were observed to have CSF dissemination by a combination of CSF cytomorphology and PCR [26].

In PCNSL, basic CSF parameters may be normal or only slightly abnormal. In a study of the CSF profile of 96 immunocompetent patients with PCNSL, a mild pleocytosis was present in only slightly more than half of patients. Specifically, CSF obtained via lumbar puncture from 70 immunocompetent patients with PCNSL showed: elevated WBC count, defined as greater than 7 cells/mm^3, in 54% of patients, with the median WBC count 8 cells/mm^3; elevated protein concentration in 67% of patients, with median value 69 mg/dl; and low glucose concentration (less than 38 mg/dl) in 10% of patients [9]. These CSF findings are non-specific and are not considered diagnostic. Moreover, although sometimes suggestive, basic CSF laboratory values will be normal in a large number of PCNSL cases.

CSF cytology is sufficient to make the diagnosis of PCNSL in only a subset of cases. The incidence of positive CSF cytology in the immunocompetent patient population with PCNSL has been reported between 7 and 42% [8]. In the largest prospective study of meningeal dissemination in PCNSL, 282 subjects had their CSF analyzed. Among the 205 subjects assessed by cytomorphology, malignant cells were observed in 33 (15%) [26].

Serial CSF samples may be required to make a diagnosis of PCNSL via CSF cytology: two-thirds of PCNSL patients with positive CSF cytology have an initial negative cytology. Even PCNSL lesions that involve the leptomeninges may not exfoliate sufficient malignant cells into the CSF to render cytology a successful diagnostic tool [9]. It is the small number of morphologically recognizable malignant cells typically observed in the CSF of PCNSL patients that accounts for the low incidence of positive CSF cytology. Similarly, the utility of DNA flow cytometry in the diagnosis of PCNSL is limited by the low cell count of most CSF specimens.

Polymerase chain reaction (PCR) examination of the CSF is an important complement to cytology, given the relatively low incidence of positive CSF cytology in PCNSL. PCR with consensus primers to the V and J regions of the immunoglobulin heavy chain gene are used to detect clonal rearrangements. Demonstration of clonal immunoglobulin gene rearrangements can establish monoclonality of a lymphocyte population in the CSF and thus, make the diagnosis of PCNSL [27–29]. From the largest prospective series cited above, 19/171 (11%) subjects had a monoclonal cell population identified by PCR. Ten of these 19 subjects had negative cytomorphology results and were determined to have CSF dissemination by PCR alone [26].

Assessment of CSF is important for all PCNSL patients in order to guide treatment and follow-up. However, in the setting of a newly diagnosed brain mass suspicious for PCNSL, it is often more practical to proceed with stereotactic brain biopsy to rapidly achieve diagnosis.

Ocular Evaluation

Approximately 15–25% of PCNSL patients will have ocular dissemination at the time of diagnosis [30]. Ocular evaluation that includes slit-lamp examination by an ophthalmologist must be performed as part of the assessment of any patient suspected of having PCNSL or the PIOL variant. Chapter 12 includes a detailed discussion of the ocular evaluation in this patient population. A cellular infiltrate in the vitreous, with or without subretinal infiltrates, is typically seen in patients with ocular lymphoma. For any patient in whom ocular complaints and slit-lamp examination findings raise the suspicion of ocular lymphoma, gadolinium-enhanced MRI of the brain and orbits should be performed. If neuroimaging shows that lumbar puncture poses no danger of herniation, CSF should be obtained for cytologic analysis. In a series of 221 PCNSL patients with ocular involvement, the CSF cytology was positive in 23% of subjects [31], and in 11% of those patients with PIOL variant [10].

If serial CSF examinations yield negative cytology results and CSF PCR studies are inconclusive, then vitrectomy may establish the diagnosis of PCNSL by demonstrating malignant lymphocytes in the eye. The vitrectomy should be performed on the eye with the worst vision or the most severe vitritis. Special handling of the vitreous specimen is required because lymphoma cells in the vitreous degenerate rapidly.

In a manner analogous to CSF analysis, the vitreous specimen can also be subjected to flow cytometry and/or immunohistochemistry in an effort to establish monoclonality. PCR can be used to detect clonal rearrangements of the VDJ regions of immunoglobulin heavy-chain genes of vitreal lymphoma cells. In addition, chorioretinal biopsy or fine-needle aspiration of a subretinal lesion may be performed to establish a diagnosis of ocular lymphoma. If the patient has received corticosteroids prior to the procedure, a false-negative result is possible. Chapter 12 contains a detailed discussion of diagnostic methods for ocular lymphoma.

Tumor Biopsy

Stereotactic Brain Biopsy (SBB) is the standard procedure for obtaining tissue adequate for pathological diagnosis of cerebral lymphoma [32]. Typically, this is the most direct and efficient method to obtain the diagnosis of PCNSL. Biopsy specimens insufficient for diagnosis can be avoided by targeting the center of the suspected lesion.

Advantages of SBB over open craniotomy include: minimal skin incision, the option of local anesthesia, short postoperative recovery period, and most importantly, relatively low morbidity and mortality [33]. Moreover, resection of cerebral parenchymal PCNSL lesions confers no survival benefit for this patient population [34]. For these reasons, the least invasive procedure that yields a diagnostic surgical specimen is preferable.

Extent of Disease Evaluation

After the diagnosis of PCNSL has been established via analysis of CSF, vitreal aspirate, or biopsy specimen, an extent of disease evaluation should be performed in every patient. Consensus guidelines regarding this evaluation have been published by the International PCNSL Collaborative Group (IPCG) and are enumerated in Table 6.1 [35]. Full ocular evaluation including a slit lamp examination should be performed in every patient, since asymptomatic ocular involvement is not uncommon, and since specific treatment may be indicated for ocular lymphoma [36]. In addition, in patients who are deemed safe for lumbar puncture, CSF should be collected for cell count, chemistry, cytopathology, flow cytometry, and possibly, PCR. Serum lactate dehydrogenase (LDH) level should be measured in every case since this parameter is a potential prognostic factor for patients with PCNSL [36]. Because PCNSL occurs so commonly in AIDS patients, HIV serology should be requested for every apparently immunocompetent patient diagnosed with PCNSL.

Table 6.1 IPCG guidelines for baseline evaluation for clinical trials (adapted from [35])

Pathology	Clinical	Laboratory	Imaging
Centralized review of pathology	Complete medical and neurological examination	HIV serology Viral BC hepatitis markers	Contrast-enhanced cranial MRI[a]
Immunophenotyping	Dilated eye examination including slit lamp evaluation	Serum LDH level	CT of chest, abdomen and pelvis
	Record prognostic factors (age, performance status)	CSF cytology, flow cytometry, IgH PCR	Bone marrow biopsy with aspirate
	Serial evaluation of cognitive function[b]	24 h urine collection for creatinine clearance[c]	Testicular ultrasound in elderly males

[a]Contrast-enhanced cranial CT in patients who have a contraindication for MRI (pacemaker) or who cannot tolerate MRI (claustrophobia).
[b]Mini-mental status examination is used commonly although improved instruments are being developed.
[c]For patients who will receive HD-MTX.

Given the rarity of spinal cord involvement, enhanced spine MRI is typically indicated only in cases in whom clinical suspicion of spinal cord tumor is high [37]. However, contrast-enhanced MRI of the entire spine should be considered in patients who cannot undergo lumbar puncture due to the presence of increased intracranial pressure. In this situation, spinal imaging may identify leptomeningeal deposits of tumor, and this could impact subsequent management.

The extent of diagnostic testing required to evaluate for systemic lymphoma after making the diagnosis of PCNSL is still a matter of investigation. However, all patients should have chest, abdomen and pelvis CT scans, and a bone marrow biopsy as recommended in the IPCG guidelines [35, 38, 39]. Testicular ultrasound should be considered in men. Body FDG-PET scans may play an increasingly important role in evaluating PCNSL patients for subclinical systemic disease. In a retrospective study of 49 PCNSL patients evaluated with body FDG-PET studies, extraneural hypermetabolic lesions were identified in 15% of subjects [40]. Subsequent tissue biopsy was performed and 11% of the lesions were found to be lymphoma, while 4% were found to represent other types of cancer.

The search for occult systemic disease has become increasingly important as recent evidence suggests that lymphoma cells may not be restricted to the CNS in a small population of patients with CNS lymphoma. Identical PCR products of clonally rearranged immunoglobulin heavy-chain (IgH) genes were identified in the bone marrow aspirates, blood samples, and brain tumor biopsy specimens in 2 of 24 patients with "primary" CNS lymphoma. In one of these patients, follow-up IgH PCR 24 months after diagnosis yielded a persistent monoclonal blood product despite a complete radiographic response in the CNS [41]. In another report, 3/3 PCNSL patients with simultaneous clonal tracking of the immunoglobulin variable (V) gene in tumor tissue and bone marrow/blood were observed to have both central and peripheral involvement [42]. Prospective, long-term follow-up studies will be necessary to further elucidate the frequency and importance of subclinical systemic disease in CNS lymphoma patients, and whether the presence of these monoclonal cell populations increase the risk of relapse.

During the course of disease, if a patient with PCNSL presents with new ocular or other nervous system symptoms/signs, re-evaluation – e.g. repeat slit-lamp examination or lumbar puncture – is indicated [31, 43]. Systemic dissemination of lymphoma is observed over time in 7–10% of "PCNSL" cases, generally in the terminal stages of the disease or at the time of post-mortem examination. In such cases, lymphoma may be found in the lymph nodes and visceral organs of the abdomen/retroperitoneum, mediastinal lymph nodes, lungs, bone marrow, or testes. The clinical significance of late-disease, systemic deposits of lymphoma is unclear.

Prognostic Scoring

The identification of prognostic markers in PCNSL enables physicians to discuss prognosis with individual patients and may eventually allow for the application of risk-adjusted therapeutic strategies. In addition, the knowledge of important prognostic markers is critical for prospective study designs.

Different prognostic scoring systems have been proposed. In a large retrospective review, the International Extranodal Lymphoma Study Group (IELSG) identified age > 60, Eastern Cooperative Oncology Group (ECOG) performance status > 1, elevated serum LDH level, high CSF protein concentration, and involvement of deep regions of the brain as independent predictors of worse prognosis in a series of 105 PCNSL patients [44]. In patients with 0–1 factors, the 2-year survival was 80%; in patients with 2–3 factors, the 2-year survival was 48%; and in patients with 4–5 factors, the 2-year survival was 15% (Fig. 6.7). Another group of investigators have proposed a prognostic model that divides PCNSL patients into 3 groups based on age and performance status: those <50 years old; those >50 years old with a KPS>70; and those >50 with a KPS <70 [45]. Based on these divisions, significant differences in overall and failure-free survival were observed (Fig. 6.8). These prognostic models are being incorporated as stratification variables in prospective randomized clinical trials of PCNSL.

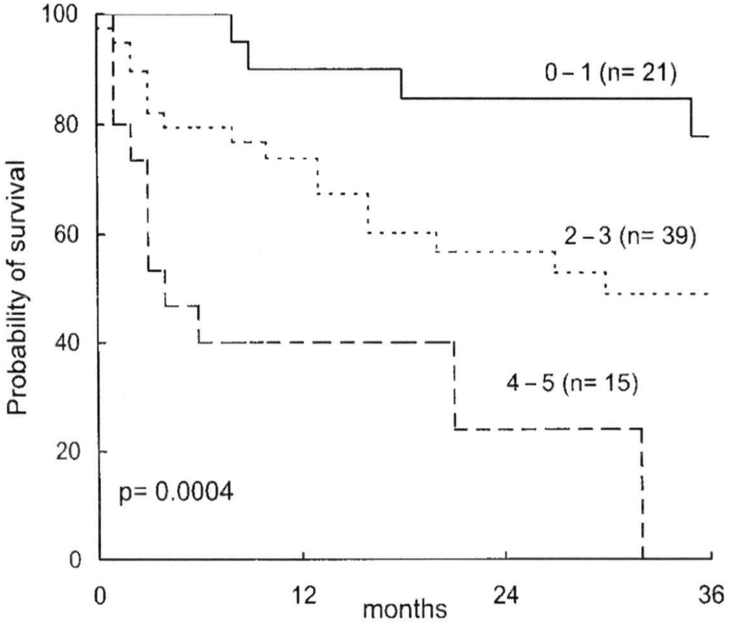

Fig. 6.7 International Extranodal Lymphoma Study Group prognostic system. This prognostic score is based on age, performance status, serum lactate dehydrogenase (LDH) level, cerebrospinal fluid protein level, and brain location of the tumor. Three different survival distributions, poor prognosis, intermediate prognosis and good prognosis, can be distinguished based on the use of this system (source: [44])

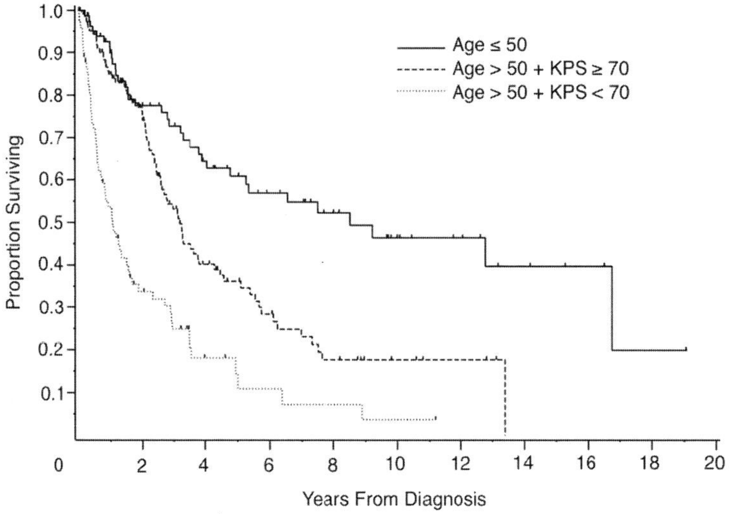

Fig. 6.8 Memorial Sloan-Kettering Cancer Center prognostic scoring system. This prognostic score is based on age and performance status and 3 survival distributions can be differentiated based on these 2 parameters (source: [45])

References

1. Schabet M (1999) Epidemiology of primary CNS lymphoma. J Neurooncol 43:199–201
2. Kadan-Lattick NS, Skluzacek MC, Gurney JG (2002) Decreasing incidence rates of primary central nervous system lymphoma. Cancer 95:193–202
3. Batchelor T, Loeffler J (2006) Primary CNS lymphoma. J Clin Oncol 24:1281–1288
4. Josephson SA, Papanastassiou AM, Berger MS et al (2007) The diagnostic utility of brain biopsy procedures in patients with rapidly deteriorating neurological conditions or dementia. J Neurosurg 106:72–75
5. Weller M (1999) Glucocorticoid treatment of primary CNS lymphoma. J Neurooncol 43: 237–239
6. Mathew BS, Carson K, Grossman SA (2006) Initial response to glucocorticoids. Cancer 106:383–387
7. Bataille B, Delwail V, Menet E et al (2000) Primary intracerebral malignant lymphoma: report of 248 cases. J Neurosurg 92:261–266
8. Kiewe P, Fischer L, Martus P et al (2010) Meningeal dissemination in primary CNS lymphoma: diagnosis, treatment, and survival in a large monocenter cohort. Neurooncology 12:409–417
9. Balmaceda C, Gaynor JJ, Sun M et al (1995) Leptomeningeal tumor in primary central nervous system lymphoma: recognition, significance, and implications. Ann Neurol 38(2):202–209
10. Grimm SA, Pulido JS, Jahnke K et al (2007) Primary intraocular lymphoma: an international primary central nervous system lymphoma collaborative group report. Ann Oncol 18: 1851–1855
11. DeAngelis LM (1990) Primary central nervous system lymphoma imitates multiple sclerosis. J Neurooncol 9:177–181
12. Buhring U, Herrlinger U, Krings T et al (2001) MRI features of primary central nervous system lymphomas at presentation. Neurology 57:393–396
13. DeAngelis LM (1993) Cerebral lymphoma presenting as a nonenhancing lesion on computed tomographic/magnetic resonance scan. Ann Neurol 33:308–311
14. Holtas S, Nyman U, Cronqvist S (1984) Computed tomography of malignant lymphoma of the brain. Neuroradiology 26:33–38
15. Jack CR Jr., O'Neill BP, Banks PM, Reese DF (1988) Central nervous system lymphoma: histologic types and CT appearance. Radiology 167:211–215
16. Johnson BA, Fram EK, Johnson PC, Jacobowitz R (1997) The variable MR appearance of primary lymphoma of the central nervous system: comparison with histopathologic features. Am J Neuroradiol 18:563–572
17. Lee YY, Bruner JM, Van Tassel P, Libshitz HI (1986) Primary central nervous system lymphoma: CT and pathologic correlation. Am J Roentgenol 147:747–752
18. Roman-Goldstein SM, Goldman DL, Howieson J et al (1992) MR of primary CNS lymphoma in immunologically normal patients. Am J Neuroradiol 13:1207–1213
19. Watanabe M, Tanaka R, Takeda N et al (1992) Correlation of computed tomography with the histopathology of primary malignant lymphoma of the brain. Neuroradiology 34: 36–42
20. Kuker W, Nagele T, Korfel A et al (2005) Primary central nervous system lymphomas (PCNSL): MRI features at presentation in 100 patients. J Neurooncol 72:169–177
21. Hochberg FH, Miller DC (1988) Primary central nervous system lymphoma. J Neurosurg 68:835–853
22. Barajas RF, Rubenstein JL, Chang JS et al (2010) Diffusion-weighted MR imaging derived apparent diffusion coefficient is predictive of clinical outcome in primary central nervous system lymphoma. Am J Neuroradiol 31:60–66

23. Hoffman JM, Waskin HA, Schifter T et al (1993) FDG-PET in differentiating lymphoma from nonmalignant central nervous system lesions in patients with AIDS. J Nucl Med 34: 567–575
24. Villringer K, Jager H, Dichgans M et al (1995) Differential diagnosis of CNS lesions in AIDS patients by FDG-PET. J Comput Assist Tomogr 19:532–536
25. Mohile NA, DeAngelis LM, Abrey LE (2008) Utility of brain FDG-PET in primary CNS lymphoma. Clin Adv Hematol Oncol 6:818–820
26. Fischer L, Martus P, Weller M et al (2008) Meningeal dissemination in primary CNS lymphoma. Neurology 71:1102–1108
27. Galoin S, Daste G, Apoil P-A et al (1997) Polymerase chain reaction on cerebrospinal fluid cells in the detection of leptomeningeal involvement by B-cell lymphoma and leukaemia: a novel strategy and its implications. Br J Haematol 99:122–130
28. Rhodes CM, Glantz MJ, Glantz L et al (1996) A comparison of polymerase chain reaction examination of cerebrospinal fluid and conventional cytology in the diagnosis of lymphomatous meningitis. Cancer 77:543–548
29. Storch-Hagenlocher B, Haas J, Vogt-Schaden ME et al (2000) Molecular analysis of the CDR3 encoding region of the immunoglobulin heavy chain locus in cerebrospinal fluid cells as a diagnostic tool in lymphomatous meningitis. Ann Neurol 47(2):211–217
30. Chan CC, Wallace DJ (2004) Intraocular lymphoma: update on diagnosis and management. Cancer Control 11:285–295
31. Grimm SA, McCannel CA, Omuro AMP et al (2008) Primary CNS lymphoma with intraocular involvement. International PCNSL collaborative group report. Neurology 71: 1355–1360
32. Sherman ME, Erozan YS, Mann RB et al (1991) Stereotactic brain biopsy in the diagnosis of malignant lymphoma. Am J Clin Pathol 95(6):878–883
33. Apuzzo ML, Sabshin JK (1983) Computed tomographic guidance stereotaxis in the management of intracranial mass lesions. Neurosurgery 12(3):277–285
34. Bellinzona M, Roser F, Ostertag H et al (2005) Surgical removal of primary central nervous system lymphomas presenting as space occupying lesions. Eur J Surg Oncol 31:100–105
35. Abrey LE, Batchelor TT, Ferreri AJ et al (2005) Report of an international workshop to standardize baseline evaluation and response criteria for primary CNS lymphoma. J Clin Oncol 23:5034–5043
36. Ferreri AJM, Reni M, Pasini F et al (2002) A multicenter study of treatment of primary CNS lymphoma. Neurology 58:1513–1520
37. DeAngelis LM (1999) Primary central nervous system lymphoma. Curr Opin Neurol 12(6):687–691
38. Nasir S, DeAngelis LM (2000) Update on the management of primary CNS lymphoma. Oncology 14(2):228–244
39. O'Neill BP, Dinapoli RP, Kurtin PJ, Habermann TM (1995) Occult systemic non-Hodgkin's lymphoma (NHL) in patients initially diagnosed as primary central nervous system lymphoma (PCNSL): How much staging is enough?. J Neurooncol 25(1):67–71
40. Mohile NA, Deangelis LM, Abrey LE (2008) The utility of body FDG PET in staging primary central nervous system lymphoma. Neurooncology 10:223–228
41. Jahnke K, Hummel M, Korfel A et al (2006) Detection of subclinical systemic disease in primary CNS lymphoma by polymerase chain reaction of the rearranged immunoglobulin heavy-chain genes. J Clin Oncol 24:4754–4757
42. McCann KJ, Ashton-Key M, Smith K et al (2009) Primary central nervous system lymphoma: tumor-related clones exist in the blood and bone marrow with evidence of separate development. Blood 113:4677–4680
43. Buggage RR, Chan C-C, Nussenblat RB (2001) Ocular manifestations of central nervous system lymphoma. Curr Opin Oncol 13(3):137–142

44. Ferreri AJ, Blay JY, Reni M et al (2003) Prognostic scoring system for primary CNS lymphomas: the international extranodal lymphoma study group experience. J Clin Oncol 21:266–272
45. Abrey LE, Ben-Porat L, Panageas KS et al (2006) Primary central nervous system lymphoma: the Memorial Sloan-Kettering Cancer Center prognostic model. J Clin Oncol 24:5711–5715

Chapter 7
Treatment of Primary Central Nervous System Lymphoma with Cranial Irradiation and Combined Modality Therapy

Lisa M. DeAngelis and Joachim Yahalom

Introduction

Primary Central Nervous System Lymphoma (PCNSL) was treated historically with cranial irradiation. The disease was considered rare and was often identified by different names such as reticulum cell sarcoma or microglioma. These factors made it extremely difficult to study alternatives to cranial irradiation, therapeutically. However, the increased incidence of PCNSL – particularly in immunocompetent patients – and the recognition that radiotherapy often produced a dramatic response, but was associated with rapid relapse, has led to continued investigation of improved therapies for PCNSL over the past 20–30 years.

Most PCNSLs are histologically comparable to diffuse large B-cell lymphomas. Like its systemic counterpart, PCNSL is an exquisitely radiosensitive tumor. Because PCNSL is usually confined to the brain, although it may also involve the CSF and ocular compartments, it can be classified as a Stage IE lymphoma, meaning it is confined to a single extranodal site of disease. In the spirit of irradiating the whole area of involvement, whole brain radiotherapy (WBRT) has been the traditional approach to treat PCNSL. However, the disease usually recurs and subsequent investigation led to the combination of chemotherapy with cranial irradiation for the treatment of this disease. In this chapter, we will explore the data on radiotherapy and combined modality treatment.

Radiation Therapy

While highly effective, the optimal dose and duration of radiotherapy (RT) has never been defined for PCNSL. There are several critical treatment parameters that determine the use of radiotherapy in the treatment of PCNSL, including the

L.M. DeAngelis (✉)
Department of Neurology, Memorial Sloan-Kettering Cancer Center, 1275 York Avenue, New York, NY 10021-6007, USA
e-mail: deangell@mskcc.org

T. Batchelor, L.M. DeAngelis (eds.), *Lymphoma and Leukemia of the Nervous System*, DOI 10.1007/978-1-4419-7668-0_7,

port of radiation and the dose. Historically, PCNSL has been treated with WBRT. This was begun decades ago when the standard treatment for any malignant brain tumor, including glioblastoma, was the use of WBRT. This was employed for several reasons. The first and most important was the highly infiltrative nature of most malignant gliomas and likewise, PCNSLs, although the latter was not appreciated at the time [1]. Secondly, WBRT was, and is, the standard treatment for brain metastases, and not all brain tumors were biopsied and pathology was not always well defined. Consequently, there were situations when the exact tumor type was unclear and it seemed prudent to incorporate treatment of the entire brain, so as to reach all areas of disease. Thirdly, high quality imaging was not available and therefore the extent of tumor was ill defined by available techniques, which made delivery of partial brain radiotherapy particularly challenging to the radiotherapist who could never be certain of the margins of disease. Finally, techniques for partial volume irradiation were crude and even when administered, continued to incorporate large areas of brain within the radiation port unnecessarily, but unavoidably. Therefore, it is easy to understand how WBRT became the standard therapeutic approach for the treatment of PCNSL, as it was for all aggressive brain tumors.

With respect to dose, no proper dose escalation study has been done for PCNSL. Earlier reports suggested that doses equal to, or in excess, of 50 Gy seemed to confer better survival than lower doses. However, it is possible that patients in worse condition or with more extensive disease received less radiotherapy than those who received higher doses, making it difficult to draw outcome conclusions. Comparable systemic lymphomas when confined to a localized area and treated with radiotherapy often required considerably less RT to achieve local control. In fact, systemic Stage IE NHL has local control rates of 90% with 40–50 Gy focal RT, with a low incidence of local relapse and prolonged survival. However, PCNSL relapsed within the RT field frequently and was associated with a much lower survival rate with comparable RT treatment. A recent retrospective analysis of 132 patients treated with WBRT alone in the 1990s reported a median survival of 18 months and a 5-year survival rate of 18%, which is higher than the typical 5-year survival rate of 3–4% reported in older comparable studies [2]. This was one of the first indications that PCNSL may have a biology that differs from its systemic counterpart, even when the histology is identical.

The first multicenter, prospective study of radiotherapy in PCNSL was conducted by the Radiation Therapy Oncology Group (RTOG) [3]. In that phase II study, 41 patients with PCNSL received 40 Gy WBRT plus a 20 Gy boost to the area of bulky disease with a 2 cm margin (Table 7.1). This produced a significant response in most patients, but unfortunately disease recurred in all. Response was measured in 26 patients using head CT scans and 16 patients (62%) had a complete response. The median survival for the entire group was 12.1 months, but the authors reported a significant difference in outcome depending upon age. Patients who were ≥ 60 years of age at the time of diagnosis had a median survival of 7 months, whereas those patients who were younger than age 60 at diagnosis had a median survival of 21 months. Short survival was related to recurrence and 61% of patients relapsed. Perhaps most importantly, the majority of relapses occurred within the region that

Table 7.1 Response rate, progression-free survival and overall survival to different treatment regimens for primary CNS lymphoma

Study	No. of patients	Chemotherapy	RT	Response rate (%) (CR and PR)	Median progression-free survival (mo)	Median overall survival (mo)
Radiotherapy alone						
Nelson et al. [3]	41	None	40 Gy WBRT + 20 Gy boost	~ 63	NA	12.2
Chemoradiotherapy CHOP-based						
Lachance et al. [8]	6	CHOD	45 Gy WBRT + 30 Gy neuraxis	17	NA	8.5
O'Neill et al. [9]	53	CHOP	50.4 Gy WBRT	60	NA	9.6
Schultz et al. [10]	52	CHOD	41.4 Gy WBRT + 18 Gy boost	67	NA	16.1
Chemoradiotherapy MTX-based						
DeAngelis et al. [5]	31	MTX (1 g/m^2) + cytarabine (3 g/m^2) – IT MTX	40 Gy WBRT with 14.4 Gy boost	94	41	42.5
Glass et al. [28]	25	MTX (3.5 g/m^2)	30–44 Gy WBRT	88	32	33
O'Brien et al. [29]	46	MTX (1 g/m^2)	45 Gy WBRT + 5.4 Gy boost	95	65% PFS at 2 yr	33
Abrey et al. [12]	52	MPV (MTX 3.5 g/m^2) + cytarabine (3 g/m^2) + IT MTX	± 45 Gy WBRT	94	NA	60

Table 7.1 (continued)

Study	No. of patients	Chemotherapy	RT	Response rate (%) (CR and PR)	Median progression-free survival (mo)	Median overall survival (mo)
Ferreri et al. [14]	13	MPV (MTX 3 g/m^2)	36–45 Gy WBRT with boost	92	NA	25+
DeAngelis et al. [13]	102	MPV (MTX 2.5 g/m^2) + IT MTX	36–45 Gy WBRT	94	24	36.9
Poortmans et al. [19]	52	MTX (3 g/m^2) + teniposide + carmustine + IT MTX + IT cytarabine	30 Gy WBRT + 10 Gy boost	81	NA	46
Omuro et al. [16]	52	MTX (1 g/m^2) + thiotepa + procarbazine + IT MTX	41.4 Gy + 14.4 Gy boost	88	18	32

Abbreviations: IT, intra-thecal; MPV, methotrexate, procarbazine, vincristine; MTX, methotrexate; NA, not available; PFS, progression-free survival; WBRT, whole-brain radiotherapy; CHOP/CHOD, cyclophosphamide, doxorubicin, vincristine, prednisone/dexamethasone.

received 60 Gy, suggesting that increasing the dose from 40 to 60 Gy did not improve local control. In a separate report of the first large prospective study combining cranial irradiation with a high-dose methotrexate (MTX)-based regimen, 40 Gy was administered to the whole brain followed by a 14.4 Gy boost to the area involved by tumor [4, 5]);. In this study, relapse occurred with equal frequency within and outside of the boosted field, suggesting a failure of a dose response above 40 Gy. Since these studies, most treating physicians have administered a dose of WBRT on the order of 45 Gy without a boost. This should suffice, but many continue to use a boost to the involved area of brain; the lack of data to support such an approach should eliminate this practice, as it also likely contributes to late neurotoxicity. In the modern era, we would like to think that RT is rarely used alone, so it may be that the addition of chemotherapy permits lower doses to be even more efficacious than was observed in the prospective RTOG study. However, population-based studies of PCNSL fail to demonstrate a widespread improvement in survival comparable to that reported from studies done in major academic centers, suggesting that advances in treatment are not being widely disseminated, that there is patient selection bias at work in these studies, or that a combination of both of these factors account for the superior outcomes reported in most phase II trials [6]. Therefore, WBRT alone may be a common approach to the treatment of PCNSL in some areas, and the data strongly suggest that 45 Gy WBRT should suffice.

With respect to the issue of whether the entire brain needs to be incorporated in the port of radiotherapy, several studies have suggested that this is a critical factor. Shibamoto et al. [7] retrospectively examined patients with PCNSL treated with focal RT using margins $\geq$4 cm margin. Patients with smaller margins had an out-of-field recurrence rate of 83% compared to 22% in those who received the wider margins. Furthermore, those who received the wider margins had better disease control and longer survival (28.5 months versus 15 months, $p = 0.057$) than those patients treated with smaller margins. This is the only study to examine this issue and it is confounded in its interpretation by the incorporation of patients with multiple lesions at diagnosis, thus making it very difficult to determine how extensive radiation therapy was in each of the treated groups.

While PCNSL may appear quite localized on MRI, and a single radiographic lesion is reported at diagnosis in approximately 70% of patients, it is often a much more infiltrative process than that appreciated on imaging. This can sometimes be observed in a biopsy specimen when tumor cells infiltrate tissue far beyond the area of bulk disease. In addition, Lai et al. [1] performed an autopsy evaluation of patients dying from PCNSL. The autopsy results were correlated with cranial MRI done before death to ascertain the radiographic extent of disease in comparison to the pathologic extent of disease. In all five patients studied, the burden of PCNSL was much greater than anticipated on the basis of imaging. Contrast-enhancing lesions represented foci of tumor, but there was frequently highly infiltrative and widespread disease throughout the brain even in areas, which were normal radiographically, including T2 and FLAIR images. These data strongly suggest that

PCNSL is not well-addressed by focal RT of any type. Therefore, the limited data available strongly suggest that if used, cranial irradiation should include the whole brain.

Combined Modality Therapy

Cranial irradiation does cause disease regression and prolongs survival over the median of about 2 months without any therapy. However, the primary problem is recurrence of disease, which usually occurs within the brain, but can also involve the CSF or ocular compartment. As patients with PCNSL were being diagnosed with increased frequency beginning in the 1980s, there was an effort to develop more effective therapies that could prolong disease control and survival. Potentially, curative chemotherapy regimens had been developed for comparable systemic non-Hodgkin lymphomas, achieving 5-year survival and cure for about 30–50% of patients. The most effective of these regimens was CHOP (cyclophosphamide, doxorubicin, vincristine and prednisone). There were 3 trials using pre-RT CHOP or CHOD, substituting dexamethasone for the prednisone, in immunocompetent patients with newly diagnosed PCNSL [8–10] (Table 7.1). At least one was terminated early because of poor outcome and survival. All three studies failed to show an improvement in the median survival over WBRT alone. Several important observations were made over the course of these efforts. Most patients receiving CHOP/CHOD had initial regression of their brain lesions during the first 1–2 cycles of therapy. However, subsequent cycles often resulted in tumor progression, frequently in areas not initially involved by tumor, suggesting that the drugs could penetrate to some degree into areas where the blood-brain barrier (BBB) was disrupted (as evidenced by contrast enhancement on CT/MRI) leading to tumor regression, but they could not reach areas where tumor cells reside behind an intact BBB, thus allowing them to grow unchecked during treatment. In addition, one study observed a high incidence of leptomeningeal relapse, perhaps for the same reason [8]. None of the critical drugs in CHOP/CHOD can traverse a normal BBB, except for the steroids, which can lead to tumor regression, but do not achieve lasting tumor control. Consequently, these regimens, and those of similar design, were abandoned because they were ineffective and caused significant systemic toxicity, particularly in the older patients diagnosed with PCNSL.

Previously, the use of high-dose MTX and cytarabine were shown to be effective in the treatment of systemic lymphoma that had metastasized to the CNS, often to the subarachnoid space. Furthermore, therapeutic concentrations of these drugs could be achieved in the CSF by high dose systemic administration. Use of leucovorin rescue to protect the bone marrow and GI tract, in particular, and development of protocols to prevent renal failure, made the use of high-dose MTX safe. Because PCNSL was often associated with CSF involvement and was characterized by infiltrative disease behind an intact BBB, it seemed reasonable to try high-dose MTX in the treatment of PCNSL. Initially, these drugs were added to WBRT because radiotherapy was the only known efficacious treatment, and the expectation was that adding the two modalities together would hopefully improve outcome.

From the beginning, there was concern about delayed neurotoxicity when adding drugs such as MTX to cranial irradiation. Studies in childhood leukemia, where systemic and intrathecal MTX were often combined with WBRT for CNS prophylaxis, had already demonstrated the synergistic toxicity of these combinations. Furthermore, it was known that using both systemic and intrathecal drug enhanced the risk. Those investigators had already observed that if the chemotherapy was given prior to the RT, the risk of permanent brain injury was less than if the drugs were administered concurrent with or after the WBRT. Therefore, in designing a regimen for PCNSL, the high dose MTX was given before RT, which also enabled an assessment of chemotherapy response. The response evaluation to MTX was critical because it had not been used previously in the initial approach to these patients.

The addition of high-dose MTX followed by WBRT has been shown in multiple phase II studies to increase survival (medians from 32 to 60 mo) compared to WBRT alone [4, 5, 11–15]. Although high-dose MTX is now widely accepted as the single most important agent in the treatment of PCNSL, the optimal dose and the best combination regimen remain unclear. One of the initial trials used only 1 gm/m^2 of single agent MTX given every 14 days and combined with intrathecal MTX to address obvious or subclinical leptomeningeal involvement; this was followed by WBRT and high-dose cytarabine [4, 5]. This study showed prolonged survival and the MTX was well-tolerated. A subsequent study of 17 patients using the same dose of MTX, plus thiotepa and procarbazine followed by WBRT, was associated with a complete response (CR) rate of 76% and a partial response (PR) rate of 12%; a median overall survival (OS) of 32 months, and 2 patients remained alive and disease-free at 12 years [16]. A multicenter trial conducted by the Trans-Tasman Radiation Oncology Group also used MTX at 1 gm/m^2; after only 2 cycles, WBRT was administered and they still achieved a median survival of 36 months despite fairly limited treatment [15]. While these studies are encouraging, and can support the use of lower doses of MTX in specific patients who may be unable to tolerate higher doses, most investigators use significantly higher doses of MTX to achieve more reliable drug levels in the CNS.

Other studies have predominately used a dose of 3–3.5 gm/m^2, which provides more reliable therapeutic drug concentrations (>1 μM) in the CSF. Given the large number of patients now treated with these doses, it is clear that even older patients can be managed safely with such doses of MTX. Abrey et al. used 3.5 gm/m^2 MTX in combination with procarbazine, vincristine, and intrathecal MTX, followed by WBRT and cytarabine [11, 12]. The response rate to pre-RT chemotherapy was 90% and median survival was 60 months. Prolonged follow-up of this cohort revealed a progression-free survival of 128 months and an OS of 51 months [17]. These data led to a multicenter study conducted by the RTOG (93–10), which enrolled 102 patients with newly diagnosed PCNSL. This study consisted of 2.5 gm/m^2 of MTX, vincristine, procarbazine, and intrathecal MTX followed by 45 Gy WBRT and high-dose cytarabine; no boost of RT was administered. There was a 94% response rate (58% CR) and the OS was 37 months [13].

Other approaches were also examined. Bessell et al. [18] reported on a systemic lymphoma regimen designed to incorporate agents capable of penetrating into the CNS. Their regimen was CHOD/BVAM, which essentially added carmustine, MTX (1.5 gm/m^2) and cytarabine to standard CHOD. These investigators reported favorable results, but it was difficult to know what contribution the CHOD made other than toxicity. Poortmans and colleagues ([19]) reported a multicenter study of 52 patients treated with 3 gm/m^2 MTX, teniposide, carmustine, and triple intrathecal therapy with MTX, cytarabine and hydrocortisone followed by 40 Gy WBRT. The overall response rate was 81% and the median OS was 46 months. However, the regimen was toxic, there was a 10% toxic death rate, and the study was limited to patients aged 65 and younger. Therefore, this regimen had unacceptable toxicity and could not be applied to almost one-half of all PCNSL patients.

It also became clear that the use of higher doses of MTX made it possible to eliminate routine intrathecal use. The only data to examine this issue is a small retrospective study, in which intrathecal chemotherapy did not improve survival, failed to reduce subsequent CSF relapse, but did not appear to contribute to neurotoxicity [20]. The sample size was small, but most investigators have eliminated intrathecal administration of drug unless a patient has significant leptomeningeal disease, as evidenced by a positive CSF cytology or unequivocal involvement in MRI.

While prolonged disease control and improved survival were seen in essentially all studies that combined a high-dose MTX-based regimen with cranial irradiation, delayed neurotoxicity became evident. Patients experienced cognitive decline and gait difficulties that were in part a consequence of prolonged disease-free survival, but also seemed to be a direct consequence of combining neurotoxic chemotherapy (MTX) and WBRT [21]. This is discussed in detail in Chapter 21. However, the growing appreciation of long-term sequelae, as a result of more effective therapy leading to durable survival, led to new studies that sought to improve tumor control while causing less harm to the brain. Most efforts have been directed towards chemotherapy-only protocols, which are discussed in Chapters 8 and 9. However, there has been some attention directed towards modifying the dose of WBRT with the expectation of preserving its clear benefit while reducing toxicity. Some may question the benefit of WBRT in the chemotherapy era. The only good data that address this issue comes from Abrey and colleagues [12, 17]. During this study of pre-RT MTX, vincristine, and procarbazine, the growing incidence of neurotoxicity was being appreciated and recognized to be primarily a problem for older patients. Therefore, midway through that study, patients aged 60 and above received the same chemotherapy regimen, but no WBRT. They then compared older patients who had received both in the first half of the study, recognizing that the patient number was small and not powered to do a direct comparison. However, the results were striking. Patients aged 60 and above had an identical median survival of 29 months whether they received WBRT or not. However, the cause of death was markedly different. Those who had received the WBRT were dying of neurotoxicity, but those who did not receive WBRT were dying of tumor progression. These data strongly point to the important role WBRT can play in contributing to tumor control; however, it has an unacceptably high cost in causing neurotoxcity.

These data led to a few studies investigating whether reducing the dose of WBRT may be feasible, and the results are mixed. Bessell et al. ([22]) conducted a second study using CHOD/BVAM in which those patients who achieved a CR received a reduced dose of 30.6 Gy WBRT compared to 45 Gy. The result of this study was that patients under age 60 experienced an increased risk of relapse and a worse survival if they received the lower dose of WBRT. There appeared to be no difference for older patients. However, two other studies suggest that reducing the dose of WBRT may not lead to an increased risk of tumor progression. The RTOG 93-10 study reduced the dose of WBRT from 45 to 36 Gy in a subset of patients who had achieved a CR after pre-RT chemotherapy [13]. There was no increase in CNS relapse observed in the 15 patients so treated; however, they also experienced a comparable rate of neurotoxicity to those who received the higher dose of WBRT [23]. The most encouraging data come from a preliminary analysis by Shah et al. [24] who described 30 patients who were treated with rituximab, high-dose MTX, vincristine, and procarbazine; if a CR was achieved following chemotherapy, these patients were then treated with 23.8 Gy WBRT. Most patients continued in complete remission and were followed with prospective, serial neuropsychological testing, which was not performed in the earlier studies. In their cohort, 77% achieved a CR and could receive low-dose WBRT. After 12 months of follow-up, none of these patients had any cognitive decline, including those over age 60, and in fact most had improved with treatment of their PCNSL. An updated report showed no decline after 24 months of follow up [25]. Therefore, these data suggest that low-dose RT may prove an excellent and safe option if the patient has a good initial response to chemotherapy. Clearly, more patients and longer follow-up are needed to clarify the role of such low WBRT doses. However, it is clear that most investigators rarely use full dose WBRT (meaning 45 Gy or greater) routinely in older patients with PCNSL and often seek to avoid it even in younger adults.

Radiotherapy as Salvage

If WBRT was not used as part of the initial treatment regimen, it is often required when a PCNSL patient experiences relapse. Even at recurrence, there has been reluctance to use WBRT, particularly because some patients can do well for a long time and can be at risk for neurotoxicity. However, it may depend upon the timing of progression. If the patient has primary progression through initial therapy with a high-dose MTX regimen, then WBRT may be the only effective option to get the disease under control. However, if relapse has occurred years after diagnosis, many will re-institute chemotherapy and withhold WBRT for a subsequent relapse. Regardless of when WBRT is employed as salvage, it appears to be effective.

There are only two studies examining this issue. Nguyen et al. [26] reported that WBRT (median dose 36 Gy) at the time of disease relapse provided a median survival of about 12 months and some patients lived for several years. Hottinger et al. [27] observed similar results (median dose 40 Gy) and were also able to demonstrate that the risk of subsequent neurotoxicity was related to the time interval between

MTX exposure and the WBRT. If the WBRT was administered more than 6 months after MTX, the risk of cognitive decline was small; however, the risk was high if administered within 6 months. Of course, this means that those patients with primary progression are at greatest risk of neurotoxicity, even though they have the strongest need for WBRT. However, these data do suggest that trying another chemotherapy regimen that is not associated with intrinsic neurotoxicity (such as temozolomide) to prolong the time interval from MTX exposure to WBRT may be beneficial. If a patient achieves a CR to salvage chemotherapy, it is unclear if WBRT at that point would consolidate the response and whether a reduced dose would be efficacious. These questions require further study to clarify the optimal and safe role of WBRT for PCNSL.

References

1. Lai R, Rosenblum MK, DeAngelis LM (2002) Primary CNS lymphoma: a whole-brain disease? Neurology 59:1557–1562
2. Shibamoto Y, Ogino H, Hasegawa M et al (2005) Results of radiation monotherapy for primary central nervous system lymphoma in the 1990s. Int J Radiat Oncol Biol Phys 62:809–813
3. Nelson DF, Martz KL, Bonner H et al (1992) Non-Hodgkin's lymphoma of the brain: can high dose, large volume radiation therapy improve survival? Report on a prospective trial by the Radiation Therapy Oncology Group (RTOG): RTOG 8315. Int J Radiat Oncol Biol Phys 23:9–17
4. DeAngelis LM, Yahalom J, Heinemann MH et al (1990) Primary CNS lymphoma: combined treatment with chemotherapy and radiotherapy. Neurology 40:80–86
5. DeAngelis LM, Yahalom J, Thaler HT, Kher U (1992) Combined modality therapy for primary CNS lymphoma. J Clin Oncol 10:635–643
6. Panageas KS, Elkin EB, Ben-Porat L et al (2007) Patterns of treatment in older adults with primary central nervous system lymphoma. Cancer 110:1338–1344
7. Shibamoto Y, Hayabuchi N, Hiratsuka J et al (2003) Is whole-brain irradiation necessary for primary central nervous system lymphoma? Patterns of recurrence after partial-brain irradiation. Cancer 97:128–133
8. Lachance DH, Brizel DM, Gockerman JP et al (1994) Cyclophosphamide, doxorubicin, vincristine, and prednisone for primary central nervous system lymphoma: short-duration response and multifocal intracerebral recurrence preceding radiotherapy. Neurology 44: 1721–1727
9. O'Neill BP, Wang CH, O'Fallon JR et al (1999) Primary central nervous system non-Hodgkin's lymphoma (PCNSL): survival advantages with combined initial therapy? A final report of the North Central Cancer Treatment Group (NCCTG) Study 86-72-52. Int J Radiat Oncol Biol Phys 43:559–563
10. Schultz C, Scott C, Sherman W et al (1996) Preirradiation chemotherapy with cyclophosphamide, doxorubicin, vincristine, and dexamethasone for primary CNS lymphomas: initial report of Radiation Therapy Oncology Group protocol 88-06. J Clin Oncol 14:556–564
11. Abrey LE, DeAngelis LM, Yahalom J (1998) Long-term survival in primary CNS lymphoma. J Clin Oncol 16:859–863
12. Abrey LE, Yahalom J, DeAngelis LM (2000) Treatment for primary CNS lymphoma: the next step. J Clin Oncol 18:3144–3150
13. DeAngelis LM, Seiferheld W, Schold SC et al (2002) Combination chemotherapy and radiotherapy for primary central nervous system lymphoma: Radiation Therapy Oncology Group Study 93-10. J Clin Oncol 20:4643–4648

14. Ferreri AJ, Reni M, Dell'Oro S et al (2001) Combined treatment with high-dose methotrexate, vincristine and procarbazine, without intrathecal chemotherapy, followed by consolidation radiotherapy for primary central nervous system lymphoma in immunocompetent patients. Oncology 60:134–140
15. O'Brien PC, Roos DE, Pratt G et al (2006) Combined modality therapy for primary central nervous system lymphoma: long-term data from a Phase II multicenter study (Trans-Tasman Radiation Oncology Group). Int J Radiat Oncol Biol Phys 64:408–413
16. Omuro AM, DeAngelis LM, Yahalom J, Abrey LE (2005a) Chemoradiotherapy for primary CNS lymphoma: an intent-to-treat analysis with complete follow-up. Neurology 64: 69–74
17. Gavrilovic IT, Hormigo A, Yahalom J et al (2006) Long-term follow-up of high-dose methotrexate-based therapy with and without whole brain irradiation for newly diagnosed primary CNS lymphoma. J Clin Oncol 24:4570–4574
18. Bessell EM, Graus F, Lopez-Guillermo A et al (2004) Primary non-Hodgkin's lymphoma of the CNS treated with CHOD/BVAM or BVAM chemotherapy before radiotherapy: long-term survival and prognostic factors. Int J Radiat Oncol Biol Phys 59:501–508
19. Poortmans PM, Kluin-Nelemans HC, Haaxma-Reiche H et al (2003) High-dose methotrexate-based chemotherapy followed by consolidating radiotherapy in non-AIDS-related primary central nervous system lymphoma: European Organization for Research and Treatment of Cancer lymphoma group phase II trial 20962. J Clin Oncol 21:4483–4488
20. Khan RB, Shi W, Thaler HT et al (2002) Is intrathecal methotrexate necessary in the treatment of primary CNS lymphoma? J Neurooncol 58:175–178
21. Omuro AM, Ben-Porat LS, Panageas KS et al (2005b) Delayed neurotoxicity in primary central nervous system lymphoma. Arch Neurol 62:1595–1600
22. Bessell EM, Lopez-Guillermo A, Villa S et al (2002) Importance of radiotherapy in the outcome of patients with primary CNS lymphoma: an analysis of the CHOD/BVAM regimen followed by two different radiotherapy treatments. J Clin Oncol 20:231–236
23. Fisher B, Seiferheld W, Schultz C et al (2005) Secondary analysis of Radiation Therapy Oncology Group study (RTOG) 9310: an intergroup phase II combined modality treatment of primary central nervous system lymphoma. J Neurooncol 74:201–205
24. Shah GD, Yahalom J, Correa D et al (2007) Combined immunochemotherapy with reduced whole-brain radiotherapy for newly diagnosed primary CNS lymphoma. J Clin Oncol 25:4730–4735
25. Correa DD, Rocco-Donovan M, DeAngelis LM et al (2009) Prospective cognitive follow-up in primary CNS lymphoma patients treated with chemotherapy and reduced-dose radiotherapy. J Neurooncol 91:315–321
26. Nguyen PL, Chakravarti A, Finkelstein DM et al (2005) Results of whole-brain radiation as salvage of methotrexate failure for immunocompetent patients with primary CNS lymphoma. J Clin Oncol 23:1507–1513
27. Hottinger AF, DeAngelis LM, Yahalom J, Abrey LE (2007) Salvage whole brain radiotherapy for recurrent or refractory primary CNS lymphoma. Neurology 69:1178–1182
28. Glass J, Gruber ML, Cher L et al (1994) Preirradiation methotrexate chemotherapy of primary central nervous system lymphoma: long-term outcome. J Neurosurg 81:188–195
29. O'Brien P, Roos D, Pratt G et al (2000) Phase II multicenter study of brief single-agent methotrexate followed by irradiation in primary CNS lymphoma. J Clin Oncol 18:519–526

Chapter 8
Chemotherapy for Primary Central Nervous System Lymphoma

Tracy Batchelor, Andrew Grigg, and Eckhard Thiel

Introduction

Chemotherapy alone is considered the standard of care for patients with newly diagnosed, systemic diffuse large B-cell lymphoma. Historically, whole brain radiation therapy (WBRT) or WBRT in combination with chemotherapy have been the most commonly accepted therapeutic regimens for PCNSL. However, the high incidence of neurotoxicity in patients >60 years of age who receive WBRT as a component of their therapeutic regimen has led to interest in the use of chemotherapy alone and deferral of WBRT in PCNSL patients. Initial efforts with chemotherapy were disappointing as the limited blood-brain barrier (BBB) penetration of the drugs in the R-CHOP (rituximab, cyclophosphamide, doxorubicin, vincristine, prednisone) regimen resulted in poor outcomes in PCNSL patients treated with this standard NHL combination [1, 2]. However, a number of chemotherapy regimens have been developed for the PCNSL population, utilizing drugs with acceptable BBB penetration and demonstrated anti-lymphoma activity. Historically, the lack of prospective, randomized controlled trials has slowed advances in chemotherapy for PCNSL. However, this situation is rapidly changing with a recent focus on the development of multicenter, randomized trials for the PCNSL patient population. This chapter will focus on chemotherapeutic approaches to PCNSL, including treatment of newly diagnosed PCNSL, elderly patients with PCNSL, relapsed or refractory PCNSL, and the role of intrathecal chemotherapy. The evolution from chemotherapy to high-dose chemotherapy and autologous stem cell transplantation is reviewed in Chapter 9.

The International PCNSL Collaborative Group (IPCG) has published consensus guidelines for the assessment of response in PCNSL patients treated on therapeutic clinical trials (Table 8.1) [3]. These guidelines are being incorporated into

---

T. Batchelor (✉)
Stephen E. and Catherine Pappas Center for Neuro-Oncology, Departments of Neurology and Radiation Oncology, Division of Hematology and Oncology, Massachusetts General Hospital, Harvard Medical School, 55 Fruit Street, Boston, MA 02114, USA
e-mail: tbatchelor@partners.org

T. Batchelor, L.M. DeAngelis (eds.), *Lymphoma and Leukemia of the Nervous System*, DOI 10.1007/978-1-4419-7668-0_8,

Table 8.1 International primary CNS lymphoma collaborative group (IPCG) guidelines for response assessment in clinical trials

Response	Brain imaging	Corticosteroid dose	Eye exam	CSF cytology
CR	No enhancing disease	None	Normal	Negative
uCR	No enhancing disease	Any	Normal	Negative
	Minimal enhancing disease	Any	Minor RPE abnormality	Negative
PR	50% decrease in enhancement	N/A	Minor RPE abnormality or normal	Negative
	No enhancing disease	N/A	Decrease in vitreous cells or retinal infiltrate	Persistent or suspicious
PD	25% increase in enhancement Any new site of disease	N/A	Recurrent or new disease	Recurrent or positive
SD	All scenarios not covered by responses above			

Adapted from Abrey et al. [3].
Abbreviation: CR, complete response; uCR, unconfirmed complete response; N/A, not applicable; PR, partial response; PD, progressive disease; RPE, retinal pigment epithelium.

prospective clinical trials of chemotherapy, which will allow some comparison across studies. The IPCG has also recommended a cognitive assessment instrument for serial use in patients treated on clinical trials as neurocognitive outcome is a critical endpoint that should be assessed in this population [4].

Corticosteroids

Although corticosteroids may rapidly reduce tumor size and decrease tumor-associated edema in PCNSL patients, these medications should be withheld prior to diagnostic biopsy in clinically stable patients who are suspected of having PCNSL based on imaging studies. Corticosteroids have a direct lymphocytolytic effect that may disrupt cellular morphology and lead to diagnostic inaccuracy at the time of microscopic analysis in patients undergoing biopsy. Despite an initial response to corticosteroids, most PCNSL patients quickly relapse and require alternate treatment strategies. Nevertheless, initial radiographic response to corticosteroids in newly diagnosed PCNSL patients is a favorable prognostic marker with an overall survival (OS) of 117 months in responders versus 5.5 months in non-responders [5].

Chemotherapy for Newly Diagnosed PCNSL

A number of cytotoxic agents have been studied in the PCNSL population either alone or in combination, and the key drugs are summarized in Table 8.2. Methotrexate, a folate antagonist that interrupts DNA biosynthesis, is the most effective and widely used drug for PCNSL. However, due to its high degree of ionization at physiologic pH methotrexate is associated with poor penetration of the BBB. Using microdialysis catheters, investigators measured the penetration of methotrexate (administered at a dose of 12 g/m^2) into high-grade brain tumor tissue [6]. The ratio of the area under the methotrexate concentration-time curve in brain extracellular fluid to plasma ranged from 0.28–0.31 in the region of contrast-enhancing tumor. Thus, high-dose systemic methotrexate is necessary for adequate CNS penetration with doses of 2–8 g/m^2 commonly administered in the PCNSL population. At these systemic doses, cytotoxic levels of methotrexate are also achieved in the CSF, and the need to use intrathecal chemotherapy to treat microscopic or macroscopic tumor in the leptomeninges can probably be avoided in most PCNSL patients [7]. In a retrospective review of 45 patients with PCNSL treated with methotrexate-based regimens, slow creatinine clearance (< 85 ml/min) and a high area-under-the-curve (AUC) for methotrexate (AUC > 1,100 $\mu mol \cdot h \cdot l^{-1}$) were two factors associated with significant improvement in survival [8]. However, slow creatinine clearance was also associated with severe toxicity. Based on these observations, it was recommended that studies of methotrexate-based chemotherapy in PCNSL patients include a methotrexate dose $\geq$ 3 g/m^2 as a 4–6 h infusion given every 3–4 weeks. However, many investigators continue to recommend administration of methotrexate over 3–4 h every 10–14 days.

In a phase II, multicenter study of methotrexate monotherapy the drug was administered at a dose of 8 g/m^2 to 25 PCNSL patients as a 4-h infusion every 14 days, as induction therapy followed by 12 maintenance cycles every 28 days at the same dose [9, 10]. The proportion of patients who achieved a complete response (CR) was 52% (13/25) and the median number of cycles and time to CR was 6 and 12 weeks, respectively. The median PFS was 12.8 months, the median OS was 55.4 months, and the median disease-specific survival had not been reached at 72.3 months. In this study, 5 of the 25 patients treated with methotrexate alone achieved a CR and had not relapsed after a median follow-up of 6.8 years. Toxicity was modest with 13/25 patients experiencing no dose-limiting adverse effects. In another study of 75 patients with PCNSL using the same dose and schedule, the CR proportion was only 29.7% with a median PFS of 10 months and median OS of 25 months [11]. However, the maximum number of induction cycles of methotrexate was capped at 6 in this study. As noted previously, 6 cycles was the median number of doses to reach CR in the previously cited methotrexate monotherapy study, and more induction cycles may have resulted in a higher proportion of patients who achieved a radiographic CR.

While methotrexate monotherapy may be effective for a subset of patients, the response proportion appears to be higher and the durability of response appears to be longer in patients who receive polychemotherapy. There have been a number

Table 8.2 Chemotherapy agents commonly used for treatment of PCNSL

Agent	Mechanism of action	Route of administration	Main toxicities	Main uses in PCNSL
Methotrexate	Anti-metabolite (folate antagonist)	i.v., i.a., i.t., i.o., p.o.	Renal, GI, bone marrow	Combinations; monotherapy, new and relapsed PCNSL; brain, CSF, ocular disease
Cytarabine	Anti-metabolite (pyrimidine antagonist)	i.v., i.t.	Bone marrow	Combinations, monotherapy, new and relapsed PCNSL; brain, CSF disease
Procarbazine	Alkylating agent	p.o.	Bone marrow	Combinations, new and relapsed PCNSL
Temozolomide	Methylating agent	p.o.	Bone marrow	Combinations, monotherapy, new and relapsed PCNSL
Cyclophosphamide	Alkylating agent	i.v., p.o.	Bone marrow, GI, bladder	Combinations, new PCNSL
Vincristine	Antimicrotubule agent	i.v.	Peripheral nerves	Combinations, new and relapsed PCNSL
Etoposide	Topoisomerase II inhibitor	i.v., p.o.	Bone marrow, GI	Combinations, new PCNSL
Ifosfamide	Alkylating agent	i.v.	Bone marrow, CNS, GI, kidney, bladder	Combinations, new PCNSL
Lomustine	Alkylating agent	p.o.	GI, bone marrow	Combinations, new and relapsed PCNSL
Topotecan	Topoisomerase I inhibitor	i.v., i.t.[a]	Bone marrow	Monotherapy, relapsed PCNSL
Rituximab	Anti-CD20 antibody	i.v., i.t.[a]	Infusion reaction, hepatitis reactivation	Combinations, new and relapsed PCNSL

Chabner and Longo [12].
[a]In experimental setting only.

of phase II trials conducted using methotrexate-based, multi-agent chemotherapy regimens without WBRT as noted in Table 8.3.

In one of the first, multicenter, randomized trials reported in the PCNSL patient population 79 subjects aged 18–75 years were randomized to receive either methotrexate alone (3.5 g/m^2) every 3 weeks versus methotrexate (3.5 g/m^2 on day 1) plus cytarabine (2 g/m^2 BID on days 2 and 3) every 3 weeks [13]. Although patients in each arm subsequently received WBRT, the radiographic response to chemotherapy was determined prior to radiation. Complete/partial radiographic responses were achieved in 18%/22% of methotrexate patients and 46%/23% of methotrexate + cytarabine patients, respectively. Grade 3–4 hematological toxicity was more common in the methotrexate + cytarabine arm (92%) versus the methotrexate arm (15%). This study confirmed observations from non-randomized trials that methotrexate-containing combination regimens achieve higher radiographic response rates compared to methotrexate monotherapy.

A multi-agent regimen consisting of methotrexate, cytarabine, vincristine, ifosfamide, cyclophosphamide, and i.t. methotrexate/cytarabine/prednisolone was studied in a phase II trial of 65 patients and was associated with a 71% overall response rate (ORR) and a median OS of 50 months [14]. Despite these promising results, 6 patients died from treatment-related complications and 12 patients experienced Ommaya reservoir infections.

In some combination regimens, rituximab, a humanized monoclonal antibody against the CD20 antigen on B-lymphoma cells, has been incorporated, although it is not yet known whether this agent will improve outcomes in PCNSL patients to the extent that it has for patients with systemic B-cell lymphomas. Rituximab concentrations in CSF are 0.1% of plasma levels when it is administered at a standard dose of 375 mg/m^2 intravenously, indicating poor BBB penetration [15]. In a report of 4 PCNSL patients administered I^{123}–labeled rituximab, there was weak tumor uptake in only 1 out of 4 patients [16]. However, in another study of the ^{90}Y-labeled anti-CD20 antibody ibritumomab tiuxetan target accumulation of the antibody was observed in 4 out of 6 PCNSL patients assessed by SPECT imaging with ^{111}In-labeled ibritumomab tiuxetan [17]. Moreover, radiographic responses were reported to rituximab alone in 5/12 patients with refractory or relapsed PCNSL in a pilot study [18]. Despite these limited data, rituximab is being incorporated into chemotherapy regimens for patients with both newly diagnosed and relapsed PCNSL under the assumption that rituximab penetration into contrast-enhancing tumor may be higher in the context of a disrupted blood brain barrier. In a single institution study, rituximab was added to a commonly used chemotherapy regimen for patients with newly diagnosed PCNSL, methotrexate, procarbazine, vincristine (MPV), and 78% of patients achieved a CR after 6 cycles [19]. While this CR proportion is higher than that historically observed for MPV, further studies are necessary to validate this result and to define the ultimate role of i.v. rituximab in the treatment of PCNSL.

Blood brain barrier disruption (BBBD) is a strategy aimed at circumventing the BBB in order to deliver higher concentrations of chemotherapeutics to the CNS (Fig. 8.1). In one report, this method was associated with complete radiographic responses in 40/53 patients with PCNSL treated with intra-arterial (i.a.)

Table 8.3 Selected chemotherapy regimens for newly diagnosed PCNSL

Study	Regimen	N	Intrathecal Rx	CR	PR	OS (mos)	PFS (mos)
[14]	MTX (5 g/m^2), vincristine, ifosfamide, dexamethasone, cyclophosphamide, cytarabine, vindesine	65	Prednisolone, MTX, cytarabine	61%	10%	50	21
[41]	MTX (1 g/m^2), lomustine, procarbazine, methylprednisolone	50	Cytarabine, MTX	42%	6%	14.3	10.6
[10]	MTX (8 g/m^2)	25	None	52%	22%	55.4	12.8
[26]	MTX, procarbazine, CCNU	30	None	44%	29.6%	–	–
[24]	MTX (3.5–8 g/m^2)	31	None	60%	36.7%	30	7.1
Intra-arterial chemotherapy							
[20]	i.a. MTX after BBBD with mannitol, i.v. cyclophosphamide, etoposide	74	None	65%	19%	40.7	–
[21]	i.a. MTX after BBBD mannitol	149	None	57.8%	24.2%	37.2	21

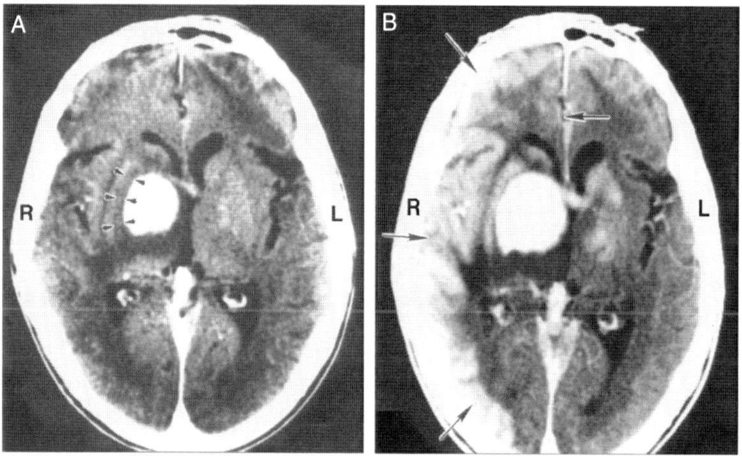

Fig. 8.1 Blood brain barrier disruption. Contrast-enhanced CT scans of the basal ganglia of a 61 year-old woman with a primary CNS lymphoma, indicating that the permeability of the blood tumor barrier is inconsistent for a given patient or even a given tumor nodule. **a** CT scan demonstrating a bright, uniformly enhancing lesion in the right basal ganglia. The hypodense signal in the brain tissue around the tumor (*arrowheads*) should be noted. **b** CT scan obtained after osmotic BBBD. CT scans were obtained 30 min after the first BBBD treatment, to confirm and assess the grade of BBBD. The patient underwent right internal carotid artery disruption in the anterior and middle cerebral artery distributions (*arrows*). Opening of the BBB around the tumor in the area of the peritumoral hypodense signal evident in the CT scan in (**a**) should be noted (courtesy of Edward Neuwelt [42] – with permission)

methotrexate (5 g), intravenous cyclophosphamide, and etoposide following BBBD with i.a. mannitol [20]. Long-term follow-up of the subjects who achieved CR in this study demonstrated maintenance of cognitive function in this population of patients treated without WBRT. In a pooled analysis of 149 patients treated with i.a. MTX following osmotic BBBD, the CR proportion was 57.8% with a median OS of 3.1 years [21]. Unique toxicities of BBBD include seizures, stroke, and venous thromboembolism. BBBD is technically complex and should only be performed in centers with expertise and experience in the technique.

Predictors of Chemotherapy Response

Since PCNSL is a densely cellular tumor, there may be restricted or low diffusion of brain water molecules within the tumor on diffusion-weighted MRI, and apparent diffusion coefficient (ADC) imaging may be useful as a biomarker of response to methotrexate. In one report of 18 immunocompetent PCNSL patients treated uniformly with methotrexate-based chemotherapy low, pre-therapeutic ADC values (increased tumor cell density) correlated with shorter progression-free survival and reduced overall survival [22]. Conversely, reduction of ADC values after start of methotrexate-based chemotherapy was associated with improved outcomes. Given that ADC maps are part of a standard MRI acquisition sequence, this observation can be readily explored in future prospective trials of chemotherapy in the PCNSL patient population.

Chemotherapy in Elderly PCNSL Patients

Chemotherapy alone is an attractive option in elderly patients with PCNSL as this group is at highest risk of neurotoxicity with regimens that contain WBRT. However, the ability of elderly patients to tolerate high doses of methotrexate or polychemotherapy regimens remains a concern. Several prospective studies have been conducted to address this issue.

In a multicenter analysis of 154 patients, 89 > 60 years and 21 > 70 years, methotrexate 4 g/m^2 administered as a 4-h intravenous infusion biweekly was safe regardless of age when the dose was adapted to the glomerular filtration rate, calculated prior to each methotrexate infusion [23].

In a single-institution study of methotrexate administered at doses of 3.5–8 g/m^2 every 2 weeks to 31 newly diagnosed PCNSL patients over the age of 70, the regimen was well-tolerated with 0, 3.2, 6.5% of patients experiencing grade III or IV renal, gastrointestinal or hematological toxicities, respectively [24]. However, 87.9% of methotrexate cycles required dose reduction due to impaired creatinine clearance. Sixty percent of patients achieved a CR and 36.7% achieved a PR. The median PFS and OS were 7.1 and 30 months, respectively.

In a phase II study, methotrexate (3 g/m^2 on days 1, 10, 20) and temozolomide (100 mg/m^2 on days 1–5) were administered to 23 patients with newly diagnosed PCNSL over the age of 60 [25]. In patients who achieved a PR or CR, 5 monthly cycles of methotrexate and temozolomide were subsequently administered. Grade III or IV nephrotoxicity and hematotoxicity were observed in 3 patients and 5 patients, respectively. However, no neurotoxicty was observed in these patients. The complete radiographic response proportion was 55%; the event-free survival was 8 months and the OS was 35 months.

A more intensive polychemotherapy regimen was studied in a phase II study of 30 elderly, newly diagnosed PCNSL patients with a median age of 70. In this study, methotrexate, procarbazine, and CCNU were administered as three 45-day cycles [26]. Twelve out of 27 patients (44%) achieved a CR and 8/27 (29.6%) achieved a PR. There were 2 treatment-related deaths. The 5-year OS was 33%, while 6 out of 8 long-term survivors had no evidence of treatment-related neurotoxicity.

A phase II trial examining methotrexate (3.5 g/m^2), vincristine, and procarbazine for newly diagnosed PCNSL patients was initially designed to administer WBRT in the post-chemotherapy setting [27]. However, for patients older than 60 years of age, the WBRT was eliminated at the mid-point of the study. At the termination of the trial, older patients treated with the chemotherapy alone had an identical median OS of 29 months to those who received both chemotherapy and WBRT. Although survival was the same, those patients who received chemotherapy alone had a higher incidence of tumor progression and they died of tumor, whereas those who received WBRT had a lower risk of tumor progression, but tended to die of neurotoxicity.

These studies in elderly PCNSL patients indicate that chemotherapy approaches are feasible, relatively non-toxic, and are associated with promising radiographic response proportions, survival, and low rates of neurotoxicity. However, subjects who meet study eligibility criteria and are enrolled into clinical trials represent a selected patient population and these results may not be generalizable to all elderly PCNSL patients.

Intrathecal Chemotherapy

A controversial issue in the management of PCNSL has been the role of intrathecal chemotherapy. Historical comparisons have determined that there appears to be no improvement in OS when intrathecal methotrexate is added to regimens that already include high doses of i.v. methotrexate [28]. By administering methotrexate systemically, the risk of Ommaya reservoir placement, extra-CSF drug delivery, chemical meningitis, and infection can be avoided. As mentioned above, the i.v. dose must be sufficiently high and administered over a rapid enough time interval for methotrexate to penetrate into the CSF and tumor. In one prospective study of 18 patients, a polychemotherapy regimen was administered without intrathecal chemotherapy [29]. Although the radiographic CR proportion was 53%, the median time to progression for responders was only 10 months, shorter than that previously reported for this same regimen when intrathecal chemotherapy was included. Although the authors contend that this early relapse was possibly due to the omission of intrathecal chemotherapy, this conclusion is speculative and should be confirmed in a larger, randomized trial. For patients with concurrent brain and leptomeningeal lymphoma, intrathecal chemotherapy may be recommended. Ommaya reservoir placement is the most efficient and safest way to deliver intrathecal chemotherapy. Repeated lumbar punctures are uncomfortable for patients and may result in inconsistent delivery of chemotherapy into the subarachnoid space. If a patient requires a ventricular-peritoneal shunt (VPS) and intrathecal chemotherapy, a VPS with an "on-off" valve is an option. Although not systematically studied, these shunts theoretically allow the treating physician to temporarily halt CSF drainage into the peritoneum after instillation of chemotherapy.

Salvage Chemotherapy

Despite aggressive treatment, most patients with PCNSL will progress or relapse and will become potential candidates for salvage therapy [30]. Optimal management of relapsed or refractory PCNSL has yet to be determined and has only been studied in small clinical trials or case series using heterogeneous therapies (Table 8.4). In

Table 8.4 Selected salvage chemotherapy regimens for relapsed or refractory PCNSL

Reference	Treatment	N	Pts with PR/CR	OS (months)
[31]	MTX	22	20	61.9
[40]	HDT/ASCT	27	26	58.6
[39]	PCV	7	6	>16
[32]	TMZ	23	6	3.5
[33]	TMZ + rituximab	15	8	14
[34]	TMZ + rituximab	7	7	8
[36]	Topotecan	27	9	8.4
[37]	Topotecan	15	6	35
[38]	VIA	16	6	41% at 12 months

Abbreviations: Pts, patients; HDT, high dose chemotherapy; ASCT, autologous stem cell transplantation; PCV, procarbazine, lomustine, vincristine; TMZ, temozolomide; VIA, etoposide, ifosfamide, cytarabine; OS, overall survival

general, prognosis for patients with relapsed or refractory PCNSL is poor with a median survival of approximately 4.5 months.

For patients who initially experienced a CR to a chemotherapy regimen that included methotrexate, re-treatment with methotrexate alone at the time of relapse may be effective [31]. Twenty-two patients who previously achieved a CR to methotrexate were treated again at relapse with methotrexate (8 g/m^2) and the ORR was 91% and the median OS was 61.9 months. While this represents a highly selected, treatment-sensitive population, this approach represents one option for this group of PCNSL patients.

Temozolomide, an alkylating agent with good CSF penetration, was associated with a 26% radiographic response proportion in 23 patients previously treated with methotrexate-containing chemotherapy with or without WBRT [32]. Rituximab was added to temozolomide in 2 studies of relapsed or progressive PCNSL, yielding median survival times of 8 and 14 months [33, 34].

Intraventricular rituximab (10–25 mg) was feasible in a Phase I study of patients with relapsed or refractory lymphomatous meningitis [35]. Toxicity was limited. Unexpected observations from this study were a radiographic response of brain parenchymal lymphoma in 1 case and 2 patients with intraocular lymphoma who experienced disease resolution or clinical improvement in vision.

Topotecan, a topoisomerase I inhibitor with good CSF penetration, was administered to 27 patients with relapsed or refractory PCNSL. The ORR was 33% with 9 patients achieving a complete or partial response, and the overall survival was 8.4 months [36]. However, 8 of 12 patients still alive at 6 months exhibited symptoms of neurotoxicity. In another study of 15 patients with relapsed or refractory PCNSL, 3/15 (20%) patients achieved a CR, 3/15 (20%) patients achieved a PR, median PFS was 2 months, and median OS was 35 months [37]. Toxicity was mainly hematological in both of these studies. Combination studies of topotecan with other agents have not been conducted in the PCNSL patient population.

Other chemotherapy salvage regimens studied include etoposide, ifosfamide, and cytarabine (VIA) and procarbazine, lomustine, and vincristine (PCV) [38, 39]. Using VIA, the 12-month OS was 41% and with PCV, it was 57%.

In a study of refractory or relapsed PCNSL or ocular lymphoma, 43 patients were treated with cytarabine and etoposide, with a subset of these patients offered subsequent high-dose chemotherapy with thiotepa, busulfan, and cyclophosphamide followed by autologous stem cell transplantation (HDT/ASCT) [40]. Twenty-seven patients received HDT/ASCT and 26/27 of these patients entered CR and achieved median PFS and OS durations of 41.1 and 58.6 months, respectively. Although this study included a highly selected salvage patient population, these results are encouraging and should be confirmed in other studies of this approach in relapsed or refractory PCNSL patients.

Future Directions

Chemotherapy alone for newly diagnosed PCNSL patients is an increasingly accepted therapeutic strategy and may reduce the incidence of neurotoxicity compared to regimens that include WBRT, especially among elderly patients. Intrathecal chemotherapy may not be necessary in PCNSL patients treated with high doses of intravenous methotrexate, although this has not been definitively established. Based on encouraging results obtained with high-dose chemotherapy followed by autologous stem cell transplantation in the relapsed and refractory PCNSL patient population, this approach is now being investigated in the newly diagnosed PCNSL population and will be reviewed in Chapter 9. However, the optimal therapeutic strategy for patients with newly diagnosed and relapsed or refractory PCNSL has yet to be defined. An increasing number of multicenter, randomized trials are being conducted in this patient population using standardized entry criteria and outcome assessment, and these investigations hold much promise in defining standards of care for PCNSL.

References

1. Lachance DH, Brizel DM, Gockerman JP et al (1994) Cyclophosphamide, doxorubicin, vincristine, and prednisone for primary central nervous system lymphoma: short-duration response and multifocal intracerebral recurrence preceding radiotherapy. Neurology 44: 1721–1727
2. O'Neill BP, Wang CH, O'Fallon JR et al (1999) Primary central nervous system non-Hodgkin's lymphoma (PCNSL): survival advantages with combined initial therapy? A final report of the North Central Cancer Treatment Group (NCCTG) Study 86-72-52. Int J Radiat Oncol Biol Phys 43:559–563
3. Abrey L, Batchelor T, Ferreri A et al (2005) Report of an international workshop to standardize baseline evaluation and response criteria for primary CNS lymphoma. J Clin Oncol 23:5034–5043
4. Correa DD, Maron L, Harder H et al (2007) Cognitive functions in primary central nervous lymphoma: literature and assessment guidelines. Ann Oncol 18:1145–1151

5. Beela MS, Carson K, Grossman SA (2006) Initial response to glucocorticoids: a potentially important prognostic factor in patients with primary CNS lymphoma. Cancer 106:383–387
6. Blakeley JO, Olson J, Grossman SA et al (2009) Effect of blood brain barrier permeability in recurrent high grade glioma on the intratumoral pharmacokinetics of methotrexate: a microdialysis study. J Neurooncol 91:51–58
7. Glantz MJ, Cole BF, Recht L et al (1998) High-dose intravenous methotrexate for patients with nonleukemic leptomeningeal cancer: is intrathecal chemotherapy necessary?. J Clin Oncol 16:1561–1567
8. Ferreri AJ, Guerra E, Regazzi M et al (2004) Area under the curve of methotrexate and creatinine clearance are outcome-determining factors in primary CNS lymphomas. Br J Cancer 90:353–358
9. Batchelor T, Carson K, O'Neill A et al (2003) Treatment of primary CNS lymphoma with methotrexate and deferred radiation therapy: a report of the NABTT 96-07. J Clin Oncol 21:1044–1049
10. Gerstner ER, Carson K, Grossman S, Batchelor TT (2008) Long-term outcome in PCNSL patients treated with high-dose methotrexate and deferred radiation. Neurology 70:401–402
11. Herrlinger U, Kuker W, Uhl M et al (2005) NOA-03 trial of high-dose methotrexate for primary central nervous system lymphoma: a final report. Ann Neurol 57:843–847
12. Chabner BA, Longo DL (eds) (2010) Cancer Chemotherapy and Biotherapy. Lippincott, Williams and Wilkins, Philadelphia/Baltimore/New York/London/Buenos Aires/Hong Kong/Sydney/Tokyo
13. Ferreri AJ, Reni M, Foppoli M et al (2009) High-dose cytarabine plus high-dose methotrexate versus high-dose methotrexate alone in patients with primary CNS lymphoma: a randomised phase 2 trial. Lancet 374:1512–1520
14. Pels H, Schmidt-Wolf IGH et al (2003) Primary central nervous system lymphoma: results of a pilot and phase II study of systemic and intraventricular chemotherapy with deferred radiotherapy. J Clin Oncol 21:4489–4495
15. Rubenstein JL, Rosenberg J, Damon L (1999) High-dose methotrexate plus rituximab (Anti-CD20) monoclonal antibody in the treatment of primary CNS lymphoma. Society for Neuro-Oncology Fourth Annual Meeting, Scottsdale, AZ, USA, November 17–21, 1999 (Abstract)
16. Dietlein M, Pels H, Schulz H et al (2005) Imaging of central nervous system lymphomas with I^{123}-labeled rituximab. Eur J Haematol 74:348–352
17. Maza S, Kiewe P, Munz DL et al (2009) First report on a prospective trial with yttrium-90-labeled ibritumomab tiuxetan (Zevalin) in primary CNS lymphoma. Neurooncol 11:423–429
18. Batchelor TT, Grossman SA, Mikkelsen T et al (2011) Rituximab monotherapy for patients with recurrent primary CNS lymphoma. Neurology 76:929–930
19. Shah G, Yahalom J, Correa D et al (2007) Combined Immunochemotherapy With Reduced Whole-Brain Radiotherapy for Newly Diagnosed Primary CNS Lymphoma. J Clin Oncol 25:4730–4735
20. McAllister LD, Doolittle ND, Guastadisegni PE et al (2000) Cognitive outcomes and long-term follow-up results after enhanced chemotherapy delivery in primary central nervous system lymphoma. Neurosurgery 46:51–60
21. Angelov L, Doolittle ND, Kraemer DF et al (2009) Blood-brain barrier disruption and intra-arterial methotrexate-based therapy for newly diagnosed primary CNS lymphoma: a multi-institutional experience. J Clin Oncol 27:3503–3509
22. Barajas RF, Rubenstein JL, Chang JS et al (2010) Diffusion-weighted MR imaging derived apparent diffusion coefficient is predictive of clinical outcome in primary central nervous system lymphoma. Am J Neuroradiol 31:60–66
23. Jahnke K, Korfel A, Martus P et al (2005) High-dose methotrexate toxicity in elderly patients with primary central nervous system lymphoma. Ann Oncol 16:445–449
24. Zhu JJ, Gerstner ER, Engler DA et al (2009) High-dose methotrexate for elderly patients with primary CNS lymphoma. Neurooncol 11:211–215

25. Omuro A, Taillandier L, Chinot O, Carnin C, Barrie M, Hoang-Xuan K (2007) Temozolomide and methotrexate for primary central nervous system lymphoma in the elderly. J Neurooncol 85:207–211
26. Illerhaus G, Marks MF et al (2009) High-dose methotrexate combined with procarbazine and CCNU for primary CNS lymphoma in the elderly: results of a pilot and prospective phase II study. Ann Oncol 20:319–325
27. Gavrilovic IT, Hormigo A, Yahalom J et al (2006) Long-term follow-up of high-dose methotrexate-based therapy with and without whole brain irradiation for newly diagnosed primary CNS lymphoma. J Clin Oncol 24:4570–4574
28. Khan R, Shi W, Thaler H, DeAngelis L, Abrey L (2002) Is intrathecal methotrexate necessary in the treatment of primary CNS lymphoma?. J Neurooncol 58:175–178
29. Pels H, Juergens A, Glasmacher A et al (2009) Early relapses in primary CNS lymphoma after response to polychemotherapy without intraventicular treatment: results of a phase II study. J Neurooncol 91:299–305
30. Jahnke K, Thiel E, Martus P et al (2006) Relapse of primary central nervous system lymphoma: clinical features, outcome and prognostic factors. J Neurooncol 80:159–165
31. Plotkin S, Betensky R, Hochberg F et al (2004) Treatment of relapsed central nervous system lymphoma with high-dose methotrexate. Clin Cancer Res 10:5643–5646
32. Reni M, Mason W, Zaja F et al (2004) Salvage chemotherapy with temozolomide in primary CNS lymphomas: preliminary results of a phase II trial. Eur J Cancer 40:1682–1688
33. Enting R, Demopoulos A, DeAngelis L, Abrey L (2004) Salvage therapy for primary CNS lymphoma with a combination of rituximab and temozolomide. Neurology 63:901–903
34. Wong ET, Tishler R, Barron L, Wu JK (2004) Immunochemotherapy with rituximab and temozolomide for central nervous system lymphomas. Cancer 101:139–145
35. Rubenstein JL, Fridlyand J, Abrey L et al (2007) Phase I study of intraventricular administration of rituximab in patients with recurrent CNS and intraocular lymphoma. J Clin Oncol 25:1350–1356
36. Fischer L, Thiel E, Klasen H et al (2006) Prospective trial on topotecan salvage therapy in primary CNS lymphoma. Ann Oncol 17:1141–1145
37. Voloschin AD, Betensky R, Wen PY et al (2008) Topotecan as salvage therapy for relapsed or refractory primary central nervous system lymphoma. J Neurooncol 86:211–215
38. Arellano-Rodrigo E, Lopez-Guillermo A, Bessell EM et al (2003) Salvage treatment with etoposide (VP-16), ifosfamide and cytarabine (Ara-C) for patients with recurrent primary central nervous system lymphoma. Eur J Haematol 70:219–224
39. Herrlinger U, Brugger W, Bamberg M (2000) PCV salvage chemotherapy for recurrent primary CNS lymphoma. Neurology 54:1707–1708
40. Soussain C, Hoang-Xuan K, Taillander L et al (2008) Intensive chemotherapy followed by hematopoietic stem-cell rescue for refractory and recurrent primary CNS and intraocular lymphoma: Societe Francaise de Greffe de Moelle Osseuse-Therapie Cellulaire. J Clin Oncol 26:2512–2518
41. Hoang-Xuan K, Taillandier L, Chinot O et al (2003) Chemotherapy alone as initial treatment for primary CNS lymphoma in patients older than 60 years: a multicenter phase II study (26952) of the European Organization for Research and Treatment of Cancer Brain Tumor Group. J Clin Oncol 21:2726–2731
42. Edward A, Neuwelt MD; Oregon Health Sciences University (2004) Neurosurgery 54: 131–142

Chapter 9
High-Dose Chemotherapy and Stem Cell Transplantation for Primary CNS Lymphoma

Carole Soussain, Patrick Johnston, and Gerald Illerhaus

Introduction

The treatment of patients with CNS lymphoma has posed a challenge since this entity was first described. Several issues have complicated the management of these patients. First, it is important to define whether the lymphoma is confined to the CNS (primary CNS lymphoma, PCNSL) or whether there is co-existent or pre-existent systemic lymphoma (stage IV or secondary CNS lymphoma, respectively). Second, it is important to define the histological subtypes of lymphoma involving the CNS since multiple histologies are known to occur in the CNS and the treatment can vary depending on the histology [1]. Because diffuse large B cell lymphoma (DLBCL) is the most common histology for PCNSL, that will be the focus of this chapter.

Any discussion of transplantation for PCNSL must be preceded by a review of the treatment for systemic DLBCL. The treatment of systemic DLBCL changed dramatically in the 1970s with the incorporation of doxorubicin into combination chemotherapy regimens, turning this fatal disease into a potentially curable malignancy [2, 3]. With introduction of the CHOP (cyclophosphamide, adriamycin, vincristine and prednisone) regimen, more than 30% of patients with DLBCL were cured with front-line chemotherapy [3]. Unfortunately, a large percentage of patients experienced relapses, which were often fatal. It was noted that more patients were cured by escalating the doses of chemotherapy, but at a price; a higher percentage of these patients experienced prolonged cytopenias, resulting in extensive transfusion requirements, and increased numbers of patients were dying of infectious and other complications of the treatment as the doses were escalated.

Early investigations into the use of related donor (allogeneic) bone marrow transplantation for lymphomas or leukemias after high dose chemotherapy and/or irradiation yielded poor results, often due to infectious complications or extensive graft versus host disease. This was in part due to the inability to achieve effective immunosuppression and due to poorly matched donors [4]. Consequently,

C. Soussain (✉)
Service d'Hématologie, Centre de Lutte Contre le Cancer René Huguenin, Saint-Cloud, France
e-mail: soussain@crh1.org

T. Batchelor, L.M. DeAngelis (eds.), *Lymphoma and Leukemia of the Nervous System*, DOI 10.1007/978-1-4419-7668-0_9,

allogeneic transplants fell out of favor and interest in autologous transplantation increased; however, the inability to store bone marrow while administering the high dose therapy was an impediment to progress in this field. A major advance occurred in the 1980s when it became feasible to cryopreserve bone marrow. With the ability to freeze stem cells, it became possible to collect and freeze bone marrow from lymphoma patients, thus alleviating the need for locating a suitable donor and for immunosuppression. Thus, when a patient relapsed with aggressive lymphoma after initial chemotherapy, he or she would be administered salvage chemotherapy to decrease the lymphoma bulk, and to show ongoing sensitivity to chemotherapy. These patients then would undergo bone marrow harvesting and cryopreservation. Patients could then receive high dose chemotherapy and/or irradiation, followed by infusion of their own frozen cells in order to abbreviate the duration of critical neutropenia (providing a shorter window for life threatening infections), to decrease the need for transfusions and eliminate graft versus host disease. This appeared to increase the cure rate of patients with systemic aggressive lymphomas, when used in a relapse setting. In a randomized phase III trial for systemic aggressive lymphoma (primarily DLBCL), patients with relapsed disease received salvage chemotherapy with DHAP (cisplatin, cytosine arabinoside and dexamethasone), and if a suitable response was achieved, were randomized to receive either high dose therapy with bone marrow transplant or additional DHAP [5]. This seminal study demonstrated the benefit of high dose therapy in relapsed disease by increasing the cure rate more than twofold. Subsequent clinical trials investigated the role of stem cell transplantation in patients considered to be at high risk for relapse from aggressive lymphomas and demonstrated a benefit in some patients [6].

Initial results with autologous bone marrow transplantation for systemic non-Hodgkin lymphoma (NHL) appeared promising; however, certain limitations were noted. The need for large volume bone marrow harvests posed a problem, as well as quantification of the "stem cell dose." The discovery of CD34 as a stem cell marker in the blood and the ability to mobilize progenitor cells from the bone marrow into the blood after chemotherapy or with the addition of growth factors was a major advance in the field. Also, advances in transfusion medicine, as well as a broader spectrum of anti-microbial agents reduced transplant related mortality from approximately 20% in the 1980s to approximately 5% currently for autologous stem cell transplants for lymphoma.

The role of stem cell transplantation in patients with CNS involvement from their systemic lymphoma has emerged over time. Early reports of patients undergoing stem cell transplant with a history of prior or active CNS lymphomatous involvement demonstrated that patients in remission from their CNS disease who underwent stem cell transplant did not have significantly higher relapse rates than a matched cohort of patients without CNS involvement undergoing transplant; however, the patients with a history of CNS involvement experienced significantly higher levels of toxicity during transplant [7]. A subsequent analysis from the Center for International Blood and Marrow Transplant Research (CIBMTR) database assessed 151 patients with a history of CNS lymphomatous involvement who underwent stem cell transplant from 1990 to 2005 [8]. When compared to 4,688 patients without lymphomatous involvement of the CNS who underwent autologous stem cell transplant (ASCT) for NHL during the same period, there was no statistically significant difference in 5-year overall or disease free survival or in the relapse rate at 5 years after transplant. Better outcomes were noted for patients who were in remission with regards to the CNS involvement prior to transplant than for those with active CNS disease at the time of transplant.

Applying these data to transplantation of PCNSL requires additional considerations. A major issue in the application of autotransplantation as initial or salvage treatment of PCNSL, is the poor blood brain barrier penetration of many of the drugs used to treat systemic lymphoma. This issue has been addressed in a prior chapter, but is important when selecting a conditioning regimen for stem cell transplantation.

As discussed in Chapters 7 and 8, radiation and chemotherapy are both effective modalities for PCNSL; however, the duration of response may be limited and the neurotoxicity, especially of radiation, may limit the maximum delivered dose. Overall, this results in a limited number of patients with CNS lymphoma being cured of their disease. Data from retrospective series and prospective clinical trials involving stem cell transplantation as a therapeutic option in the treatment of PCNSL, including intraocular lymphoma, suggests that this therapy appears promising and has the potential to increase the cure rate for this often fatal disease.

High-Dose Chemotherapy Followed by Autologous Stem Cell Transplantation in Relapsed or Refractory PCNSL

Approximately half of patients with PCNSL who are in complete remission after conventional combined modality therapy, will relapse, and 15% of the patients are classified as a primary refractory group [9]. Without treatment, patients with relapsed PCNSL have a median overall survival (OS) of approximately 5 months [10]. There is no consensus treatment for relapsed or refractory disease. Optimal salvage treatment should be determined according to the first-line treatment history, time of recurrence, and patient characteristics. Conventional chemotherapies including temozolomide, topotecan, intra-arterial carboplatin, high-dose cytarabine, and ifosfamide are active in recurrent PCNSL with response rates of 26–37% and a 1-year PFS between 13 and 22% [11]. Treatment with high-dose methotrexate can be successful in patients who obtained a sustained CR after previous methotrexate. Whole brain radiotherapy at recurrence can induce a response in 70% of patients, but median survival does not exceed 16 months [11]. The efficacy of radioimmunotherapy with ^{90}Y ibritumomab is limited [12].

Results of High-Dose Chemotherapy and Stem Cell Transplantation in Refractory or Relapsed PCNSL

The use of high-dose chemotherapy (HDT) followed by autologous stem cell transplantation (ASCT) in PCNSL is based on its efficacy in recurrent systemic NHL [5] (Table 9.1). In the specific setting of PCNSL, the aim of intensive chemotherapy is also to increase penetration of the blood brain barrier, which otherwise restricts drug delivery to the brain [13].

Table 9.1 Published cases and series of intensive chemotherapy and autologous hematopoietic stem cell rescue for refractory and relapsed PCNSL

Ref	N	Relapse/refractory	Treatment of relapse	Status before intensive chemotherapy	Intensive chemotherapy	Status after HDT	Survival
Hong SJ et al [36]	1 PCNSL	Relapse	Rituximab in Ommaya reservoir + VIA	CR	BEAM	CR	Alive in CR 28 months after HDT
Khalfallah S et al [14]	1 PCNSL	Relapse	DIAME	PR	BEAM-derived HDT followed by radiotherapy (14 Gy to brain and spinal cord to C2 level)	CR	Alive 6 years after HDT
Cheng T et al [23],	7 PCNSL	• 5 PR after first-line treatment • 1 PD after first-line treatment • 1 relapse after BEAM + HCR		5 PR 2PD	Thiotepa-busulfan-cyclophosphamide	7 CR	Median survival = 24 months
Soussain et al [15],	11 IOL	11 refractory		Refractory	Intensification in 5 patients Thiotepa-busulfan-cyclophosphamide	5 CR	3 patients alive in CR 15, 15 and 14 months after ABMT
Soussain et al [37],	22	• 10 relapses (2 IOL; 8 PCNSL) • 12 refractory (9 IOL; 3 PCNSL)	No treatment in 7 patients; high dose MTX in one; CYVE regimen in 14 patients.	HDT in 20 patients: 8 CR; 4 PR; 1 SD; 7 refractory IOL	Thiotepa-busulfan-cyclophosphamide	16 CR; 2 PR; 1 SD IOL; 1 PD	3 y OS = 63.7%

Table 9.1 (continued)

Ref	N	Relapse/refractory	Treatment of relapse	Status before intensive chemotherapy	Intensive chemotherapy	Status after HDT	Survival
Soussain et al [17],	43 PCNSL	Partial response 4 Relapse 22 Refractory 17	CYVE	Intensive chemotherapy in 27 patients: 12 CR; 3 PR; 1 SD; 11 PD.	Thiotepa-busulfan-cyclophosphamide	26 CR; 1 PD	2-y OS= 45% in the whole population and 69% among the 27 patients who received HDT – HCR. 2-y PFS = 43% among all the patients and 58% in the HDT + HC subpopulation.
Varadi et al [26],	1	Relapse	VP16 – MTX – CCNU – CDDP – Cytarabine	PD	Allogeneic transplantation *Conditioning regimen*: ATG + CPM	CR at 3 months	Alive in CR 30 months after transplantation

VIA, etoposide, ifosfamide, cytarabine; BEAM, BCNU 300 mg/m^2 on day –7, Etoposide 200 mg/m^2 on days –6 through –3, cytarabine 200 mg/m^2 on days –6 through –3, and melphalan 140 mg/m^2 on day –2; HDT, Intensive chemotherapy; HCR, hematopoietic cell rescue; OS, overall survival; PFS, progression-free survival; CR, complete response; PR, partial response; SD, stable disease; PD, progressive disease; MTX, methotrexate; CYVE, high dose etoposide and cytarabine; PCNSL, primary central nervous system lymphoma; IOL, intraocular lymphoma; CDDP, cisplatin; ATG, anti-thymocyte globulin; CPM, cyclophosphamide; DIAME, dexamethasone 40 mg/D D1 to D4, Ifosfamide 1,500 mg/m^2/D D1 to D5, Cytarabine 2 g/m^2 D1, Methotrexate 3 g/m^2 D1, Etoposide 100 mg/m^2/D D1 to D3; BEAM-derived HDT, BCNU 400 mg/m^2 D8, Etoposide 200 mg/m^2/D D-7 to D-4, Cytarabine 2 g/m^2/D D-7 to D-4, Melphalan 140 mg/m^2 D3, Dexamethasone 20 mg/m^2/D D-7 to D-4

The first case of HDT + ASCT for a recurrent PCNSL patient was published in 1996 [14], and the patient was alive 6 years after treatment. A second study used HDT + ASCT to treat five patients who had refractory intraocular lymphoma (IOL) [15]. HDT consisted of a combination of thiotepa, busulfan, and cyclophosphamide (TBC). All five patients achieved a complete response after HDT, and three were still disease-free at a median follow-up of 26 months. Based on this experience, an additional 22 patients with recurrent or refractory PCNSL or IOL were treated with TBC and ASCT, either initially at the time of relapse (7) or following induction chemotherapy (15) [16]. The probability of 3-year overall and event-free survival was 63.7 and 53%, respectively. However, half of the patients had IOL and the slower progression of this CNS lymphoma variant, might partly explain these positive results.

A prospective multicenter phase II study was conducted in 43 patients with refractory or relapsed PCNSL [17]. The second-line treatment, aimed at cytoreduction before HDT + ASCT, consisted of high dose cytarabine and etoposide (CYVE) [18]. Twenty-seven of the forty-three patients received the HDT + ASCT. The median PFS and OS were 41 and 58 months, respectively, after HDT. The outcome of patients who were chemosensitive prior to HDT was excellent: their median OS and PFS times were not reached. Patients who neither responded to CYVE nor received HDT + ASCT had the worst outcome, with a median OS of only 3 months. Responders to CYVE who did not receive HDT + ASCT, and non-responders to CYVE who still received HDT + ASCT had intermediate survival rates, with a median OS of approximately 18 months in both cases (Fig. 9.1). Improved PFS was associated with chemosensitivity to the CYVE regimen and the use of HDT + ASCT. Response to first-line chemotherapy at the time of the initial PCNSL diagnosis was not associated with subsequent response to CYVE or outcome after HDT + ASCT. Interestingly, HDT + ASCT demonstrated activity in patients resistant to conventional salvage chemotherapy. Twelve patients received HDT + ASCT in the setting of progressive disease and 11/12 achieved CR. Eight of these patients relapsed at a median of 5.4 months after HDT + ASCT (range, 2.5–42 months). Five of these patients were alive at last follow-up at 20, 23, 36, 68, and 81 months, respectively. Although comparative studies are lacking, these results suggest a potential role of intensification in refractory or relapsed PCNSL. The findings also underline the need to achieve a higher response rate to second-line treatment before HDT + ASCT. The choice of the combination of TBC as intensive chemotherapy was based on the high CSF and brain diffusion of thiotepa and busulfan [19–22], although the inclusion of cyclophosphamide was debatable.

The benefit of TBC-intensive chemotherapy and ASCT in patients with active disease was also suggested by Cheng et al. [23] These investigators reported 7 cases of poor prognosis PCNSL: one patient with relapsed PCNSL 7 months after initial HDT + ASCT with the BEAM conditioning regimen, one patient with progressive disease, and five patients with partial responses after a combination of methotrexate and cytarabine. All seven of the patients entered a CR after TBC with a median survival of 24 months. The TBC regimen used by Cheng et al [23] differed slightly from that used by Soussain et al [17] (Table 9.2).

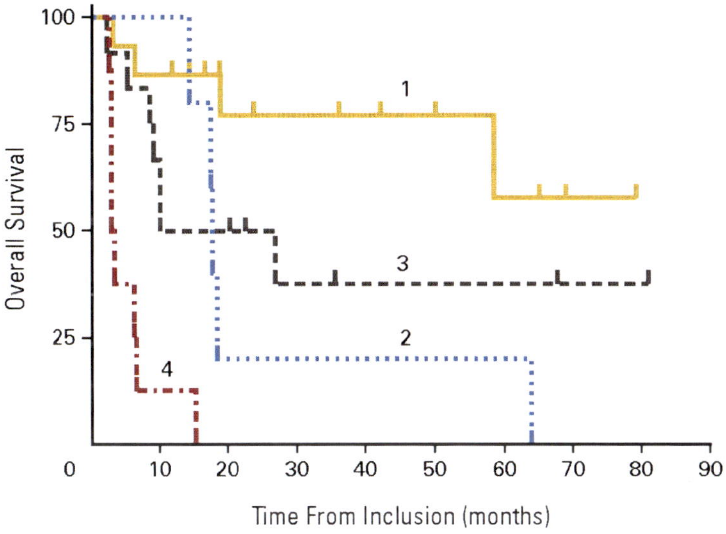

Fig. 9.1 Overall survival according to the response to high-dose cytarabine and etoposide (CYVE) and the use of intensive chemotherapy followed by autologous hematopoietic stem-cell rescue (HDT – HCR). Group 1: patients who responded to CYVE and received HDT – HCR (n = 15). Group 2: patients who responded to CYVE but did not receive HDT – HCR (n = 5). Group 3: patients who did not respond to CYVE but received HDT – HCR (n = 12). Group 4: patients who did not respond to CYVE and did not receive HDT – HCR (n = 8). Significant statistical difference was observed between groups 1 and 2 ($P = 0.0183$) and between group 3 and 4 ($P = 0.0023$) (Reproduced with permission from J Clin Oncol)

Table 9.2 High dose thiotepa- busulfan- cyclophosphamide (TBC) used as intensive chemotherapy before hematopoietic stem cell rescue

	In Soussain et al [17]		In Cheng et al [23]	
Thiotepa	250 mg/m^2/D	D-9 to D-7	300 mg/m^2/D	D-8; D-7
Busulfan	10 mg/kg/total dose PO or 0.8 mg/kg total dose IV[a] in 4 divided doses	D-6 to D-4	3.2 mg/kg/D once daily	D-6 to D-4
Cyclophosphamide	60 mg/kg/D	D-3; D-2	2 g/m^2/D	D-3; D-2
Reinfusion of hematopoietic stem cells		D0		D0

[a]Reduced dose in patients over 60: 8 mg/kg total dose PO or 0.6 mg/kg total dose IV

Toxicity of Intensive Chemotherapy and Hematopoietic Cell Rescue

HDT + ASCT is often restricted to patients under 65, although certain older patients might be suitable for HDT. The main toxicity of the TBC regimen is hematologic with grade 4 neutropenia and thrombocytopenia for a median duration of 11 and 18 days, respectively [17]. The use of granulocyte-colony-stimulating factor (G-CSF) is recommended by some authorities. Although grade 3 or 4 infectious complications were limited, late neurotoxicity was observed in 5 of 27 patients after HDT + ASCT. The role of TBC for the observed adverse effects in these cases is difficult to establish, since the late neurotoxicity could possibly have resulted from the cumulative, combined toxicity of first-line treatment, possibly including cranial radiotherapy, as well as the salvage treatment prior to HDT + ASCT and to the HDT itself.

Allogeneic Transplantation

Central nervous system graft-versus-host disease has been reported in a few cases, but remains a controversial entity [24]. Cases of graft-versus leukemia effect in the CNS have been reported in patients with acute myeloid leukemia [25]. Varadi et al published the only case of a patient with a recurrent PCNSL who underwent allogeneic bone marrow transplantation from an HLA-identical sibling after non-myeloablative conditioning [26]. The patient experienced acute, grade II graft-versus-host disease. The cerebral tumor shrank progressively after transplantation, and the patient was alive 30 months after transplant, free of disease. No other experience with allogeneic bone marrow transplantation has been reported since this case report.

Conclusions: Intensive Chemotherapy and Stem Cell Transplantation in Refractory or Relapsed PCNSL

Thiotepa-based intensive chemotherapy followed by ASCT is a therapeutic option for relapsed or refractory PCNSL in the appropriate patient population. Although long-term survival has been observed in some patients with progressive disease at the time of intensive chemotherapy, chemosensitive patients have better outcomes.

High-Dose Chemotherapy Followed by Hematopoietic Stem Cell Transplantation as First Line Treatment of PCNSL

Induction Chemotherapy

The optimal induction treatment regimen for PCNSL has not yet been defined. All the published trials on HDT and ASCT have included high-dose methotrexate as monotherapy, or in combination with cytarabine, thiotepa, ifosphamide, or VP 16 [16, 17, 23, 27–32]. The doses of methotrexate ranged from 3 to 8 g/m^2 for up to 5 cycles. Various chemotherapy regimens for mobilizing stem cells and for intensifying treatment have been reported. Cytarabine alone [23, 27] or in combination with thiotepa [30, 31] or ifosfamide [28, 29], as well as the use of methotrexate alone [33] in combination with G-CSF have all been reported to result in a sufficient harvest of CD34+ cells.

HDT in First-Line PCNSL Therapy

The first report on HDT and ASCT as a component of first-line treatment was published by Abrey et al. in 2003 [27]. Twenty-eight patients received induction chemotherapy with systemic methotrexate (3.5 g/m^2) and cytarabine (3 g/m^2 daily for 2 days). At the time, systemic NHL transplant regimens often used the combination "BEAM" (BCNU 300 mg/m^2 day –7, etoposide 100 mg/m^2 every 12 h days –6 to –3, cytarabine 200 mg/m^2 every 12 h days –6 to –3, melphalan 140 mg/m^2 day –2), as the conditioning regimen before ASCT and thus, it was selected in this trial because it is well tolerated by older individuals. The objective response rate to the induction phase chemotherapy was 57% (32% CR, 25% PR). Only 50% of the patients completed HDT and ASCT, resulting in 8/14 CR and 2/14 PR. Response improvement from PR to CR occurred in 2 patients. With a high relapse rate and a median event-free survival of 5.6 months, these results were disappointing. Two further ASCT trials with BEAM conditioning and consolidating WBRT [28, 29] demonstrated higher remission rates and long-term disease control, but a substantial proportion of patients developed neurotoxicity.

Other HDT + ASCT strategies have been used as part of front-line treatment in PCNSL patients with more encouraging results, mostly when thiotepa-based conditioning regimens were used (Table 9.3) [30]. In one report, thirty patients with PCNSL under 65 years of age (median, 54 years; range, 27–64 years) were enrolled in a phase II HDT + ASCT clinical trial. Sequential induction chemotherapy included three cycles of MTX (8 g/m^2); cytarabine (two doses of 3 g/m^2), and thiotepa (40 mg/m^2) followed by stem-cell harvest. The transplant conditioning regimen consisted of carmustine (400 mg/m^2) and thiotepa (two doses of 5 mg/kg body weight), followed by ASCT. WBRT (45 Gy) was administered as consolidation therapy. Induction treatment resulted in 10 CR and 14 PR. Twenty-three of the thirty patients proceeded to HDT + ASCT, resulting in 15 patients in CR and 8 in PR. Twenty-one patients subsequently underwent WBRT, all achieving CR. One patient died of liver failure after methotrexate. Overall, the HDT was well tolerated, apart from WHO grade 3/4 cytopenias. With a median follow-up of 63 months (range, 4–84 months), the 5-year overall survival was 69% for all patients and 87% for those patients completing HDT + ASCT (Fig. 9.2). The 5-year probability of relapse-related death was 21% for all patients (n = 30) and 8.7% for patients treated with HDT + ASCT (n = 23).

Table 9.3 Published clinical trials of intensive chemotherapy and autologous hematopoietic stem cell rescue for front-line therapy of PCNSL

Author	No of pts.	Median Age	Induction regimen	Conditioning regimen	WBRT	CRR [%]	FU [mo]	Survival	TRM
Colombat et al [29]	25	51	MVBP +i.th. AraC	BEAM	Yes	44%	34	4-y EFS: 46%	4%
Abrey et al [27]	28	53	MTX AraC	BEAM	No	18%	27	mEFS: 9 mo	0%
Stewart et al [35]	11	56	MTX	Thiotepa Busulfan Cy	Yes	82%	22	3-yr OS: 61%	18%
Illerhaus et al [30]	30	54	MTX (8 g) AraC/TT	Thiotepa (10 mg/kg) BCNU	Yes[a]	76%	63	5-yr OS: 69%	3%
Montemurro et al [32]	23	55	MTX (8 g)	Bu/TT (10 mg/kg)	Yes[a]	69%	15	2-yr OS: 48%	13%
Illerhaus et al [31]	13	54	MTX (8 g) AraC/TT	TT (20 mg/kg)/ BCNU + WBRT	No	54%	25	3-yr OS: 77%	0%

araC, cytarabine; ASCT, autologous stem cell transplantation; BCNU, carmustine; BEAM (regimen), carmustine, etoposide, cytarabine, and melphalan; Bu, busulfan; Cy, cyclophosphamide; IFO, ifosfamide; i.th., intrathecal; MBVP (regimen), methotrexate, carmustine, etoposide, and methylprednisolone; OS, overall survival; TRM, treatment-related mortality; TT, thiotepa WBRT, whole-brain-radiotherapy.

[a]Only for patients not achieving a complete remission

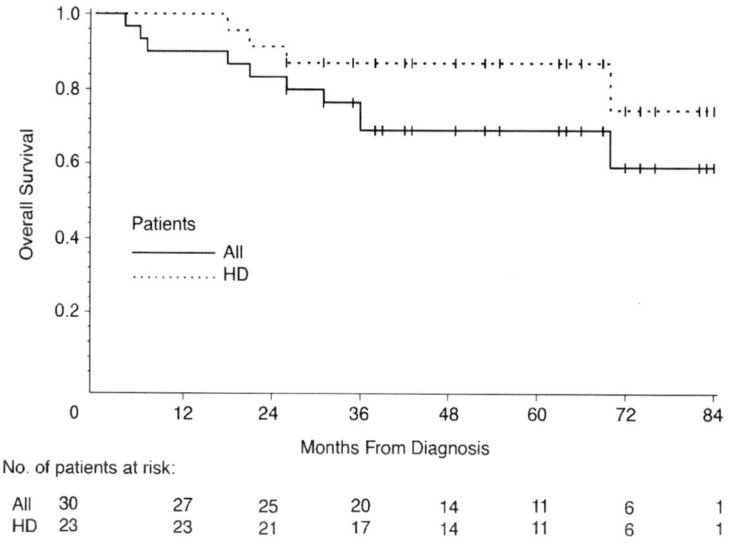

Fig. 9.2 Kaplan-Meier plot: overall survival from time of initial diagnosis of all patients (–) and of the 23 patients (- - -) who completed high-dose chemotherapy (HD) (Reproduced with permission from J Clin Oncol)

In a follow-up pilot study conducted by the same group, the induction chemotherapy was intensified and consolidating WBRT was restricted only to patients not achieving a CR after the induction (HD-MTX followed by cytarabine and thiotepa) [31]. Seven of eleven patients were in CR following ASCT, and 3 in PR after ASCT received radiotherapy as consolidative treatment. After a median follow-up of 25 months, 3-year disease-free and overall survival was 77%. None of the patients suffered from severe neurotoxicity during the follow-up period. Both trials demonstrated a curative effect from HD chemotherapy in young patients.

The discrepancies in the effectiveness between the BEAM and the thiotepa-based conditioning regimens may be related to the variable ability of these drugs to cross the blood brain barrier (BBB). In particular, busulfan, thiotepa, and BCNU exhibit excellent CNS penetration, with CSF levels in excess of 80% of serum levels for busulfan and thiotepa, and 50–80% for BCNU, while the CNS penetration rates of agents in the BEAM regimen are very low, i.e. 5% for etoposide, 6–22% for cytarabine, and 10% for melphalan [34]. These data suggest that thiotepa-based conditioning regimens are likely to be more efficacious in PCNSL than BEAM, one of the most effective conditioning regimens in systemic NHL.

Conclusions: Intensive Chemotherapy and Stem Cell Transplantation in Front-Line Therapy of PCNSL

The effectiveness of HDT + ASCT in PCNSL appears to depend on successful induction chemotherapy, leading to maximum cytoreduction prior to HDT.

However, the choice of drugs within the conditioning regimen may play an important role in determining the potential curative effect of this approach in the front-line therapy of PCNSL. To date, only small series and phase II trials have demonstrated the feasibility and high level of efficacy of HDT + ASCT in PCNSL. To further investigate the potential benefit of HDT + ASCT in the treatment of PCNSL, the International Extranodal Lymphoma Study Group (IELSG) and the German Freiburg Collaborative Study Group are enrolling patients in a randomized phase II trial, in which patients receive one of three induction chemotherapy regimens and those without progressive disease are randomized to WBRT versus HDT + ASCT.

References

1. Miller DC, Hochberg FH, Harris NL et al (1994) Pathology with clinical correlations of primary central nervous system non-Hodgkin's lymphoma. The Massachusetts General Hospital experience 1958–1989. Cancer 74:1383–1397
2. Bonadonna G, De Lena M, Lattuada A et al (1975) Combination chemotherapy and radiotherapy in non-Hodgkin's lymphoma. Br J Cancer Suppl 2:481–488
3. Skarin AT, Frei E 3rd, Moloney WC et al (1975) New agents and combination chemotherapy of non-Hodgkin's lymphoma. Br J Cancer Suppl 2:497–504
4. Thomas ED, Buckner CD, Rudolph RH et al (1971) Allogeneic marrow grafting for hematologic malignancy using HLA matched donor-recipient sibling pairs. Blood 38:267–287
5. Philip T, Guglielmi C, Hagenbeek A et al (1995) Autologous bone marrow transplantation as compared with salvage chemotherapy in relapses of chemotherapy-sensitive non-Hodgkin's lymphoma. N Engl J Med 333:1540–1545
6. Haioun C, Besson C, Lepage E et al (2000) Incidence and risk factors of central nervous system relapse in histologically aggressive non-Hodgkin's lymphoma uniformly treated and receiving intrathecal central nervous system prophylaxis: a GELA study on 974 patients. Ann Oncol 11:685–690
7. van Besien K, Przepiorka D, Mehra R et al (1996) Impact of preexisting CNS involvement on the outcome of bone marrow transplantation in adult hematologic malignancies. J Clin Oncol 14:3036–3042
8. Maziarz RT, Wang Z, Zhang M-J et al (2010) CNS Remission Predicts Survival After Autologous Hematopoietic Stem Cell Transplantation (AHCT) for non-Hodgkin Lymphoma (NHL) with Pre-existing CNS Involvement: a CIBMTR Analysis. Biol Blood Marrow Transplant 16:s166 (abstract 31)
9. Morris PG, Abrey LE (2009) Therapeutic challenges in primary CNS lymphoma. Lancet Neurol 8:581–592
10. Jahnke K, Thiel E, Martus P et al (2006) Relapse of primary central nervous system lymphoma: clinical features, outcome and prognostic factors. J Neurooncol 80:159–165
11. Sierra del Rio M, Rousseau A, Soussain C et al (2009) Primary CNS lymphoma in immunocompetent patients. Oncologist 14:526–539
12. Iwamoto FM, Schwartz J, Pandit-Taskar N et al (2007) Study of radiolabeled indium-111 and yttrium-90 ibritumomab tiuxetan in primary central nervous system lymphoma. Cancer 110:2528–2534
13. Muldoon LL, Soussain C, Jahnke K et al (2007) Chemotherapy delivery issues in central nervous system malignancy: a reality check. J Clin Oncol 25:2295–2305
14. Khalfallah S, Stamatoullas A, Fruchart C et al (1996) Durable remission of a relapsing primary central nervous system lymphoma after autologous bone marrow transplantation. Bone Marrow Transplant 18:1021–1023
15. Soussain C, Merle-Beral H, Reux I et al (1996) A single-center study of 11 patients with intraocular lymphoma treated with conventional chemotherapy followed by high-dose

chemotherapy and autologous bone marrow transplantation in 5 cases. Leuk Lymphoma 23:339–345
16. Soussain C, Suzan F, Hoang-Xuan K et al (2001) Results of intensive chemotherapy followed by hematopoietic stem-cell rescue in 22 patients with refractory or recurrent primary CNS lymphoma or intraocular lymphoma. J Clin Oncol 19:742–749
17. Soussain C, Hoang-Xuan K, Taillandier L et al (2008) Intensive chemotherapy followed by hematopoietic stem-cell rescue for refractory and recurrent primary CNS and intraocular lymphoma: societe Francaise de Greffe de Moelle Osseuse-Therapie Cellulaire. J Clin Oncol 26:2512–2518
18. Patte C, Michon J, Frappaz D et al (1994) Therapy of Burkitt and other B-cell acute lymphoblastic leukaemia and lymphoma: experience with the LMB protocols of the SFOP (French Paediatric Oncology Society) in children and adults. Baillieres Clin Haematol 7:339–348
19. Egorin MJ, Akman SR, Gutierrez PL: (1984) Plasma pharmacokinetics and tissue distribution of thiotepa in mice. Cancer Treat Rep 68:1265–1268
20. Hassan M, Oberg G, Ericson K et al (1992) In vivo distribution of [11C]-busulfan in cynomolgus monkey and in the brain of a human patient. Cancer Chemother Pharmacol 30:81–85
21. Heideman RL, Cole DE, Balis F et al (1989) Phase I and pharmacokinetic evaluation of thiotepa in the cerebrospinal fluid and plasma of pediatric patients: evidence for dose-dependent plasma clearance of thiotepa. Cancer Res 49:736–741
22. Vassal G, Gouyette A, Hartmann O et al (1989) Pharmacokinetics of high-dose busulfan in children. Cancer Chemother Pharmacol 24:386–390
23. Cheng T, Forsyth P, Chaudhry A et al (2003) High-dose thiotepa, busulfan, cyclophosphamide and ASCT without whole-brain radiotherapy for poor prognosis primary CNS lymphoma. Bone Marrow Transplant 31:679–685
24. Kamble RT, Chang CC, Sanchez S et al (2007) Central nervous system graft-versus-host disease: report of two cases and literature review. Bone Marrow Transplant 39:49–52
25. Classen CF, Debatin KM, Friedrich W et al (2003) Long-term remission of APL with a second allogeneic BMT after CNS relapse following HLA-identical allogeneic BMT. Bone Marrow Transplant 32:843–846
26. Varadi G, Or R, Kapelushnik J et al (1999) Graft-versus-lymphoma effect after allogeneic peripheral blood stem cell transplantation for primary central nervous system lymphoma. Leuk Lymphoma 34:185–190
27. Abrey LE, Moskowitz CH, Mason WP et al (2003) Intensive methotrexate and cytarabine followed by high-dose chemotherapy with autologous stem-cell rescue in patients with newly diagnosed primary CNS lymphoma: an intent-to-treat analysis. J Clin Oncol 21(22):4151–4156
28. Brevet M, Garidi R, Gruson B et al (2005) First-line autologous stem cell transplantation in primary CNS lymphoma. Eur J Haematol 75:288–292
29. Colombat P, Lemevel A, Bertrand P et al (2006) High-dose chemotherapy with autologous stem cell transplantation as first-line therapy for primary CNS lymphoma in patients younger than 60 years: a multicenter phase II study of the GOELAMS group. Bone Marrow Transplant 38:417–420
30. Illerhaus G, Marks R, Ihorst G et al (2006) High-dose chemotherapy with autologous stem-cell transplantation and hyperfractionated radiotherapy as first-line treatment of primary CNS lymphoma. J Clin Oncol 24:3865–3870
31. Illerhaus G, Muller F, Feuerhake F et al (2008) High-dose chemotherapy and autologous stem-cell transplantation without consolidating radiotherapy as first-line treatment for primary lymphoma of the central nervous system. Haematologica 93:147–8
32. Montemurro M, Kiefer T, Schuler F et al (2007) Primary central nervous system lymphoma treated with high-dose methotrexate, high-dose busulfan/thiotepa, autologous stem-cell

transplantation and response-adapted whole-brain radiotherapy: results of the multicenter Ostdeutsche Studiengruppe Hamato-Onkologie OSHO-53 phase II study. Ann Oncol 18:665–671
33. Kiefer T, Kruger WH, Montemurro M et al (2008) Mobilization of hemopoietic stem cells with high-dose methotrexate plus granulocyte-colony-stimulating factor in patients with primary central nervous system lymphoma. Transfusion 48:2624–2628
34. Wiebe VJ, Smith BR, DeGregorio MW et al (1992) Pharmacology of agents used in bone marrow transplant conditioning regimens. Crit Rev Oncol Hematol 13:241–270
35. Stewart DA, Forsyth P, Chaudhry A et al High Dose Thiotepa, Busulfan, Cyclophosphamide (TBC) and Autologous Hematopoietic Stem Cell Transplantation (ASCT) without Whole Brain Radiotherapy (WBRT) for Primary Central Nervous System Lymphoma (PCNSL). ASH Annual Meeting Abstracts 104:9112004
36. Hong SJ, Kim JS, Chang JH et al (2009) A successful treatment of relapsed primary CNS lymphoma patient with intraventricular rituximab followed by high-dose chemotherapy with autologous stem cell rescue. Yonsei Med J 50:280–283
37. Soussain C, Hoang-Xuan K, Levy V (2004) Results of intensive chemotherapy followed by hematopoietic stem-cell rescue in 22 patients with refractory or recurrent primary CNS lymphoma or intraocular lymphoma. Bull Cancer 91:189–192

Part IV
Variants of CNS Lymphoma

Chapter 10
CNS Lymphoma in the Immunocompromised Host

Silvia Montoto

Introduction

Immunosuppression is a well-known risk factor for the development of lymphoproliferative disorders, with the incidence of lymphoma being higher in immunocompromised patients than in the general population, regardless of the underlying cause of the immunosuppression (i.e. congenital, iatrogenic as in post-transplant lymphoproliferative disorders or acquired as in patients with human immunodeficiency virus (HIV) infection). Not surprisingly, therefore, the incidence of PCNSL has been reported to be significantly increased in patients with either congenital or acquired immunodeficiencies [1–5], and is highest in those infected with HIV. The pathogenesis of AIDS-related lymphoma (ARL) [which includes diffuse large B-cell lymphoma (DLBCL), Burkitt's lymphoma (BL) and primary CNS lymphoma (PCNSL)], seems to be related to the HIV infection itself [6], but also to the degree of immunodeficiency, especially in PCNSL, which is typically diagnosed in patients with advanced HIV infection and extremely low CD4 counts. Since the introduction of highly active anti-retroviral therapy (HAART), the incidence of HIV-related PCNSL has decreased [7, 8]. The prognosis of PCNSL in HIV patients in the pre-HAART era was dismal, leading some authorities to advocate for a palliative approach. After the advent of HAART, the outcome of HIV-associated PCNSL (HIV-PCNSL) significantly improved in some series [9, 10], although not in others [8, 11]. However, because of the decline in the incidence of PCNSL, the data are sparse and definitive conclusions are difficult to reach. Moreover, in spite of the suggestion of a better outcome in more recent years, many (of the few) patients diagnosed with PCNSL in the HAART era are still managed in a palliative fashion, rather than with a more aggressive approach incorporating high-dose methotrexate (HD-MTX) as used in the non-HIV

S. Montoto (✉)
CR-UK Medical Oncology Unit, Barts and the London School of Medicine and Dentistry, St Bartholomew's Hospital, EC1A 7BE London, UK
e-mail: s.montoto@qmul.ac.uk

T. Batchelor, L.M. DeAngelis (eds.), *Lymphoma and Leukemia of the Nervous System*, DOI 10.1007/978-1-4419-7668-0_10,

population. Therefore, the prognosis of patients with HIV-PCNSL remains significantly worse than the prognosis of comparable immunocompetent patients with PCNSL [9].

Epidemiology

In the pre-HAART era, the incidence of PCNSL, the second most frequent cause of a brain mass in HIV patients after toxoplasmosis, was 4.7/1,000 person-years, contrasting with an incidence of 0.28/100,000 person-years in the immunocompetent population [12]. HIV-PCNSL is associated with very low CD4 counts at diagnosis: the median CD4 count ranges in different series from 7 to 91/mm^3 [8, 9, 13–17]. Since the introduction of HAART into the standard HIV treatment regimen in Western countries, its incidence has dropped significantly [7–9, 15, 16, 18, 19]; it is now diagnosed more frequently as an AIDS-defining illness than in the past [7–9, 11]. A European multicenter study (the EuroSIDA Study Group) reported an incidence of 8.3 cases/1,000 person-years of prospective follow-up (PYF) before 1995, contrasting with 0.4 cases/1,000 PYF after 1999 [20]. Other than the low CD4 count, no significant risk factors for HIV-PCNSL have been defined. An Italian study analyzed the causes of focal brain lesions in HIV patients, both in the pre- and post-HAART era, and concluded that the risk of being diagnosed with HIV-PCNSL was only associated with the calendar year [7], a surrogate for the availability of HAART. Investigators from the EuroSIDA Study Group described the characteristics of patients with AIDS-related lymphomas (ARL) in the HAART era and observed that patients with PCNSL were significantly younger and had lower CD4 counts than patients with other types of lymphoma; there were no statistically significant differences in terms of gender, race, or mode of HIV transmission [20]. In contrast, in a recent, multicenter European cohort study, diagnosis of PCNSL versus nodal lymphoma was associated with heterosexual transmission; however, this may have been a spurious association as no multivariate analysis was performed [17].

Pathogenesis

HIV-PCNSL is usually a NHL of B-cell origin, most frequently, a DLBCL, as in immunocompetent patients. The mechanisms leading to the accumulation of malignant lymphocytes in the CNS are not completely understood, but the fact that it is a viral sanctuary in patients with HIV is believed by some to play a significant role in the pathogenesis of HIV-PCNSL [9, 21]. There are contradictory data regarding the B-cell of origin of PCNSL in the general population, some studies describing characteristics compatible with a germinal center origin (i.e. BCL-6 expression and ongoing somatic mutation) [22, 23], and other studies consistent with a "late" germinal or post-germinal center origin [24]. In patients with HIV-related PCNSL, 2 patterns of protein expression have been recognized: one similar to that seen in HIV negative patients, with expression of BCL-6, but not LMP-1 or BCL-2, and a second pattern characteristic of HIV patients, with expression of LMP-1 and BCL-2, but without BCL-6 expression [22, 25]. In fact, a feature that distinguishes HIV-PCNSL (and, in general, PCNSL in immunocompromised patients) [2, 3, 5, 26] from PCNSL in the general population is the almost universal detection of Epstein-Barr virus (EBV) in the tumor tissue of patients with HIV-PCNSL, suggesting a role for EBV in the pathogenesis of HIV-PCNSL [26]. One study reported that rather than the actual CD4 count, it is the lack of EBV-specific T-cell function that predisposes patients to HIV-PCNSL [27]. It has been hypothesized that EBV up regulates BCL-2, leading to its over-expression in the absence of gene rearrangement. However, the relationship between EBV and BCL-2 is unclear. To gain further insight into the pathogenesis of HIV-PCNSL, Camilleri-Broët and colleagues studied the expression of different members of the BCL-2 family in patients with PCNSL and found that BCL-2, BCL-X and BAX were over-expressed in immunocompromised patients (mostly with HIV) in comparison with immunocompetent patients, although this did not translate into differences in the rate of apoptosis [28].

Pathological and Clinical Features

HIV-PCNSL is histologically a DLBCL in most cases, although immunoblastic features with plasmacytic differentiation are frequently observed [29]. Other pathological characteristics more common in HIV-PCNSL than in PCNSL in immunocompetent patients are the presence of necrosis, reactive astrogliosis and macrophages [29]. BCL-2 oncoprotein is expressed more frequently in HIV-PCNSL than in PCNSL in the general population, and than in systemic ARL, but no BCL-2 gene rearrangement has been detected [26]. EBV is found in 91–100% of cases, depending on whether immunohistochemistry is used to detect LMP-1 or PCR/in situ hybridization to detect EBNA-1 or EBER. Other pathological features distinguishing HIV-PCNSL from PCNSL in the general population are shown in Table 10.1.

From a clinical standpoint, most of the HIV-PCNSL patients have a poor performance status at diagnosis (ECOG>2: 60–72%) [9, 15, 16] with the following presenting symptoms or signs: focal neurological deficits (38–61%) [13, 15, 16, 30], confusion, cognitive decline and personality changes (48–56%) [13, 15, 16], headache (35–43%) [13, 15, 16], seizures (22–41%) [13, 15, 16, 30], and ataxia (18–35%) [13, 15, 16]. Thus, the same types of symptoms are observed in HIV-PCNSL patients as in the general PCNSL population, although seizures seem to be more frequent in the former [31]. Information on cerebrospinal fluid (CSF) and ocular involvement is scarce, as not many studies include these data. Forsyth et al detected CSF involvement in 30% of patients with HIV-PCNSL and ocular infiltration in 1 of 10 patients [32], whereas Newell and colleagues did not detect CSF involvement in the 9 patients assessed [15].

Table 10.1 Differential clinical and pathological characteristics of PCNSL in immunocompromised and immunocompetent patients

	HIV-PCNSL	PCNSL in immunocompetent patients
Clinical characteristics		
Median age (years)	38–39 [8, 15]	61 [37]
Male gender	94% [29]	43–58% [24, 37]
Multiple lesions	43–59% [16, 29]	34–49% [24, 37]
CSF involvement	0–30 [15, 32]	3–16% [24, 37]
Ocular involvement	10 [32]	13% [37]
Pathological characteristics		
EBV	91–100 [22, 26, 29]	0 [22, 24]
BCL-2 expression	44–94% [22, 26, 29]	14–56% [22, 24]
BCL-6 expression	36–56% [22, 25]	56–100% [22, 24]
GC	–	4% [24]
MUM-1	68% [25]	84–93% [24, 57]

Diagnosis

Definitive diagnosis of PCNSL requires histological confirmation. However, biopsy was often avoided in the pre-HAART era because of patients' poor performance status, the dismal prognosis of HIV-PCNSL, and the higher frequency of biopsy-related hemorrhage. Thus, such patients were diagnosed retrospectively on post-mortem examination, or treated based on a "presumptive" diagnosis more frequently than in the HAART era when biopsy is performed more routinely [9].

The radiological investigation of choice in HIV patients with neurological symptoms and presumed PCNSL is a contrast-enhanced cranial MRI. This typically shows ring-enhancing lesions [30], in contrast to the homogeneous, non-ring-enhancing pattern of enhancement observed in PCNSL in non-HIV patients [33, 34]. Occasionally, the lesions are non-enhancing. The lesions are most frequently located in supratentorial areas [29, 32, 35] and in the cortex [30], with a characteristic periventricular distribution [15, 36]. Multiple lesions are seen in approximately half the patients [13, 15, 29, 30], more frequently than in the general PCNSL population [33, 34, 37]. The lesions tend to be hemorrhagic and necrotic, more often than in non-HIV patients, frequently with tumor-associated edema causing mass effect [30]. The main differential diagnosis is with toxoplasmosis, from which it may be indistinguishable on MRI scan. However, focal uptake on a single photon emission computerized tomography (SPECT) scan with thallium-201 (^{201}Tl) is more frequently associated with lymphoma than with toxoplasmosis [36], and studies in the pre-HAART era reported that FDG-PET is capable of discriminating PCNSL from toxoplasmosis [38, 39]. Because of the universal association of HIV-PCNSL with EBV infection, some authors have suggested that the detection of EBV by PCR in the CSF in the setting of a brain mass suspicious for PCNSL on MRI, would allow the diagnosis of HIV-PCNSL without a biopsy [40, 41]. Another study reported that the combination of a positive PCR for EBV with increased uptake on a ^{201}Tl-SPECT scan has a positive predictive value of 100%, and a negative PCR with no uptake on ^{201}Tl-SPECT has a negative predictive value of 100% [42], which would make a brain biopsy unnecessary. However, the same authors have recently questioned the validity of the diagnostic value of ^{201}Tl-SPECT in patients on HAART [43], and other authors have reported lower positive predictive values of the detection of EBV in the CSF [44–46]. Therefore, biopsy remains the only certain method of establishing the diagnosis as in the general population; it is optimally performed before the administration of steroids. Despite these data, the British HIV Association (BHIVA) still recommends a 2-week course of empiric anti-toxoplasma therapy, performing a biopsy only in those patients not responding or progressing on anti-toxoplasma therapy [47]. This was the approach in the pre-HAART era in the United States, but has largely been abandoned because of the rapidity of the patient's deterioration during the 2 weeks of antibiotics when the diagnosis is PCNSL. Thus, immediate biopsy is the preferred approach.

Once the diagnosis is confirmed, conventional staging should be undertaken, including CSF examination (if feasible), slit-lamp examination, as well as body CT scan, and bone marrow biopsy [48].

Treatment

The median overall survival (OS) for HIV-PCNSL patients in the pre-HAART era was approximately 1–3 months, whole-brain radiotherapy (WBRT) being the treatment modality of choice [30, 31, 49]. Although treatment with WBRT is associated with a clinical benefit, often including improvement in neurological symptoms and performance status, and is associated with a longer survival (both in the pre HAART [30, 31] era and in the post HAART [13]), it has also been associated with long-term neurotoxicity in 15–30% of patients [13, 14, 30, 32]. A few small studies and case reports have been published on the use of systemic chemotherapy (plus or minus WBRT) in the pre-HAART era [32, 50]. Forsyth and colleagues treated 10 patients with HIV-PCNSL with combination chemotherapy, including HD-MTX (3 g/m^2), followed by WBRT [32]. In this study, the response rates after chemotherapy and WBRT were 57 and 86%, respectively, with a median OS of 7 months for patients who completed all treatment. Of note, 3 "long-term" survivors developed dementia with MRI changes consistent with WBRT-associated neurotoxicity [32]. In another small study, 15 patients with HIV-PCNSL were treated with HD-MTX, WBRT being given only to those who did not respond or to those who relapsed. The complete response rate was 47% and the median OS was 10 months [35]. Following the observation that EBV lytic cycle mRNA is present in the CSF of patients with PCNSL [51], several studies explored the use of ganciclovir (plus or minus zidovudine and interleukin-2) in the management of HIV-PCNSL [52, 53]. Moreover, Bossolasco and colleagues reported that EBV-viral load was significantly lower in patients with HIV-PCNSL receiving ganciclovir for concomitant cytomegalovirus infection, and that treatment with ganciclovir was associated with a longer survival [54].

Two studies reported no differences in the median OS for HIV-PCNSL, according to whether patients were diagnosed in the pre or post HAART era [8, 11]; however, one of the studies only included patients through 1997 [8]. In contrast, other studies have demonstrated that being on HAART is associated with prolonged survival [13–15, 55]. Furthermore, there are anecdotal reports of patients with HIV-PCNSL responding to HAART as the sole treatment for PCNSL [56]. However, there are only occasional reports of patients treated with HD-MTX in the HAART era [9, 13], as most patients are still treated with WBRT alone. Hoffmann and colleagues reported a series of 29 patients with HIV-PCNSL, of whom 5 of 6 patients receiving HAART were treated with WBRT. The median OS for these patients was 36 months, contrasting with 4 months for those treated with WBRT without HAART, and 1 month for patients receiving no treatment. Of note, there was one confirmed and one suspicious case of radiation-induced neurotoxicity among the 12 patients who received WBRT [13]. Skiest and colleagues reported a better outcome for 7 patients treated with WBRT and HAART, in comparison to those treated with WBRT without HAART or no treatment. Long-term neurotoxicity secondary to WBRT was also described in this study [14].

The introduction of HAART into the standard management of patients with ARL has significantly improved their survival, such that their outcomes approach that of the general population with lymphoma when treated with the same protocols. The exception is HIV-PCNSL, which is decreasing in incidence in the HAART era, but is still associated with a poor outcome, some of which derives from the reluctance to use aggressive treatment in these patients. However, when employed, aggressive therapies are often well tolerated, and improve both neurological function and outcome. This emphasizes the importance of early and accurate diagnosis and treatment in HIV patients and the need to adopt a similar approach to that used in the general population.

Acknowledgment The author would like to thank Professor TA Lister for his helpful comments on the chapter. Silvia Montoto was kindly supported by grants from the Olivia Walduck family and the Ridgwell family.

References

1. Schabet M (1999) Epidemiology of primary CNS lymphoma. J Neurooncol 43:199–201
2. O'Neill BP, Vernino S, Dogan A et al (2007) EBV-associated lymphoproliferative disorder of CNS associated with the use of mycophenolate mofetil. Neurooncol 9:364–369
3. Kaufman DA, Hershfield MS, Bocchini JA et al (2005) Cerebral lymphoma in an adenosine deaminase-deficient patient with severe combined immunodeficiency receiving polyethylene glycol-conjugated adenosine deaminase. Pediatrics 116:e876–e879
4. Phan TG, O'Neill BP, Kurtin PJ (2000) Posttransplant primary CNS lymphoma. Neurooncol 2:229–238
5. Kleinschmidt-DeMasters BK, Damek DM, Lillehei KO et al (2008) Epstein Barr virus-associated primary CNS lymphomas in elderly patients on immunosuppressive medications. J Neuropathol Exp Neurol 67:1103–1111
6. Baeuerle M, Schmitt-Haendle M, Taubald A et al (2005) Severe HIV-1 encephalitis and development of cerebral non-Hodgkin lymphoma in a patient with persistent strong HIV-1

replication in the brain despite potent HAART – case report and review of the literature. Eur J Med Res 10:309–316
7. Ammassari A, Cingolani A, Pezzotti P et al (2000) AIDS-related focal brain lesions in the era of highly active antiretroviral therapy. Neurology 55:1194–1200
8. Besson C, Goubar A, Gabarre J et al (2001) Changes in AIDS-related lymphoma since the era of highly active antiretroviral therapy. Blood 98:2339–2344
9. Bower M, Powles T, Nelson M et al (2006) Highly active antiretroviral therapy and human immunodeficiency virus-associated primary cerebral lymphoma. J Natl Cancer Inst 98: 1088–1091
10. Kreisl TN, Panageas KS, Elkin EB et al (2008) Treatment patterns and prognosis in patients with human immunodeficiency virus and primary central system lymphoma. Leuk Lymphoma 49:1710–1716
11. Robotin MC, Law MG, Milliken S et al (2004) Clinical features and predictors of survival of AIDS-related non-Hodgkin's lymphoma in a population-based case series in Sydney, Australia. HIV Med 5:377–384
12. Cote TR, Manns A, Hardy CR et al (1996) Epidemiology of brain lymphoma among people with or without acquired immunodeficiency syndrome. AIDS/Cancer Study Group. J Natl Cancer Inst 88:675–679
13. Hoffmann C, Tabrizian S, Wolf E et al (2001) Survival of AIDS patients with primary central nervous system lymphoma is dramatically improved by HAART-induced immune recovery. AIDS 15:2119–2127
14. Skiest DJ, Crosby C (2003) Survival is prolonged by highly active antiretroviral therapy in AIDS patients with primary central nervous system lymphoma. AIDS 17:1787–1793
15. Newell ME, Hoy JF, Cooper SG et al (2004) Human immunodeficiency virus-related primary central nervous system lymphoma: factors influencing survival in 111 patients. Cancer 100:2627–2636
16. Haldorsen IS, Krakenes J, Goplen AK et al (2008) AIDS-related primary central nervous system lymphoma: a Norwegian national survey 1989-2003. BMC Cancer 8:225
17. Collaboration of Observational HIV Epidemiological Research Europe (COHERE) Study Group (2009) Prognosis of HIV-associated non-Hodgkin lymphoma in patients starting combination antiretroviral therapy. AIDS 23(15):2029–2037
18. Diamond C, Taylor TH, Aboumrad T et al (2006) Changes in acquired immunodeficiency syndrome-related non-Hodgkin lymphoma in the era of highly active antiretroviral therapy: incidence, presentation, treatment, and survival. Cancer 106:128–135
19. International Collaboration on HIV and Cancer (2000) Highly active antiretroviral therapy and incidence of cancer in human immunodeficiency virus-infected adults. J Natl Cancer Inst 92(22):1823–1830
20. Kirk O, Pedersen C, Cozzi-Lepri A et al (2001) Non-Hodgkin lymphoma in HIV-infected patients in the era of highly active antiretroviral therapy. Blood 98:3406–3412
21. Stebbing J, Gazzard B, Douek DC (2004) Where does HIV live? N Engl J Med 350: 1872–1880
22. Larocca LM, Capello D, Rinelli A et al (1998) The molecular and phenotypic profile of primary central nervous system lymphoma identifies distinct categories of the disease and is consistent with histogenetic derivation from germinal center-related B cells. Blood 92:1011–1019
23. Montesinos-Rongen M, Kuppers R, Schluter D et al (1999) Primary central nervous system lymphomas are derived from germinal-center B cells and show a preferential usage of the V4-34 gene segment. Am J Pathol 155:2077–2086
24. Camilleri-Broet S, Criniere E, Broet P et al (2006) A uniform activated B-cell-like immunophenotype might explain the poor prognosis of primary central nervous system lymphomas: analysis of 83 cases. Blood 107:190–196
25. Carbone A, Gloghini A, Larocca LM et al (2001) Expression profile of MUM1/IRF4, BCL-6, and CD138/syndecan-1 defines novel histogenetic subsets of human immunodeficiency virus-related lymphomas. Blood 97:744–751

26. Camilleri-Broet S, Davi F, Feuillard J et al (1995) High expression of latent membrane protein 1 of Epstein-Barr virus and BCL-2 oncoprotein in acquired immunodeficiency syndrome-related primary brain lymphomas. Blood 86:432–435
27. Gasser O, Bihl FK, Wolbers M et al (2007) HIV patients developing primary CNS lymphoma lack EBV-specific CD4+ T cell function irrespective of absolute CD4+ T cell counts. PLoS Med 4:e96
28. Camilleri-Broet S, Camparo P, Mokhtari K et al (2000) Overexpression of BCL-2, BCL-X, and BAX in primary central nervous system lymphomas that occur in immunosuppressed patients. Mod Pathol 13:158–165
29. Camilleri-Broet S, Davi F, Feuillard J et al (1997) AIDS-related primary brain lymphomas: histopathologic and immunohistochemical study of 51 cases. The French Study Group for HIV-Associated Tumors. Hum Pathol 28:367–374
30. Goldstein JD, Dickson DW, Moser FG et al (1991) Primary central nervous system lymphoma in acquired immune deficiency syndrome. A clinical and pathologic study with results of treatment with radiation. Cancer 67:2756–2765
31. Ling SM, Roach M 3rd, Larson DA et al (1994) Radiotherapy of primary central nervous system lymphoma in patients with and without human immunodeficiency virus. Ten years of treatment experience at the University of California San Francisco. Cancer 73:2570–2582
32. Forsyth PA, Yahalom J, DeAngelis LM (1994) Combined-modality therapy in the treatment of primary central nervous system lymphoma in AIDS. Neurology 44:1473–1479
33. Batchelor T, Loeffler JS (2006) Primary CNS lymphoma. J Clin Oncol 24:1281–1288
34. Fine HA, Mayer RJ (1993) Primary central nervous system lymphoma. Ann Intern Med 119:1093–1104
35. Jacomet C, Girard PM, Lebrette MG et al (1997) Intravenous methotrexate for primary central nervous system non-Hodgkin's lymphoma in AIDS. AIDS 11:1725–1730
36. Miller RF, Hall-Craggs MA, Costa DC et al (1998) Magnetic resonance imaging, thallium-201 SPET scanning, and laboratory analyses for discrimination of cerebral lymphoma and toxoplasmosis in AIDS. Sex Transm Infect 74:258–264
37. Ferreri AJ, Blay JY, Reni M et al (2003) Prognostic scoring system for primary CNS lymphomas: the International Extranodal Lymphoma Study Group experience. J Clin Oncol 21:266–272
38. Hoffman JM, Waskin HA, Schifter T et al (1993) FDG-PET in differentiating lymphoma from nonmalignant central nervous system lesions in patients with AIDS. J Nucl Med 34:567–575
39. O'Doherty MJ, Barrington SF, Campbell M et al (1997) PET scanning and the human immunodeficiency virus-positive patient. J Nucl Med 38:1575–1583
40. De Luca A, Antinori A, Cingolani A et al (1995) Evaluation of cerebrospinal fluid EBV-DNA and IL-10 as markers for in vivo diagnosis of AIDS-related primary central nervous system lymphoma. Br J Haematol 90:844–849
41. Cingolani A, De Luca A, Larocca LM et al (1998) Minimally invasive diagnosis of acquired immunodeficiency syndrome-related primary central nervous system lymphoma. J Natl Cancer Inst 90:364–369
42. Antinori A, De Rossi G, Ammassari A et al (1999) Value of combined approach with thallium-201 single-photon emission computed tomography and Epstein-Barr virus DNA polymerase chain reaction in CSF for the diagnosis of AIDS-related primary CNS lymphoma. J Clin Oncol 17:554–560
43. Giancola ML, Rizzi EB, Schiavo R et al (2004) Reduced value of thallium-201 single-photon emission computed tomography in the management of HIV-related focal brain lesions in the era of highly active antiretroviral therapy. AIDS Res Hum Retroviruses 20:584–588
44. Ivers LC, Kim AY, Sax PE (2004) Predictive value of polymerase chain reaction of cerebrospinal fluid for detection of Epstein-Barr virus to establish the diagnosis of HIV-related primary central nervous system lymphoma. Clin Infect Dis 38:1629–1632
45. Wang J, Ozzard A, Nathan M et al (2007) The significance of Epstein-Barr virus detected in the cerebrospinal fluid of people with HIV infection. HIV Med 8:306–311

46. Corcoran C, Rebe K, van der Plas H et al (2008) The predictive value of cerebrospinal fluid Epstein-Barr viral load as a marker of primary central nervous system lymphoma in HIV-infected persons. J Clin Virol 42:433–436
47. Bower M, Collins S, Cottrill C et al (2008) British HIV Association guidelines for HIV-associated malignancies 2008. HIV Med 9:336–388
48. Abrey LE, Batchelor TT, Ferreri AJ et al (2005) Report of an international workshop to standardize baseline evaluation and response criteria for primary CNS lymphoma. J Clin Oncol 23:5034–5043
49. Bower M, Fife K, Sullivan A et al (1999) Treatment outcome in presumed and confirmed AIDS-related primary cerebral lymphoma. Eur J Cancer 35:601–604
50. Chamberlain MC (1994) Long survival in patients with acquired immune deficiency syndrome-related primary central nervous system lymphoma. Cancer 73:1728–1730
51. Weinberg A, Li S, Palmer M et al (2002) Quantitative CSF PCR in Epstein-Barr virus infections of the central nervous system. Ann Neurol 52:543–548
52. Raez L, Cabral L, Cai JP et al (1999) Treatment of AIDS-related primary central nervous system lymphoma with zidovudine, ganciclovir, and interleukin 2. AIDS Res Hum Retroviruses 15:713–719
53. Aboulafia DM, Ratner L, Miles SA et al (2006) Antiviral and immunomodulatory treatment for AIDS-related primary central nervous system lymphoma: AIDS Malignancies Consortium pilot study 019. Clin Lymphoma Myeloma 6:399–402
54. Bossolasco S, Falk KI, Ponzoni M et al (2006) Ganciclovir is associated with low or undetectable Epstein-Barr virus DNA load in cerebrospinal fluid of patients with HIV-related primary central nervous system lymphoma. Clin Infect Dis 42:e21–e25
55. Diamond C, Taylor TH, Im T et al (2006) Highly active antiretroviral therapy is associated with improved survival among patients with AIDS-related primary central nervous system non-Hodgkin's lymphoma. Curr HIV Res 4:375–378
56. Aboulafia DM, Puswella AL (2007) Highly active antiretroviral therapy as the sole treatment for AIDS-related primary central nervous system lymphoma: a case report with implications for treatment. AIDS Patient Care STDS 21:900–907
57. Lin CH, Kuo KT, Chuang SS et al (2006) Comparison of the expression and prognostic significance of differentiation markers between diffuse large B-cell lymphoma of central nervous system origin and peripheral nodal origin. Clin Cancer Res 12:1152–1156

Chapter 11
CNS Post-Transplant Lymphoproliferative Disorder

Samar Issa, M. Beatriz S. Lopes, and David Schiff

Epidemiology

Post-transplant lymphoproliferative disorders (PTLDs) were first recognized in 1968 and central nervous system (CNS) PTLD in 1970 [1]. They arise in both solid organ and bone marrow/stem cell transplant recipients. The causative role of Epstein-Barr virus (EBV) was quickly recognized, although not all PTLD is EBV-driven.

PTLD afflicts < 2% of transplant recipients [2]. It represents the most common cause of post-transplant malignancy in children and the second most common (after skin cancer) in adults [3]. Its incidence varies with the transplanted organ; the highest incidence is seen with multiple organ and small bowel transplants. Lung, liver, and heart transplants have a higher incidence of PTLD than renal transplants; bone marrow transplants are associated with the lowest risk (0.5–1%), and unlike solid organ recipients, tend to develop PTLD of donor origin. Increased risk likely relates in part to the intensity of immunosuppression; the amount of transplanted lymphoid tissue (e.g. in the lung) may also convey risk by increasing the likelihood of EBV infection. EBV seronegativity at the time of transplantation greatly increases the risk, and children are two to three times more likely to develop PTLD than adults, both circumstances relating to the increased risk of acquiring EBV infection.

PTLD may involve the CNS in isolation, or CNS involvement may co-exist with systemic PTLD. CNS involvement was observed in 15% of solid organ transplant recipients with PTLD in the Israel Penn International Transplant Tumor Registry [4, 5]. Approximately half of all CNS PTLD is restricted to the CNS [4, 5]. Herein, we will focus principally on CNS PTLD *without* systemic PTLD, which is better described, despite having fewer than 100 cases reported in detail [6].

D. Schiff (✉)
Departments of Neurology, Neurological Surgery and Medicine, School of Medicine, University of Virginia, Charlottesville, VA 22908-0214, USA
e-mail: davidschiff@virginia.edu

T. Batchelor, L.M. DeAngelis (eds.), *Lymphoma and Leukemia of the Nervous System*, DOI 10.1007/978-1-4419-7668-0_11,

Pathogenesis

The great majority of CNS PTLDs are associated with EBV infection and represents EBV-induced disorders, ranging from monoclonal B-cell lymphomas to less common polyclonal B-cell or monoclonal T-cell proliferations. It is believed that immunosuppressive therapy after transplantation leads to uncontrolled proliferation of EBV-infected B cells. After normal primary EBV infection, usually during childhood or adolescence, the virus remains present as a life-long latent infection in B-lymphocytes under stringent EBV-specific T-cell surveillance. The immunosuppression required by organ transplantation results in decreased T-cell function, allowing unrestricted expansion of EBV-infected B cells, EBV oncogene expression, and ultimately, malignant transformation [7]. This theory is partially supported by the observation that some patients with PTLD respond to reconstitution of the immune response by either decreased immunosuppression or adoptive immunotherapy with infusion of anti-EBV cytotoxic T-lymphocytes (see Treatment).

However, approximately 30% of the systemic PTLDs are EBV-negative [8]. In the CNS, these numbers are less accurate with reports of only a minority of documented cases of EBV-negative primary CNS PTLD [6, 9]. The etiology of EBV-negative PTLD is unknown [8]. Some hypotheses for these cases include undetectable EBV, other unknown causative viruses, and continuous chronic antigenic stimulation including by the transplant itself. Gene expression profiling of EBV-positive and EBV-negative systemic PTLD has demonstrated that these two types of the disease may be distinct biologically, and that EBV-negative monomorphic PTLD is not virally related [10]. In addition to the absence of expression of any EBV-related genes, EBV-negative PTLD cases do not express any virally induced immune response genes [10].

Pathology and Classification

PTLDs are defined by the World Health Organization (WHO) as any lymphoid or plasmacytic proliferation that develops in immunosuppressed recipients of solid organ, bone marrow, or stem cell allografts [8]. The lesions are pathologically characterized by a spectrum of diseases ranging from EBV-related infectious mononucleosis-type polyclonal proliferations to EBV-positive or EBV-negative malignant lymphomas (Table 11.1). In contrast to systemic PTLDs, which are heterogeneous and may include low-grade proliferations like the early lesions and polymorphic PTLD (Table 11.1), PTLDs arising in the CNS are more advanced and aggressive, and in general, are malignant lymphomas.

Monomorphic B-Cell PTLD

The great majority of PTLDs are of B-cell lineage with monoclonal transformed B cells that fulfill the WHO criteria for a diffuse large B-cell lymphoma (DLBCL),

Table 11.1 Pathological classification of post-transplant lymphoproliferative disease (PTLD) according to the WHO classification (2009)

Early lesions
Plasmacytic hyperplasia
Infectious mononucleosis-like lesion
Polymorphic PTLD
Monomorphic PTLD[a]
B-cell neoplasms
Diffuse large B-cell lymphoma
Burkitt lymphoma
Plasma cell neoplasm
Plasmacytoma-like lesion
Other
T-cell neoplasms
Peripheral T-cell lymphoma, NOS
Hepatosplenic T-cell lymphoma
Other
Classical Hodgkin lymphoma-type PTLD

[a]classified according to the lymphoma they resemble

and less frequently for Burkitt lymphoma, plasmacytoma, or other plasmacytic dyscrasias (Table 11.1). Primary CNS PTLDs are usually DLBCL. The lesions are microscopically characterized by large cells, with round or lobated nuclei with vesicular chromatin and prominent nucleoli that are typically admixed with variable numbers of reactive T-cell lymphocytes, histiocytes, and microglia. The lymphomatous infiltrates are poorly delineated, diffusely infiltrate the parenchyma, and show an angiocentric growth pattern, including both perivascular infiltrates and angioinvasion (Fig. 11.1). The transmural invasion of tumor cells with expansion of the vessel wall is highlighted by reticulin stains (Fig. 11.1). Necrosis is commonly seen in lesions with an accentuated angioinvasive pattern. The lesions are distinguished by the expression of B-cell associated antigens, including CD19, CD20 (Fig. 11.1), and CD79a, demonstrate monotypic immunoglobulin light chain (kappa or lambda) restriction, and immunonoglobulin heavy chain gene rearrangement. The presence of EBV can be detected by immunohistochemical analysis for EBV nuclear antigen (EBVNA) or latent membrane protein-1 (LMP-1); however, the most sensitive method is EBV-encoded small RNA in situ hybridization (EBER-ISH) [8] (Fig. 11.1).

Monomorphic T-Cell PTLD

T-cell PTLDs are monoclonal proliferations of T-cells that fulfill the WHO criteria of a T-cell leukemia or lymphoma. The majority of the lesions are peripheral T-cell lymphomas that rarely involve the CNS. In a review of 130 reported cases of combined T- and NK (natural killer)-PTLD, the CNS was involved in only 5% of cases [11]. T-cell PTLDs typically occur late compared to other PTLDs, especially EBV-positive PTLDs. Only one-third of the T-cell PTLDs are EBV-positive proliferations [8].

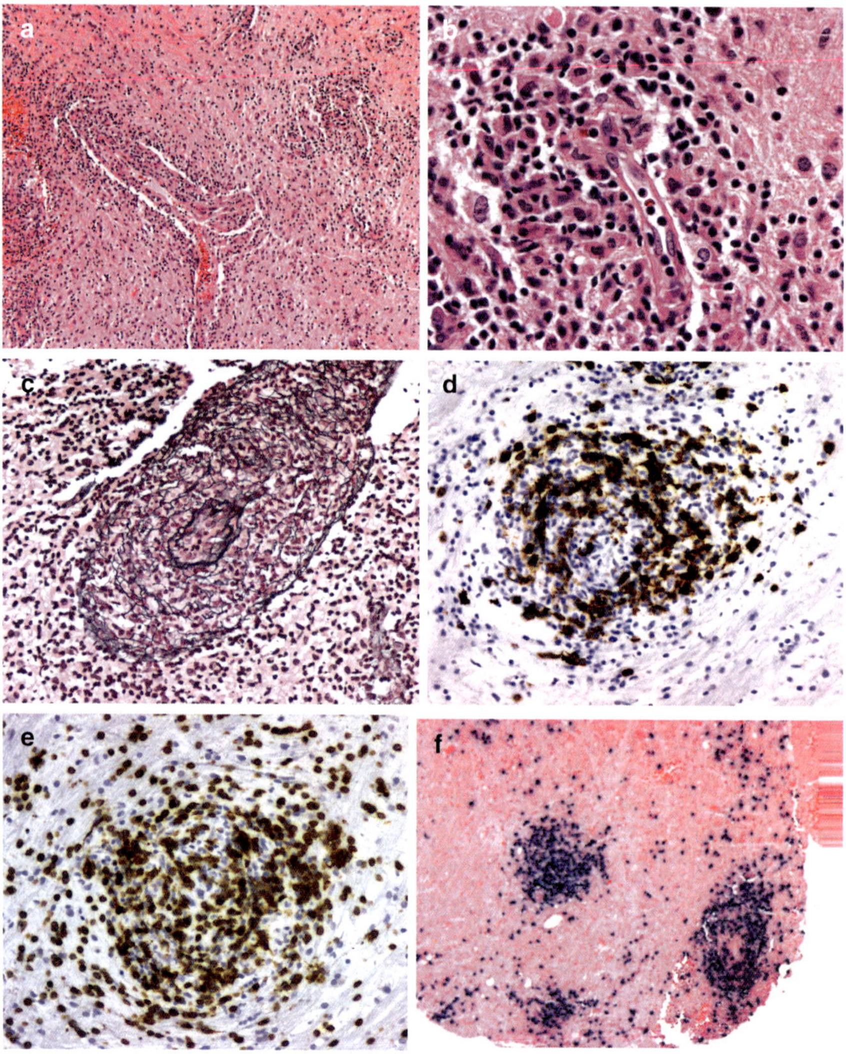

Fig. 11.1 Monomorphic B-cell PTLD – Diffuse large B-cell lymphoma (DLBCL) in a 46-year-old female 5 years following kidney transplantation. **a, b** Large immunoblastic-like cells with prominent nucleoli diffusely infiltrate the brain parenchyma and the perivascular areas. **c** Prominent angioinvasive pattern of the tumor cells with expansion of the vascular wall seen also by reticulin stain. **d** Neoplastic cells are strongly immunoreactive for CD20 suggestive of B-cell population. Monoclonality was confirmed by gene rearrangement assays. **e** Reactive CD5 immunoreactive cells can be prominent. **f** EBER-ISH confirms an EBV infection. [**a:** H&E, ×100; **b:** H&E, ×400; **c:** Wilder's reticulin, ×200; **d:** CD20, ×200; **e:** CD5, ×200; **f:** EBER-ISH, ×100]

Histologically, these lesions are similar to T-cell lymphomas in systemic organs and are characterized by infiltrates of small lymphocytes with irregular nuclear contours. Immunophenotypic analysis shows expression of pan T-cell antigens CD3 and CD5, and the tumors may also express the T-cell subset-associated antigens CD4 or CD8. Clonality is demonstrated by T-cell receptor chain gene rearrangement.

Polymorphic PTLD

Polymorphic PTLDs are histologically characterized by a proliferation of heterogeneous populations of atypical lymphoid cells, ranging from immature B-cells (immunoblasts) to more prominent plasmacytic populations intermixed with small and medium-sized lymphocytes (Fig. 11.2). These infiltrates are destructive of the underlying tissues with focal or diffuse areas of necrosis. Bizarre cells resembling Reed-Sternberg cells may be observed occasionally. Immunophenotypic analysis demonstrates a mixture of B-cells and T-cells in variable proportions. Light chain restriction may be focally demonstrated, and these cases must be distinguished from monomorphic DLBCL-like PTLD. EBV is detected in the great majority of polymorphic PTLD [8] (Fig. 11.2).

The incidence of polymorphic PLTD among primary CNS cases is low, except as reported by Snanoudj et al where they represented 79% of cases [6, 12]. In this series, however, analysis of clonal population lineage was performed in only 13 of the 25 cases.

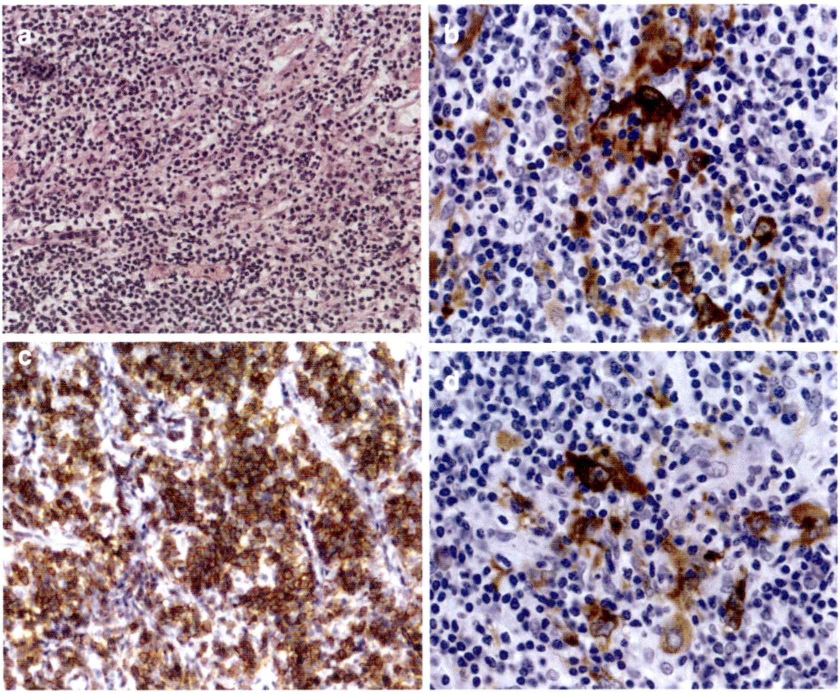

Fig. 11.2 Polymorphic PTLD – Polymorphic, mononucleosis-like lesion in a 23-year-old female 10 years following heart transplantation. **a** Mixed proliferation of immunoblasts, medium-sized lymphocytes and plasma cells diffusely infiltrating the brain parenchyma. Reed-Sternberg-like cells may also be present in the inflammatory infiltrate. **b, c** CD20 (**b**) and CD5 (**c**) immunolabeling demonstrates a heterogeneous population of B- and T-cells, respectively. **d** EBV positive cells are labeled by immunohistochemistry for LMP-1. [**a:** H&E, ×100; **b:** CD20, ×400; **c:** CD5, ×400; **d:** LMP-1 IHC, ×400]

Clinical Manifestations

CNS PTLD can arise anytime following transplantation. While it has been observed in patients less than 3 months following transplantation, approximately 20% of cases occur more than 10 years after transplant [6, 12]. About one-third of cases arise within the first year, and the median time from transplant to CNS PTLD ranges from just over 1–4.4 years in different case series [6, 9, 12, 13].

Neurological presentations of CNS PTLD are variable. Most patients (>80%) have localizable symptoms and signs, such as aphasia, hemiparesis, or ataxia; approximately one-third has seizures [6, 12]. Headache affects 34%, but fevers and other systemic symptoms are exceptional in patients with CNS PTLD restricted to the nervous system. Symptoms typically arise over weeks. Clinical features of vitreal or retinal involvement, as seen in primary CNS lymphoma affecting immunocompetent hosts, are not recognized as part of CNS PTLD [6].

Diagnostic Evaluations

Neuroimaging, preferably MR imaging, is the initial diagnostic test in most patients with suspected CNS PTLD. Neuroimaging is invariably abnormal, and parenchymal brain lesions from CNS PTLD usually demonstrate pathological contrast enhancement that may either be homogenous, heterogeneous, or ring-enhancing [6, 12]; however, some patients have non-enhancing lesions identified best on T2-weighted or FLAIR sequences. The majority of patients (61–83%) have multifocal lesions, commonly in the periventricular regions or deep gray nuclei [6, 9, 12, 13]. One-quarter to one-third of patients has infratentorial lesions; spinal cord lesions are very uncommon. On brain CT, lesions may be either hypo- or hyperdense [12].

CSF is commonly abnormal in CNS PTLD, but rarely in a definitive fashion. A majority of patients have mild pleocytosis and protein elevation [6, 12]. However, an unequivocal demonstration of malignant lymphocytes in CSF is exceptional (one out of 30 patients in the two largest series) [6, 12]. Serum LDH is generally normal or marginally elevated in CNS PTLD. Finally, slit lamp examination, which demonstrates ocular lymphoma in approximately 15% of patients with immunocompetent primary CNS lymphoma, is rarely useful in CNS PTLD [6], although one case of uveitis in a patient with biopsy-proven CNS PTLD has been reported [14].

Differential Diagnosis

The principal diagnostic considerations in a transplant recipient with focal neurological symptoms and signs, with parenchymal brain lesions on CT or MRI, are infection and neoplasm. Organ transplant recipients have impairment of cell-mediated immunity, predisposing to bacterial, fungal, and viral infections. The ten main organisms producing space-occupying lesions in transplant recipients include four fungi (Aspergillus, Zygomyces, Cryptococcus, and Candida), three viruses (varicella-zoster virus, EBV, and JC virus), two bacteria (Mycobacterium tuberculosis and Nocardia), and one parasite (Toxoplasma gondi) [15]. The timing of development of intracranial pathology relative to transplantation may provide valuable clues to a causative infectious agent [16]. Among neoplasms, CNS PTLD is the major consideration, but there is some evidence to suggest that the immunosuppression associated with organ transplantation may predispose to gliomas [17, 18].

Ultimately, most patients with suspected CNS PTLD will undergo a neurosurgical procedure (stereotactic biopsy or craniotomy) unless CSF analysis or biopsy of a non-neural specimen is diagnostic of lymphoma. CNS PTLD is no more predisposed to hemorrhage after stereotactic biopsy than other intracranial lesions [13], and stereotactic biopsy is a safe and effective diagnostic approach [6, 12].

Prognosis

Isolated CNS involvement is rare and is associated with a poor prognosis [19]. CNS PTLDs are more aggressive as a group than PTLDs involving other organ systems [9]. Median survival is short, around 13 weeks, but long-term survival of up to 93 months has been reported [13]. CNS localization of the tumor is, in itself, a poor prognostic factor in both the adult and pediatric populations [9, 20, 21]. Mortality is as high as 60% and 90% of patients who develop CNS PTLD post bone marrow transplantation die, despite treatment [22]. However, survival is still longer in patients with CNS PTLD, compared to PCNSL.

In the systemic PTLD setting, some poor prognostic factors have been identified including: advanced age, elevated LDH [23], recipient EBV seronegativity at the time of transplantation [24], poor performance status [20], presence of B symptoms, severe organ dysfunction, high tumor burden due to multiple extra-nodal sites of involvement ($\geq$4) or advanced stage disease (III&IV), low platelet count and low segmented neutrophil count at diagnosis [25], hematopoietic stem cell transplantation (HST) versus solid organ transplant [25, 26], especially if it is done for hematological malignancies versus immunodeficiency disorders. Grafted organ involvement was a poor prognostic factor in one study [27], and favorable in another [28]. EBV negative tumor and late onset PTLD are both poor prognostic factors. One report demonstrated that hepatitis B or C infections conferred a poor prognosis. PTLDs following allogeneic stem cell transplants have a worse outcome than PTLDs following solid organ transplant with an overall mortality of up to 92% [25, 28]. Treatment with azathioprine carried a higher risk of death among CNS PTLD patients in one study [28]. In the rituximab era, CD20 positivity of the tumor tissue has a positive influence on survival for all PTLD patients [29], however, no data are published thus far on its prognostic value in CNS PTLD.

A prognostic model has been developed by Choquet et al for PTLD patients without CNS involvement using the performance status (PS) $\geq$2, and number of involved sites >1. Three risk groups can be identified using this system: low risk (PS≤2 & 1 site), intermediate risk (PS ≥ 2 or > 1 site), high risk (PS ≥ 2 & > 1 site), the median survival has not been reached in the low-risk group, is 34 months in the intermediate-risk group, and is 1 month in the high-risk group.

Although factors that confer a poor prognosis have been identified in patients with PCNSL (age >60 year, poor performance status (ECOG >1), elevated LDH, high CSF protein concentration and deep brain location), no specific prognostic scoring system has been established for CNS PTLD [31, 32].

In the Israel Penn International Transplant Tumor Registry (IPITTR), 136 (15%) of 910 PTLD cases reported had CNS PTLD. Approximately half of the CNS PTLD cases were restricted to the CNS. Better survival was noted in patients with isolated CNS involvement versus multiple site involvement including the brain, particularly in children [4].

There are few published data on the prognostic factors that determine survival in CNS PTLD. Age does not appear to be a negative prognostic factor [9], unlike the situation in the PCNSL population, in which age >60, or even 50, years is a negative prognostic factor. Patient outcome is dependent on the histological grade with monomorphic histology conferring worse prognosis compared to the polymorphic subtype (78% versus 0% PTLD-related mortality) [33]. CNS PTLD prognosis is dependent on the type of transplant as well. CNS PTLD that develops after bone marrow transplantation may be more prevalent and has a worse outcome compared to PTLD that develops after solid organ transplant, as the former is driven by the allografted stem cells [9, 22]. HLA mismatch, T cell depletion and Anti-Thymocyte Globulin (ATG) conditioning increase the risk of developing CNS PTLD after bone marrow transplantation due to the lack of a T cell response to the EBV infection/reactivation [9, 34]. In the setting of solid organ transplantation, younger age, cytomegalovirus (CMV) infection, EBV negative recipient (and positive donor), and high intensity immunosuppressant therapy are all risk factors for developing CNS PTLD [34].

The prognosis also depends on the response to the reduction in the immunosuppressive treatment, with better survival achieved in patients who respond to this modality [9]; this is likely a reflection of the histological subtype as polymorphic disease is usually responsive to a reduction in immunosuppression, suggesting the PTLD has not transformed to a monoclonal malignancy.

A Mayo Clinic review [35] of 381 non-renal transplant patients demonstrated that the risk of PTLD increased by a factor of 654 if patients had all the following risk factors: EBV seronegative recipients, OKT3 therapy and CMV seromismatch, compared with a low incidence if none of these factors were present (0.458 cases per 100 person years). The use of azathioprine-based therapies may lead to a higher risk of CNS PTLD while cyclosporine-based regimens were more closely associated with non-CNS PTLD involving the lymph nodes. There is evidence that since the introduction of cyclosporine in the post- renal transplant setting, there has been a reduction in the incidence of CNS PTLD [9] [19, 30].

In the pediatric population, stage IV PTLD (with bone marrow and/or CNS involvement) was an independent risk factor for poor survival after solid organ transplantation [21].

Increased LDH might be a poor prognostic factor [23].

Treatment

There are limited data on the treatment of CNS PTLD. Many treatment modalities have been attempted alone or in combination. These include: reduction in immunosuppression; surgery; steroids; radiation therapy; chemotherapy; chemoradiotherapy; monoclonal antibodies; cellular therapy; antivirals and alpha interferon. It is difficult to recommend one modality over another based on the limited experience published thus far. Multimodality treatment tailored to the special needs of each CNS PTLD is recommended. The treatment should be instituted as soon as the diagnosis is made to minimize the risk of irreversible neurological injury.

Reduction in Immunosuppression

PTLD usually results from impaired immune-mediated activity of the cytotoxic T cell population due to immunosuppressant drugs. Consequently, there is a proliferation of EBV infected B cells that may result in PTLD. Reduction or cessation of the immunosuppressant drugs is typically recommended in patients with PTLD. It is also suggested that the risk of PTLD is related to the intensity of the immunosuppression.

Reduction of immunosuppression is generally insufficient as an effective treatment in the case of CNS PTLD for many reasons. First, the location of the disease in the immune-privileged CNS with its relative paucity of lymphocyte trafficking makes it difficult for a strategy dependent on reconstitution of the immune system to work. Thus, in the CNS, EBV infection can drive the neoplastic progression more efficiently. The lack of a lymphatic drainage system and low numbers of mononuclear cells in the CNS may contribute to an inability to control the proliferation of neoplastic cells that have either arisen locally or disseminated into the CNS from an extraneural location [5]. Second, the pathologic characterization of this disease in the CNS, which is monomorphic in most instances, is unfavorable. Published data indicate that the majority of polymorphic PTLD responds to reduction of immunotherapy, but those with monomorphic disease have a more aggressive course and respond poorly to treatment [36]. Third, the course of CNS PTLD is rapidly progressive with neurological impairment and thus, requires immediate treatment to ensure rapid response, something that reduction in immunosuppression cannot provide [37, 38].

Reduction of immunosuppression as the sole treatment for CNS PTLD has resulted in low remission rates. One of 18 patients achieved complete remission with this modality alone, and the only responding patient relapsed 40 months later and then died [12]. In another study, 4/12 patients recovered with decreased immunosuppression in combination with other modalities (including multiagent chemotherapy, steroids, rituximab, radiotherapy, and cytotoxic T cell infusions). These patients had no evidence of disease at 12, 14, 23 and 62 months of follow-up [9]. There are reports of CNS PTLD responding to reduction of immunosuppression and antiviral therapy early in the disease course. This is possibly due to early treatment prior to the neoplastic transformation, suggesting that early diagnosis and prompt treatment hold the best chance of remission in CNS PTLD [39]. T-cell PTLD is rarely associated with EBV infection; hence reduction in immunosuppression is not effective [40].

Surgical Resection

Complete remission has been reported post surgical excision of solitary lesions in the brain [12]. Two of 25 patients with localized CNS PTLD underwent gross total resection, but one patient died 1 month post surgery of infection, and the other relapsed 10 months later. Thus, surgical resection is reserved for the rare patient who requires immediate debulking of mass effect and must be followed by some other form of therapy (Fig. 11.3).

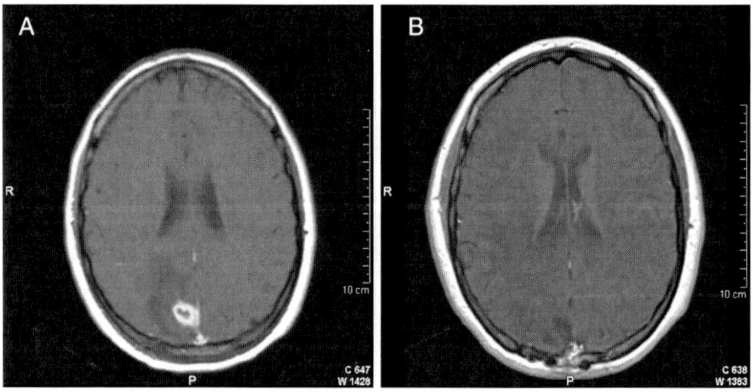

Fig. 11.3 A 23-year old woman with a history of cardiac transplantation a decade earlier for anthracycline-related cardiomyopathy presented with a left hemiparesis. T1-weighted post-contrast MRI demonstrated a right parietal mass (Fig. 11.3a); systemic staging was negative. Gross total resection was performed, revealing an EBV-positive PTLD (shown in Fig. 11.2). Postoperatively, she received five cycles of high-dose intravenous methotrexate, vincristine and procarbazine followed by two cycles of intravenous cytarabine. She remains in remission six-plus years later (Fig. 11.3b)

Steroids

PCNSL in immunocompetent hosts is steroid-responsive, but is incurable using this treatment alone [41]. Most CNS PTLD patients are already on corticosteroids post-transplant, and typically the dose is increased when CNS PTLD is diagnosed. Dexamethasone is commonly administered once the diagnosis is made to reduce brain edema. Complete response has been reported following a single pulse of methylprednisolone [12]. However, steroids as the sole modality of therapy are not recommended.

Radiotherapy

Whole brain radiotherapy (WBRT) alone in immunocompetent PCNSL achieves a median survival of only 11–21.5 months [42]. Since CNS PTLD was first described, WBRT has been used effectively as first line treatment because of the high rate and rapidity of response.

A review of the IPITTR suggested that radiotherapy appeared to provide the best outcome; 3 year survival was achieved in 7 of 28 (25%) patients [4]. In a review by Penn et al of 30 CNS PTLD patients who achieved CR following treatment, radiotherapy (as a single agent modality in most patients) again appeared to be the most effective treatment [5]. A case report documents successful use of WBRT (40 Gy) in EBV- associated T/NK cell type CNS PTLD in a renal transplant patient [43]. Durable survival can be achieved with fractionated radiotherapy (alone, or in combination with other modalities like chemotherapy). In the Penn series, 10/30 (33%) patients were alive for >5 years, 6 of whom survived for more than 10 years. However, the risk of post-treatment neurotoxicity and death was significant. Although 39/198 patients achieved a complete remission (20%), 17 of them subsequently died, including 3 deaths due to cerebrovascular accidents [5].

High-Dose Methotrexate

High-dose methotrexate (HDMTX), alone or in combination, has considerable activity in immunocompetent patients with PCNSL, as MTX crosses the blood brain barrier at high doses [44]. Despite concern regarding the development of MTX toxicity in renal and liver transplant patients because of its direct renal and hepatic toxicity [36], HDMTX alone (dose 1–5 g/m^2) has been used effectively and without hepatotoxicity in pediatric patients with CNS PTLD in the post liver transplant setting.

A recent published report described six patients with renal allografts and histologically proven isolated CNS PTLD [45]. All six patients were treated with high-dose intravenous methotrexate (HDMTX) 8 g/m^2, with dose adjustments for creatinine clearance. Four patients achieved a complete response. These results suggest that as in PCNSL, CNS PTLD is sometimes highly responsive to single agent HDMTX. Caution should be taken when HDMTX is given to patients with low glomerular filtration rate. In high-risk patients, in addition to dose adjustment, more aggressive use of folinic acid rescue may be necessary. It is critical to remember that MTX cannot be removed with conventional dialysis.

Other Chemotherapy

Despite concerns that combination chemotherapy may be undesirable in CNS PTLD due to potentially severe immunosuppressive effects in heavily immunosuppressed patients [5], such an approach has been utilized with acceptable morbidity (Fig. 11.4). Typically, as in PCNSL, such regimens include a backbone of HDMTX, with other agents that cross the blood-brain barrier, including temozolomide, procarbazine, vincristine, doxorubicin, cytarabine, ifosfamide, etoposide, and cyclophosphamide [6, 12].

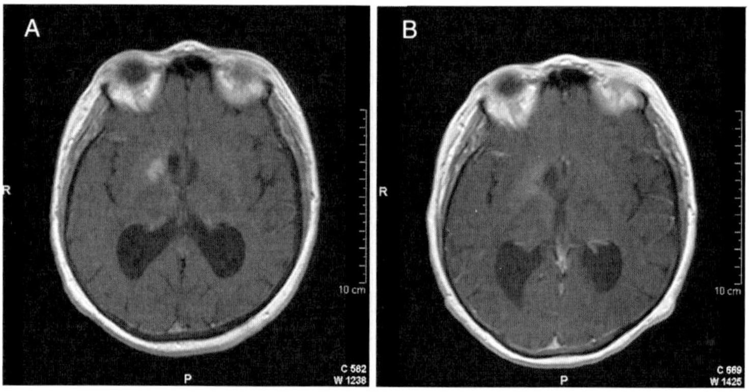

Fig. 11.4 A 46 year old woman with diabetic nephropathy, status post renal transplantation, developed headaches and a *left* hemiparesis. Stereotactic biopsy of a *right* basal ganglia mass that demonstrated T1 hyperintensity on post-contrast images (Fig. 11.4a) demonstrated EBV-positive B-cell PTLD (shown in Fig. 11.1). She received 5 cycles of rituximab, high-dose intravenous methotrexate, procarbazine and vincristine. She achieved a complete response and remains in remission 18 months later (Fig. 11.4b – the slight peripheral hyperintensity was present on pre-contrast T1-weighted images)

Chemoradiotherapy

The addition of HDMTX or cytarabine to radiation therapy improved survival in one CNS PTLD report (median survival 42 versus 21 months); however, it is associated with increased risk of treatment-related leukoencephalopathy [12]. Three severe postradiation leukoencephalopathies were observed among patients lacking the usual risk factors for treatment toxicity (cumulative radiotherapy dose of 50 Gy and age >60 years). As such, the combination of radiotherapy and chemotherapy appears to be associated with radiographic response, but neurotoxicity is prohibitive.

Immunotherapy

Treatment of CNS NHL by local infusion of B cell specific monoclonal antibodies was attempted in the early 1990s [46]; since then, there have been many published reports on the use of anti-CD 20 in PCNSL. However, CNS involvement is a predictor of poor response to anti-CD 20 antibodies [22].

Rituximab

Rituximab is a chimeric murine/human anti-CD20 monoclonal antibody effective in the treatment of CD20-positive systemic NHL [47]. It works by depleting the circulation of CD20-positive B lymphocytes via complement-dependent cytotoxicity. Its use in PCNSL represents a therapeutic challenge since its large molecular weight limits CNS penetration. Its value in immunocompetent PCNSL remains to be proven, although there are anecdotal reports of responses in the literature [48]. During the early phases of PCNSL treatment, the blood brain barrier is disrupted with increased vascular permeability [49]. Rituximab can be reproducibly detected in the CSF of patients with PCNSL who are treated systemically with this drug [50, 51]. Rituximab has improved survival in CD20 positive systemic PTLD with an overall response rate of 60–70% [6, 22, 29, 52]. A few case reports on the successful use of rituximab in the setting of PTLD with CNS involvement have been published [6, 53, 54]. An intensive, dose-escalated biweekly schedule has been used because of concerns of limited rituximab penetration into the CNS [14], but it also has been used as weekly infusions of 375 mg/m^2 for 5 weeks with good response [55].

Intrathecal rituximab has been used successfully in a small number of patients with relapsed CNS lymphoma; more data are required before it is recommended for use in CNS PTLD.

Anti-CD21 and Anti-CD24 Monoclonal Antibodies

The results on the use of anti-CD21 and anti-CD24 murine antibodies in CNS PTLD have been disappointing [22]; only 4/14 patients (29%) achieved remission when these antibodies were used. This is likely due to the inaccessibility of these antibodies to the CNS when they are injected intravenously. Two patients treated with intraventricular anti-CD21 infusions died early of disease progression [12].

Cellular Therapy

There are reports indicating successful use of EBV-specific cytotoxic T lymphocyte (CTL) infusions in patients with PTLD that developed after hematopoietic stem cell transplantation [56]. This treatment has not been used in CNS PTLD, and is also not readily available. Donor lymphocyte infusion (DLI) may be used with the same effect in the setting of post bone marrow transplant lymphoproliferative disorder [55]. The use of EBV-specific CTLs might not be restricted to the setting of bone marrow transplantation; a child with CNS PTLD, following lung transplant, achieved complete remission after receiving a CTL infusion from an HLA-matched sibling [57]. Seven solid organ transplant recipients with PTLD received autologous lymphokine activated killer cells (LAK); peripheral blood mononuclear cells were collected from these patients, cultured with recombinant human IL-2, and reinfused. All four EBV-positive tumors regressed, but two patients suffered organ rejection [58].

Antiviral Treatment

As most PTLDs are associated with EBV infections, a strategy of EBV surveillance might be of value. In the high-risk patient setting [34], these markers tend to rise prior to PTLD development and peak at diagnosis [59]; however, the use of antivirals was ineffective in preventing PTLD in EBV-negative patients [60].

There are reports on the prophylactic use of antivirals to prevent EBV reactivation in high-risk patients, but no randomized trials on its effectiveness. A case report successfully incorporating use of the antiviral drug cidofovir in the setting of EBV reactivation and CNS PTLD has been published [55]. Phan et al have shown that antiviral treatment with acyclovir or valacyclovir has no effect on CNS PTLD progression [13].

Cytokine Therapy

Deletions of the interferon alpha gene have been observed in PTLD patients. Treatment with alpha interferon has led to clinical improvement in some PTLD patients through an effect on type 2 helper T lymphocytes [13]. Interferon alpha is also known to have antiviral and antiproliferative effects, but its use could lead to organ rejection due to its immunostimulatory effects [5]. Several case reports describe the successful use of interferon alpha in combination with intravenous immunoglobulins in the setting of PTLD [61]. IL-6 could be a target, as it promotes the growth of B cells.

Intrathecal Treatments

These have generally been used in combination with systemic chemotherapy or anti-CD20 antibodies. Intrathecal methotrexate, methylprednisolone, and rituximab were used in combination with systemic chemotherapy in a patient with CNS PTLD, with leptomeningeal lymphomatosis [55]. As most CNS PTLDs involve the brain parenchyma alone, justification for routine use of intrathecal therapy is lacking.

References

1. Schneck SA, Penn I (1970) Cerebral neoplasms associated with renal transplantation. Arch Neurol 22:226–233
2. Dharnidharka VR, Tejani AH, Ho PL, Harmon WE (2002) Post-transplant lymphoproliferative disorder in the United States: young Caucasian males are at highest risk. Am J Transplant 2:993–998
3. Taylor AL, Marcus R, Bradley JA (2005) Post-transplant lymphoproliferative disorders (PTLD) after solid organ transplantation. Crit Rev Oncol Hematol 56:155–167
4. Buell JF, Gross TG, Hanaway MJ et al (2005) Posttransplant lymphoproliferative disorder: significance of central nervous system involvement. Transplant Proc 37:954–955
5. Penn I, Porat G (1995) Central nervous system lymphomas in organ allograft recipients. Transplantation 59:240–244
6. Cavaliere R, Petroni G, Lopes MB, Schiff D (2010) Primary CNS post-transplant lymphoproliferative disorder. The International PCNSL Collaborative Group Experience. Cancer 116:863–870
7. Tanner JE, Alfieri C (2001) The Epstein-Barr virus and post-transplant lymphoproliferative disease: interplay of immunosuppression, EBV, and the immune system in disease pathogenesis. Transpl Infect Dis 3:60–69
8. Swerdlow SH, Webber SA, Chadburn A, Ferry JA (2008) Post-transplant lymphoproliferative disorders. In: Swerdlow SH (ed) WHO Classification of Tumours of Haematopoietic and Lymphoid Tissues, International Agency for Research on Cancer, Lyon, pp 343–349
9. Castellano-Sanchez AA, Li S, Qian J et al (2004) Primary central nervous system posttransplant lymphoproliferative disorders. Am J Clin Pathol 121:246–253
10. Craig FE, Johnson LR, Harvey SA et al (2007) Gene expression profiling of Epstein-Barr virus-positive and -negative monomorphic B-cell posttransplant lymphoproliferative disorders. Diagn Mol Pathol 16:158–168
11. Swerdlow SH (2007) T-cell and NK-cell posttransplantation lymphoproliferative disorders. Am J Clin Pathol 127:887–895
12. Snanoudj R, Durrbach A, Leblond V et al (2003) Primary brain lymphomas after kidney transplantation: presentation and outcome. Transplantation 76:930–937
13. Phan TG, O'Neill BP, Kurtin PJ (2000) Posttransplant primary CNS lymphoma. Neuro Oncol 2:229–238
14. Traum AZ, Rodig NM, Pilichowska ME, Somers MJ (2006) Central nervous system lymphoproliferative disorder in pediatric kidney transplant recipients. Pediatr Transplant 10:505–512
15. Pruitt AA (2008) Central nervous system infections in cancer patients. In: Schiff D, Kesari S, Wen PY (eds) Cancer Neurology in Clinical Practice, 2nd edn. Humana Press, Totowa, NJ, pp 353–380
16. Rubin RH, Wolfson JS, Cosimi AB, Tolkoff-Rubin NE (1981) Infection in the renal transplant recipient. Am J Med 70:405–411

17. Schiff D, O'Neill B, Wijdicks E et al (2001) Gliomas arising in organ transplant recipients: an unrecognized complication of transplantation? Neurology 57:1486–1488
18. Schiff D (2004) Gliomas following organ transplantation: analysis of the contents of a tumor registry. J Neurosurg 101:932–934
19. Opelz G, Henderson R (1993) Incidence of non-Hodgkin lymphoma in kidney and heart transplant recipients. Lancet 342:1514–1516
20. Leblond V, Dhedin N, Mamzer Bruneel MF et al (2001) Identification of prognostic factors in 61 patients with posttransplantation lymphoproliferative disorders. J Clin Oncol 19:772–778
21. Maecker B, Jack T, Zimmermann M et al (2007) CNS or bone marrow involvement as risk factors for poor survival in post-transplantation lymphoproliferative disorders in children after solid organ transplantation. J Clin Oncol 25:4902–4908
22. Benkerrou M, Jais JP, Leblond V et al (1998) Anti-B-cell monoclonal antibody treatment of severe posttransplant B-lymphoproliferative disorder: prognostic factors and long-term outcome. Blood 92:3137–3147
23. Crawford DH, Mulholland N, Iliescu V et al (1986) Epstein-Barr virus infection and immunity in bone marrow transplant recipients. Transplantation 42:50–54
24. Knight JS, Tsodikov A, Cibrik DM et al (2009) Lymphoma after solid organ transplantation: risk, response to therapy, and survival at a transplantation center. J Clin Oncol 27:3354–3362
25. Dror Y, Greenberg M, Taylor G et al (1999) Lymphoproliferative disorders after organ transplantation in children. Transplantation 67:990–998
26. Gross TG, Steinbuch M, DeFor T et al (1999) B cell lymphoproliferative disorders following hematopoietic stem cell transplantation: risk factors, treatment and outcome. Bone Marrow Transplant 23:251–258
27. Ghobrial IM, Habermann TM, Maurer MJ et al (2005) Prognostic analysis for survival in adult solid organ transplant recipients with post-transplantation lymphoproliferative disorders. J Clin Oncol 23:7574–7582
28. Caillard S, Lelong C, Pessione F, Moulin B (2006) Post-transplant lymphoproliferative disorders occurring after renal transplantation in adults: report of 230 cases from the French Registry. Am J Transplant 6:2735–2742
29. Ghobrial IM, Habermann TM, Ristow KM et al (2005) Prognostic factors in patients with post-transplant lymphoproliferative disorders (PTLD) in the rituximab era. Leuk Lymphoma 46:191–196
30. Choquet S, Mamzer BM, Hermine O et al (2002) Identification of prognostic factors in post-transplant lymphoproliferative disorders. Recent Results Cancer Res 159:67–80
31. Ferreri AJ, Blay JY, Reni M et al (2003) Prognostic scoring system for primary CNS lymphomas: the International Extranodal Lymphoma Study Group experience. J Clin Oncol 21:266–272
32. Abrey LE, Ben-Porat L, Panageas KS et al (2006) Primary central nervous system lymphoma: the Memorial Sloan-Kettering Cancer Center prognostic model. J Clin Oncol 24:5711–5715
33. Miller WT Jr, Siegel SG, Montone KT (1997) Posttransplantation lymphoproliferative disorder: changing manifestations of disease in a renal transplant population. Crit Rev Diagn Imaging 38:569–585
34. Loren AW, Porter DL, Stadtmauer EA, Tsai DE (2003) Post-transplant lymphoproliferative disorder: a review. Bone Marrow Transplant 31:145–155
35. Walker RC, Marshall WF, Strickler JG et al (1995) Pretransplantation assessment of the risk of lymphoproliferative disorder. Clin Infect Dis 20:1346–1353
36. Taj MM, Messahel B, Mycroft J et al (2008) Efficacy and tolerability of high-dose methotrexate in central nervous system positive or relapsed lymphoproliferative disease following liver transplant in children. Br J Haematol 140:191–196
37. Chadburn A, Chen JM, Hsu DT et al (1998) The morphologic and molecular genetic categories of posttransplantation lymphoproliferative disorders are clinically relevant. Cancer 82:1978–1987

38. Armitage JM, Kormos RL, Stuart RS et al (1991) Posttransplant lymphoproliferative disease in thoracic organ transplant patients: ten years of cyclosporine-based immunosuppression. J Heart Lung Transplant 10:877–886; discussion 886–877
39. Patchell RA (1988) Primary central nervous system lymphoma in the transplant patient. Neurol Clin 6:297
40. Waller EK, Ziemianska M, Bangs CD et al (1993) Characterization of posttransplant lymphomas that express T-cell-associated markers: immunophenotypes, molecular genetics, cytogenetics, and heterotransplantation in severe combined immunodeficient mice. Blood 82:247–261
41. DeAngelis LM (1999) Primary central nervous system lymphoma. Curr Opin Neurol 12:687–691
42. Deangelis LM, Hormigo A (2004) Treatment of primary central nervous system lymphoma. Semin Oncol 31:684–692
43. Omori N, Narai H, Tanaka T et al (2008) Epstein-Barr virus-associated T/NK cell-type central nervous system lymphoma which manifested as a post-transplantation lymphoproliferative disorder in a renal transplant recipient. J Neurooncol 87:189–191
44. Batchelor T, Carson K, O'Neill A et al (2003) Treatment of primary CNS lymphoma with methotrexate and deferred radiotherapy: a report of NABTT 96-07. J Clin Oncol 21: 1044–1049
45. Nabors LB, Palmer CA, Julian BA et al (2009) Isolated central nervous system posttransplant lymphoproliferative disorder treated with high-dose intravenous methotrexate. Am J Transplant 9:1243–1248
46. Stephan JL, Le Deist F, Blanche S et al (1992) Treatment of central nervous system B lymphoproliferative syndrome by local infusion of a B cell-specific monoclonal antibody. Transplantation 54:246–249
47. Coiffier B, Lepage E, Briere J et al (2002) CHOP chemotherapy plus rituximab compared with CHOP alone in elderly patients with diffuse large-B-cell lymphoma. N Engl J Med 346:235–242
48. Shah GD, Yahalom J, Correa DD et al (2007) Combined immunochemotherapy with reduced whole-brain radiotherapy for newly diagnosed primary CNS lymphoma. J Clin Oncol 25:4730–4735
49. Rubenstein J, Fischbein N, Aldape K et al (2002) Hemorrhage and VEGF expression in a case of primary CNS lymphoma. J Neurooncol 58:53–56
50. Rubenstein JL, Combs D, Rosenberg J et al (2003) Rituximab therapy for CNS lymphomas: targeting the leptomeningeal compartment. Blood 101:466–468
51. Stern JI, Raizer JJ (2005) Primary central nervous system lymphoma. Expert Rev Neurother 5:S63–S70
52. Ifthikharuddin JJ, Mieles LA, Rosenblatt JD et al (2000) CD-20 expression in post-transplant lymphoproliferative disorders: treatment with rituximab. Am J Hematol 65:171–173
53. Reshef R, Tsai DE (2008) Rituximab for PTLD of the CNS: is it a "no-brainer"? Onkologie 31:650–651
54. Kordelas L, Trenschel R, Koldehoff M et al (2008) Successful treatment of EBV PTLD with CNS lymphomas with the monoclonal anti-CD20 antibody rituximab. Onkologie 31:691–693
55. Nozzoli C, Bartolozzi B, Guidi S et al (2006) Epstein-Barr virus-associated post-transplant lymphoproliferative disease with central nervous system involvement after unrelated allogeneic hematopoietic stem cell transplantation. Leuk Lymphoma 47:167–169
56. Pakakasama S, Eames GM, Morriss MC et al (2004) Treatment of Epstein-Barr virus lymphoproliferative disease after hematopoietic stem-cell transplantation with hydroxyurea and cytotoxic T-cell lymphocytes. Transplantation 78:755–757
57. Emanuel DJ, Lucas KG, Mallory GB Jr et al (1997) Treatment of posttransplant lymphoproliferative disease in the central nervous system of a lung transplant recipient using allogeneic leukocytes. Transplantation 63:1691–1694

58. Nalesnik MA, Rao AS, Zeevi A et al (1997) Autologous lymphokine-activated killer cell therapy of lymphoproliferative disorders arising in organ transplant recipients. Transplant Proc 29:1905–1906
59. Kenagy DN, Schlesinger Y, Weck K et al (1995) Epstein-Barr virus DNA in peripheral blood leukocytes of patients with posttransplant lymphoproliferative disease. Transplantation 60:547–554
60. Aris RM, Maia DM, Neuringer IP et al (1996) Post-transplantation lymphoproliferative disorder in the Epstein-Barr virus-naive lung transplant recipient. Am J Respir Crit Care Med 154:1712–1717
61. Davis CL, Wood BL, Sabath DE et al (1998) Interferon-alpha treatment of posttransplant lymphoproliferative disorder in recipients of solid organ transplants. Transplantation 66:1770–1779

Chapter 12
Intraocular Lymphoma

Andrés J.M. Ferreri, Silvia Govi, and José S. Pulido

Introduction

Intraocular lymphoma (IOL) is an uncommon malignancy with three different clinical forms, according to the presence or absence of concomitant lymphomatous lesions in other central nervous system (CNS) areas or in distant organs. In the present chapter, disease exclusively involving ocular structures will be termed primary intraocular lymphoma (PIOL; ~17% of all cases of lymphoma involving the eyes), intraocular involvement concomitant with involvement of other CNS areas, the most common form of IOL (~60% of cases), will be termed primary CNS lymphoma with intraocular disease (PCNSL+IOL) and involvement of the eyes by a disseminated lymphoma, the rarest form of IOL (5–15% of lymphomas involving the eyes) [1], will be termed secondary intraocular lymphoma (SIOL). The definition of these forms is often difficult due to variable clinical presentation and behavior. For example, intraocular involvement can be detected during clinical staging in 15–25% of patients presenting with brain lymphomatous lesions [2–4]; while 50–80% of patients with IOL will develop parenchymal brain lesions, in a period ranging from weeks to years from the onset of ocular symptoms [3–5]. Moreover, IOL may be detected only at relapse in PCNSL patients, with or without concomitant brain disease; intraocular recurrence is observed in ~25% of patients with PCNSL without ocular involvement at the initial diagnosis [6]. IOL can be stratified also on the basis of the ocular structures infiltrated; the vitreoretinal form is the most common presentation of IOL, while lymphomas arising in the iris or the choroid are less common forms, with particular clinical and histopathological characteristics.

Because of its rarity, heterogeneous presentation and, as described later, relatively poor prognosis, IOL represents a complex diagnostic and therapeutic challenge for a multidisciplinary group of physicians. In this chapter, risk factors,

A.J.M. Ferreri (✉)
Unit of Lymphoid Malignancies, Medical Oncology Unit, Department of Oncology, San Raffaele Scientific Institute, Milan, Italy
e-mail: andres.ferreri@hsr.it

T. Batchelor, L.M. DeAngelis (eds.), *Lymphoma and Leukemia of the Nervous System*, DOI 10.1007/978-1-4419-7668-0_12,

epidemiology, presentation, molecular and morphological features, treatment, and prognosis of IOL will be reviewed. Most concepts in this chapter pertain to vitreoretinal lymphoma, while other rare forms of IOL are reviewed in the last part of the chapter.

Incidence and Risk Factors

Studies focused on epidemiological trends in PIOL do not exist. Data on the incidence of this condition can be indirectly obtained from epidemiological studies on PCNSL patients. PCNSL and IOL constitute approximately 1% of all non-Hodgkin lymphomas, 1% of intracranial tumors, and less than 1% of intraocular tumors [7]. The increase in the overall incidence of PCNSL is a matter of debate (see Chapter 4). Discrepancies in reported studies are mainly due to the data source, the period of analysis and the inclusion, or not of HIV-positive individuals. According to the National Cancer Institute Surveillance, Epidemiology and End Results (SEER) program [6, 8], the incidence of PCNSL rose from 0.027 per 100,000 in 1973 to 0.075 in 1983 and 1.0 per 100,000 in early 1990s, indicating more than a 30-fold increase over these three decades. The main cause of the increased incidence of PCNSL is related to the growing prevalence of immunodeficiency and immunosuppression, in particular, the HIV pandemic [6, 9]. In fact, the risk of development of PCNSL among patients with AIDS was 3,600-fold higher compared to the general population in the pre-highly active antiretroviral therapy (HAART) era [10]. With more disseminated use of HAART, the incidence of PCNSL in AIDS patients has been significantly reduced [11]. Other conditions of immune deficiency, such as congenital immune deficiency and systemic autoimmune disease, also confer a higher risk of PCNSL [10, 12].

In Japan, a nationwide survey on uveitis was conducted at 41 university hospitals. A total of 151,299 new patients with various ocular diseases presented to the outpatient clinics of the eye departments of these university hospitals in 2002, and 3,060 [2.2%] of these patients were affected by various clinical forms of uveitis, including 32 patients with IOL. These data indicate that IOL consists of ~1% of uveitis patients and ~0.021% of all patients with ocular diseases at referral eye centers in Japan. Based on these data, the incidence of PIOL can be estimated to be ~21 per 100,000 patients with ocular disorders presenting to referral eye centers each year.

The median age of onset of PCNSL+IOL/PIOL in immunocompetent patients is the late 50's and 60's, with a reported range of 15–85 years of age for PIOL [13, 14]. However, rare cases in young children have also been reported [15]. IOL is slightly more common in men with a male to female ratio, ranging from 1.2 to 1.7, with a single small retrospective study, suggesting a higher prevalence among women [16]. A survey of incidence of PCNSL in American whites and blacks has shown no racial differences [17], though a more recent study has shown a racial preference [18]. In this study, the PCNSL incidence for black patients ages 20–49 years was twice that of whites, while the incidence of PCNSL in white patients over age 49 years was twice that for blacks.

Risk factors for IOL have not been clearly identified. The role of infectious agents in the development of PCNSL, and consequently in IOL, is a matter of debate. The association between lymphotropic viruses, such as HIV and Epstein-Barr Virus (EBV), and PCNSL development has been well-documented in immunodeficient patients [19], while a role for other viruses, like polyomaviruses [SV40, BK, JC], has been excluded, both in AIDS-related and immunocompetent patients with PCNSL [20]. Interestingly, DNA from human herpesvirus-8 (HHV-8), EBV and *Toxoplasma gondii* was detected in 19, 10 and 13% of IOL cases, respectively in one series [21, 22], while another series did not find similar results for HHV-8 infection.

Clinical Presentation

Within the eyes, lymphoma cells usually infiltrate the vitreous, retina, subretinal pigment epithelium, and/or the optic nerve [23]. Thus, IOL is associated with a wide variety of clinical manifestations, masquerading as many other diseases. Retinal lymphomas account for most cases of IOL [24], usually being associated with vitreous involvement. Rarely, retinal tumor deposits may occur without any vitreous cells, and vice versa [25]. These different clinical varieties are based on ophthalmoscopy, which may not allow detection of minimal retinal tumor deposits. Lymphoma infiltrates present as diffuse vitreous opacities and multiple retinal or subretinal creamy-white lesions, which can be either small or large and diffuse [26]. These lesions resemble uveitis and are often misdiagnosed. The disease is bilateral in 80% of cases [27, 28]. Patients often complain of blurred vision and floaters [13, 29]. Less commonly, they present with red eye, photophobia, and ocular pain [5, 30]. Initially, patients with IOL may respond to corticosteroid therapy and their symptoms may improve. Ultimately, the disease progresses and becomes refractory to corticosteroids [31]. The neoplastic process has several secondary effects on the eye, including retinal vasculopathy, which can cause exudation, macular edema, and serous retinal detachment. The diffuse retinitis can resemble acute retinal necrosis. Iris neovascularization develops rarely, resulting in glaucoma, secondary hyphema, and a painful, red eye. These appearances can be mistaken for uveitis and neovascular glaucoma, especially if it is not possible to adequately examine the fundus.

The average interval between the onset of symptoms and definitive diagnosis is ~2 years. Differential diagnoses include sarcoidosis, intermediate uveitis, multifocal choroiditis, toxoplasmosis, birdshot chorioretinopathy, ocular tuberculosis, and acute retinal necrosis. In patients with IOL and concomitant brain involvement, neurological symptoms are undistinguishable from those reported for patients with PCNSL [32]. More than one-third of patients with IOL do not have ocular symptoms. This highlights the importance of a complete diagnostic evaluation, including a slit lamp and detailed ophthalmic examination in all patients with PCNSL.

Diagnostic Approach

The diagnosis of IOL is challenging. Patients for whom there is a clinical suspicion of IOL should be assessed with ophthalmologic examination, fluorescein angiography, and color photography. The most common findings on ophthalmic examination include vitreous cells and haze, which progresses to form large cellular clumps, sheets and strands in the vitreous with mild to moderate haze [3, 5, 16, 29–31, 33–36]. Compared with cases of actual uveitis, iritis is rarely noted [26]. Furthermore, macular edema is absent or less severe that what one might expect, considering the degree of vitreous opacity, and the visual acuity may be surprisingly good. The patients often develop multiple orange-yellowish, subretinal infiltrates, resulting in small overlying retinal pigment epithelium detachments that are pathognomonic for IOL (Fig. 12.1a). Lymphoma infiltration under the retinal pigment epithelium is recognized by the presence of "leopard skin" pigmentation overlying the mass [29]. The retinal infiltrates may appear as whitish punctate lesions and retinal pigment epithelium atrophy [26]. Larger deposits may be mistaken for metastases, or, if only a single lesion is present, amelanotic melanoma. These tumors occur most commonly in the equatorial region, where they can become confluent, forming a long, narrow, white/yellow, ring-shaped mass, which is pathognomonic [37]. Tumor formation at the macula may resemble a disciform scar. Optic nerve infiltration causes disc swelling and eventually, optic atrophy [38]. This must be distinguished from papilledema caused by raised intracranial pressure, secondary to intracranial disease. Sometimes, IOL may mimic a viral retinitis, showing large areas of yellow creamy infiltrates, retinal hemorrhages, vasculitis, detachment, and necrosis [39, 40]. Less frequent ocular findings include iris infiltration, isolated subretinal masses, endophthalmitis, keratic precipitates on the cornea, and mild anterior cell and flare [41]. A few cells in the anterior chamber may be present in up to 50% of patients, though peripheral synechiae are seen only in those with prior intraocular intervention [7, 26].

Fluorescein angiograms and indocyanine green angiograms may demonstrate window defects that appear to correspond to tumor infiltrates of the retinal pigment epithelium [26, 30, 42] (Fig. 12.1a, b). Half of patients have punctate hyperfluorescent window defects, which seems to be preceded by hypofluorescence in an early phase, while round hypofluorescent lesions and leakage can be observed in 34 and 14%, respectively [16]. Extensive retinal pigment epithelial changes demonstrated by fluorescein, combined with the absence of perivascular staining or leakage and macular edema may be associated with and distinctive of IOL [26, 30].

Ultrasound may be a helpful diagnostic tool. Ultrasonographic findings in IOL patients include vitreous debris (77%), as opposed to choroidal lymphomas, which tend to have choroidal thickening and thickening of subtenon's space.

The subgroup of patients with suspected IOL without concomitant brain lesions should be assessed with vitrectomy or ocular biopsy [43]. Steroid treatment prior to the diagnostic procedure may lead to false negative results, and these drugs should be discontinued several days before the biopsy is performed [5]. Even when

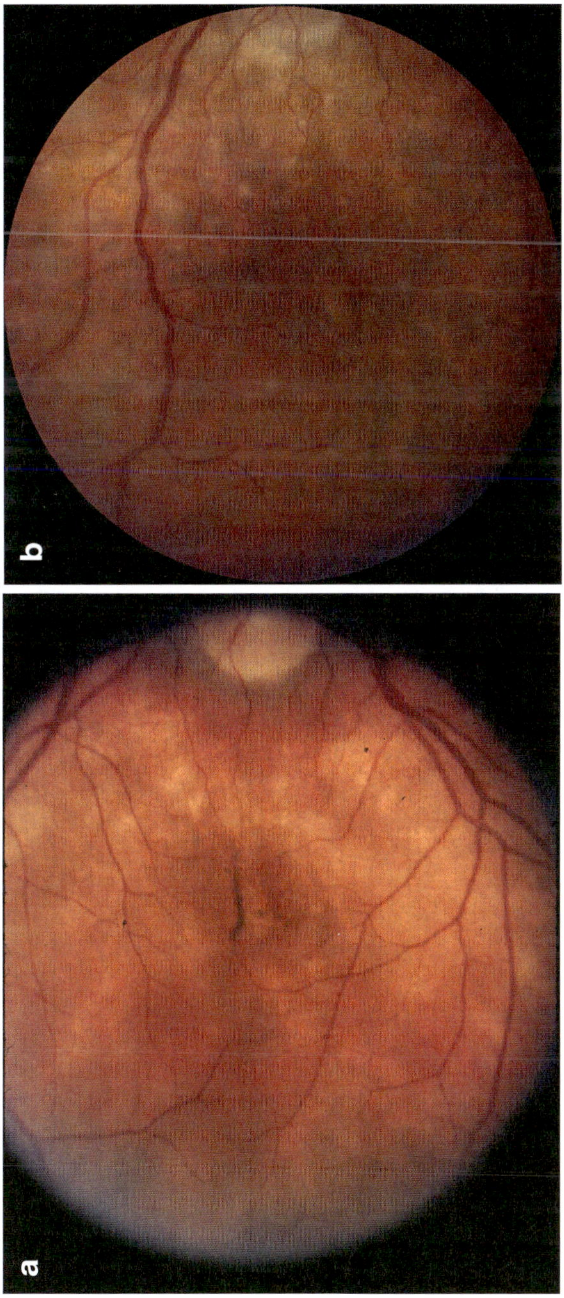

Fig. 12.1 Fundus photograph of two patients with primary intraocular lymphoma showing *yellow* subretinal infiltrates that appear slightly hazy due to an overlying vitreitis

lymphoma is suspected, it can be difficult to confirm the diagnosis cytologically because of the fragility of lymphoma cells, and also because laboratory techniques are demanding [44]. Biopsy is invaluable in the management of patients with IOL because it usually confirms the diagnosis, also providing information of prognostic importance. Unfortunately, lymphoma cells are fragile and undergo morphological changes within 60 min of collection [45], so that the biopsy can easily fail if the specimen is not handled properly. It is therefore important for the surgeon to consult with the pathologist before any surgical intervention is undertaken, so as to ensure that the correct collection procedures are followed and to transport the samples without delay to the relevant laboratories (e.g. pathology, bacteriology and cytogenetics).

It is useful to obtain as much undiluted vitreous as possible [i.e., 1–2 mL], indenting the eye to maintain pressure. The cutting rate should be low and occasionally the vitreous infusion is turned on to reform the globe and then turned off to continue to get as concentrated a sample as possible. Placing the sample into RPMI solution and immediately placing it on ice is also helpful. The remaining vitreous cassette fluid should also be treated in the same way. In addition to obtaining the largest possible vitreous specimen, it is necessary to consider sampling the retinal or subretinal deposits. Again, using low cut rates and taking as much, as safely as possible, is helpful. In eyes with liquid vitreous or those that have already undergone prior vitrectomy, vitreous aspiration needle tap may also be used for diagnostic purposes: this technique can be completed in an outpatient setting [46]. Malignant lymphoma cells found in the vitreous are usually large and pleomorphic with scanty basophilic cytoplasm [47]. However, the identification of malignant cells in vitrectomy samples is often confounded by the presence of reactive immune cells, necrotic cells, debris, and fibrin. Biopsy may need to be repeated more than once to establish the diagnosis of lymphoma. When attempts to obtain a vitrectomy specimen have been unsuccessful, chorioretinal biopsies may be considered.

Cytological, Histological and Molecular Features

Diagnosis of IOL is usually performed on cytospin specimens obtained by spinning vitreous specimens at 500 rpm for 5 min, and concentrating the cells onto glass slides. These are subsequently air dried and treated with conventional stains and immunocytochemistry techniques. Standard smear techniques are inadequate. The sensitivity of cytology is relatively low compared with other investigations, but it provides the basic morphological information upon which all other data are interpreted [48].

Similarly to PCNSL, diffuse large B-cell lymphoma (CD20+) is the most common histotype arising in the eyes (95% of cases). Lymphoma cells are recognized by their large size, the folded nuclei, prominent, sometimes multiple, nucleoli, pleomorphism, and scanty basophilic cytoplasm; multiple mitoses are very common (Fig. 12.2). Interestingly, reactive lymphocytes (CD3+) may be more numerous

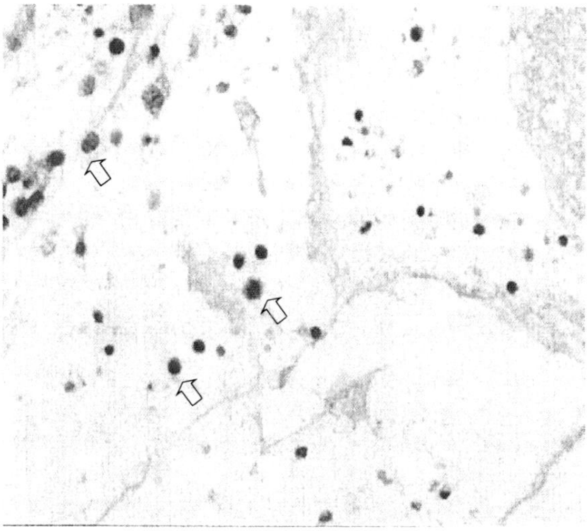

Fig. 12.2 Cytological examination of vitreous humor sample in a patient affected by intraocular large B-cell lymphoma. Several large cells with lymphoid morphology can be observed (*arrows*)

than lymphoma cells. Rare ocular lymphoma subtypes, such as T-cell-rich B-cell lymphoma, as well as T-cell lymphoma [49], have also been described.

In chorioretinal biopsies, multiple, tiny, cream-colored deposits can develop, resembling peripheral drusen, or a white-dot syndrome may be seen. These may result in punched-out, atrophic retinal pigment epithelial lesions. With disease progression, the lymphomatous infiltrations become more extensive, eventually replacing the entire thickness of the retina, which on ophthalmoscopy becomes opaque in areas. The tumor cells seem to permeate the retinal pigment epithelium, accumulating in large numbers on the retinal side of Bruch's membrane. The lymphoma cells closest to Bruch's membrane tend to remain viable, whereas the more superficial deposits become necrotic, forming amorphous masses. The overlying retinal pigment epithelium undergoes atrophy, leaving a fine pigment dusting over the tumor surface. Infiltrates of reactive T-lymphocytes can accumulate in the adjacent choroid. On ophthalmoscopy, these tumor deposits appear initially as tiny, creamy white flat spots, which grow and become confluent to form elevated, yellow-white, discrete tumors. In the early stages, the appearance may resemble fundus flavimaculatus [50].

Lymphoma cells infiltrating the vitreous cavity form visible clumps and a hazy vitreous. These rarely extend into the anterior chamber, resulting occasionally in aqueous cells, flare and keratic precipitates, but not posterior synechiae. Deposits may form on the iris and the anterior chamber angle [30, 51]. Reactive inflammatory cells accumulate in the vitreous and these may predominate over the lymphoma cells. Scavenging macrophages are also present. These features are often mistaken for uveitis and have therefore been termed the "masquerade syndrome" [45]. Necrosis and apoptosis, with scavenging macrophages in the background, are frequently present, making the diagnosis of monoclonal lymphoma difficult [52].

Immunocytochemistry

Cells on glass slides are stained with a panel of antibodies directed at markers identifying B-lymphocytes [CD19, CD20, CD22, CD79a], T-lymphocytes [CD2, CD3, CD4, CD5, CD7, CD8], natural killer cells [CD56] and macrophages [CD68PG], as well as kappa and lambda light chains [34]. If the vitreous sample is small, or if only few cells are available for analysis, it is possible to screen only a few prioritized markers. Usually, IOL is constituted by a monoclonal populations of B lymphocytes (CD19+, CD20+, CD22+), with restricted expression of κ or λ chains. Reactive inflammation in the vitreous is usually T-cell dominant; for example, CD4+ lymphocytes tend to predominate over CD8+ lymphocytes in autoimmune uveitis. In contrast, retinal lymphomas show a dominance of B-lymphocytes [usually atypical in morphology] on a background of macrophages and lysis. It has been appreciated that statins alter the conformation of the CD20 receptor, so that it may become undetectable with standard CD20 antibodies [53]. Therefore, staining with CD79a or PAX5 antibody could be useful in patients receiving this class of medications. Similar to most diffuse large B-cell lymphomas, IOL expresses BCL-6 and MUM-1 [54]. BCL-6 is a B-cell marker that is normally turned off as B cells move from the germinal center into the marginal zone during B-cell differentiation. MUM1 is a protein involved in the control of plasma cell differentiation. While B cells usually express only one of these proteins at a time, concomitant expression of these proteins has been observed in systemic diffuse large B-cell lymphoma.

Flow Cytometry

Flow cytometry may be a helpful addition in the diagnosis of IOL. Cells are simultaneously stained with a panel of antibodies and separated using a fluorescence-activated cell-sorter. Flow cytometry may confirm monoclonality in IOL, and exhibits greater sensitivity versus conventional cytological examination. This method requires fewer cells than slide-based immunocytochemistry, so that it is possible to screen more markers [55]. Flow cytometry and analysis of cytokine levels in the vitreous may help to confirm the diagnosis in patients with suspicious cytology [56].

Polymerase Chain Reaction

DNA extracted from B-lymphocytes is amplified by the polymerase chain reaction (PCR) using primers corresponding to the CDR3 (third complementarity-determining region) variable region immunoglobulin heavy chain (IgH) genes. The use of improved primers has increased the yield in detecting clonal rearrangements of the IgH gene in lymphoma samples [57, 58], with a 100% detection rate in one IOL series [6]. PCR shows monoclonality characteristic of neoplasia in retinal lymphoma, even when reactive cells are present. In inflammatory disease, pseudo-monoclonality can occur if DNA from a single cell is amplified; this is particularly a risk in studies using microdissection. If initial investigations indicate that the lymphoma is of T-cell type, PCR is performed with primers for the γ chain of the T-cell receptor. Translocation t(14;18) has been detected in IOL, involving the bcl-2 gene and genes for IgH [59]. *Bcl-2*, a gene involved in the regulation of apoptosis, is located on chromosome 18, while IgH is located on chromosome 14. The t(14;18) translocation brings the *Bcl-2* gene under the control of the *IgH* promoter, thus deregulating the *Bcl-2* gene and resulting in *Bcl-2* expression. This translocation is found in one quarter of systemic diffuse large B-cell lymphomas [60]. The role of *Bcl-2* expression in IOL remains to be defined.

Lymphoma cells express chemokine receptors selective for B cells, such as CXCR4 and CXCR5, while the ligands for these receptors, such as SDF-1 (CXCL12) and BLC (CXCL13), are frequently expressed in the retinal pigment epithelium of involved eyes [61]. This suggests a pathogenetic role for B-cell chemokines in the homing of lymphoma cells to the retinal pigment epithelium [61].

Interleukin Levels in Vitreous

Biochemical analysis of the vitreous specimen for interleukin ratios may also support the diagnosis of IOL, and it is useful in distinguishing PIOL from uveitis [62]. While interleukin 6 (IL-6) is produced in high levels by inflammatory cells in uveitis, IL-10 is produced by malignant B-lymphocytes in intraocular and CNS lymphoma [62–64]. Thus, IOL is associated with an increased IL-10:IL-6 ratio, with a sensitivity and specificity of ~75% [62]. It is a helpful adjunct, but it is not advisable to make a diagnosis only from an increased ratio.

Extent of Disease Evaluation

Extent of disease evaluation for patients with IOL at presentation is similar to that proposed for PCNSL [65, 66]. It includes complete blood cell count, erythrocyte sedimentation rate, beta microglobulin and lactate-dehydrogenase (LDH) levels, routine blood chemistries, neuroimaging of the brain, CSF cytology examination and physicochemical tests, whole-body computed tomography scan, bone marrow biopsy, and ophthalmological examination including slit lamp evaluation (Fig. 12.3) (more information in Chapter 6). In elderly patients, testicular ultrasonography is suggested, considering that testicular lymphomas may disseminate to the CNS and eyes. CSF cytology is positive at diagnosis in ~25% of tested IOL patients [67]. Neuroimaging plays an important role in the diagnosis of PCNSL and in cases of PIOL [68]. Follow-up neuroimaging should be performed periodically following the diagnosis of PIOL to assess for potential brain dissemination.

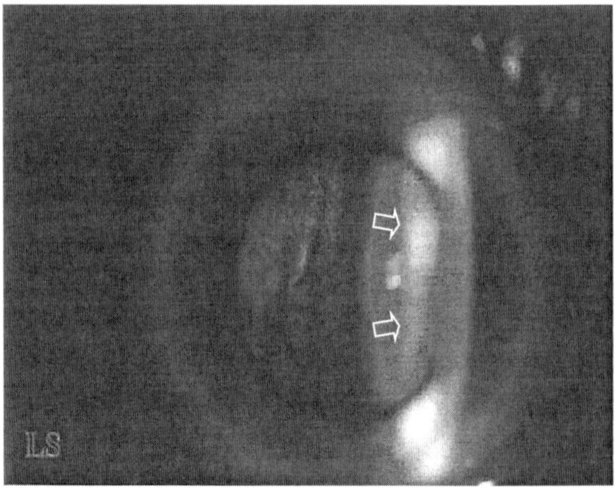

Fig. 12.3 Slit-lamp examination in a patient with intraocular lymphoma. Lymphomatous cells are present in the vitreous humour (*arrows*)

Treatment

The treatment of IOL requires collaboration between ophthalmologists, oncologists, radiation oncologists, and neuro-oncologists. The optimal therapeutic approach for this uncommon condition remains to be defined, and the lack of a uniform assessment and definition of therapeutic response and failure constitutes an important pitfall in the estimation of treatment efficacy. However, there is no evidence in the literature to suggest that IOL should be treated in a different way from other presentations of PCNSL; only minor differences in radiation fields and doses have been recommended for IOL patients. In the past, patients with symptomatic disease were treated with radiotherapy alone, but nearly all of the patients developed early CNS progression and died. A few case reports and small retrospective studies suggested the efficacy of chemotherapy, and anecdotal results using high-dose cytarabine, high-dose methotrexate, procarbazine, and nitrosoureas were reported [34, 69]. The efficacy of these cytostatics is dependent on intraocular pharmacokinetics, which are not well understood. Limitation of drug penetration through the blood-ocular barrier is a major challenge in the treatment of IOL. This anatomic barrier is formed by tight junctions located between vascular endothelial cells and between epithelial cells of the anterior uvea (blood-aqueous barrier) and retina (blood-retinal barrier) [70]. Preliminary data [71] suggest that vitreous drug concentrations of methotrexate following intravenous administration are 100-fold lower than those achieved in the patient's serum. However, micromolar concentrations of methotrexate are achieved in the aqueous and vitreous when the drug is given at a dose of 8 g/m^2. Nevertheless, these concentrations are erratic, do not predict response, and are lower in the vitreous, where lymphomatous cells usually grow, than in the aqueous [71]. As a consequence, persistence of ocular disease has been reported in patients treated with chemotherapy alone.

Better disease control, combining ocular irradiation with high-dose methotrexate-based chemotherapy has been reported [27]. The irradiation of the posterior two thirds of the ocular globes with a dose between 35 and 45 Gy has been recommended, although some authorities suggest irradiation of the entire orbit up to 20 Gy, followed by an additional 10 Gy after shielding the anterior chamber of the eyes. Even in the presence of unilateral disease, both eyes should be irradiated, considering the high frequency of bilateral microscopic involvement.

The poor results obtained with conventional strategies have led investigators to search for new therapeutic approaches. Encouraging results with high-dose chemotherapy supported by autologous peripheral blood stem-cell transplantation (ASCT) [72] and intravitreal chemotherapy [73] in patients with relapsed or refractory IOL have been reported. The first experience with high-dose chemotherapy supported by ASCT was started in 1992, in France, firstly among patients with relapsed intraocular lymphoma and, subsequently, applied to every patient with recurrent PCNSL [72]. Twenty-two patients, half of them with relapse limited to the eyes, were treated with two courses of cytarabine and etoposide, and patients with chemosensitive lymphoma were subsequently treated with a combination of thiotepa, busulfan, and cyclophosphamide followed by ASCT. The complete remission rate after the entire treatment program was 80%, with grade 4 neutropenia and thrombocytopenia in all patients, septic complications in 86% of cases and 23% treatment-related mortality, mostly among patients >60 years old [72]. With this strategy, the 3-year event-free survival and overall survival were 53 and 64%, respectively. Interestingly, the outcome was different among patients with failure limited to the eyes (n=11) versus the rest of the patients (n=11); lethal events were observed in two and six patients, respectively, with a median OS of 33+ and 12 months, respectively [72]. Discrepancies in outcome between these subgroups suggest biological differences and a potential interpretation bias. Importantly, 32% of patients developed neurologic toxicity, which was lethal in one-third of affected patients. This complication, consisting of severe chronic leukoencephalopathy with cognitive dysfunction, had been observed equally in elderly patients (>60 years old) who did not receive WBRT and in previously irradiated younger patients [72].

Some protocols using intravitreal injections of methotrexate, with or without thiotepa, are currently ongoing. A weekly intravitreal injection of 400 μg/0.1 ml of methotrexate, for 4 weeks, and once a month thereafter, has been associated with encouraging results and acceptable morbidity [73]. Importantly, intravitreal methotrexate is able to maintain therapeutic concentrations in the vitreous humour for 5 days [73–75], with a high proportion of complete remissions and the induction of a second remission in patients re-treated with intravitreal methotrexate after first relapse.

The experience with intravitreal rituximab, an anti-CD20 monoclonal antibody is limited, but it may become a valid alternative in IOL. In Dutch-belted rabbits, intravitreal rituximab penetrated the retina [76]. This strategy has been associated with good remission in patients with IOL, although recurrence is common. Two cases of intravitreous injections of rituximab in patients with recurrent CNS lymphoma are reported. In case 1, a woman received intravitreous rituximab at her second relapse, with response after the first administration. Case 2 was a patient with a CD-20 positive lymphoma in the anterior chamber and vitreous cavity bilaterally, which had relapsed after methotrexate. She received intravitreous rituximab weekly for 4 weeks with complete remission [77]. Prospective studies in larger groups of patients are necessary to adequately assess intravitreous rituximab as a potential therapy for IOL. Anecdotal and unexplained cases of intraocular responses have been observed following intraventricular administration of rituximab and methotrexate [78].

Iatrogenic Ocular Toxicity

Treatment of IOL with external beam radiotherapy is usually associated with adverse side effects, including cataract formation, radiation retinopathy, an ischemic retinopathy that appears weeks to years after exposure, optic neuropathy, dry eye syndrome, and corneal epithelial defects. The antilymphoma activity of radiation therapy is associated with retinal pigment epithelial atrophy due to the regression of the subretinal tumor deposits [79].

Methotrexate administered by intravitreal route can cause a variety of complications, including keratopathy, corneal epitheliopathy, hypotony, optic atrophy periorbital edema, blepharitis, macular edema, conjunctival hyperemia, increased lacrimation, and photophobia [80]. Most of these complications seem to be reversible with reduced drug dose, and no systemic complications have been reported in the small case series. Intravitreal rituximab seems to be well tolerated, with a risk of ocular complications related mostly to the invasive procedure, such as endophthalmitis, hemorrhage, and cataract though the possibility of intraocular inflammation following its use has not been well-determined [81].

The risk of ocular complications in IOL patients treated with systemic chemotherapy or rituximab are similar to those reported for patients with systemic lymphomas treated with the same therapies; these are mostly opportunistic ocular infections and other ocular manifestations due to chemotherapy-related hematotoxicity and immunosuppression. Neurotoxicity and treatment-related mortality seem to be higher, especially in elderly patients treated with high-dose chemotherapy supported by autologous stem cell transplant. Patients undergoing blood–brain barrier disruption as part of their treatment for CNS lymphoma can develop maculopathy consisting of an irregular retinal pigment epithelium disturbance, with or without visual loss [82].

Prognosis

The prognosis of patients with IOL remains poor, although the outcome of these patients is usually included in retrospective and prospective studies consisting mainly of patients with PCNSL and only a minority of those with IOL. Thus, the prognosis and natural history of IOL remain to be defined and are only suggested from large retrospective series.

In an international retrospective study of 83 immunocompetent patients with PIOL treated with varied approaches, 56% of patients experienced relapse, in the brain (47% of relapses), eyes (30%) or both (15%), with a median time to relapse of 19 months [14]. Meningeal dissemination of lymphomatous cells was detected in 11% of PIOLs [14], but the prognostic role and impact on therapeutic choice of this feature remain to be defined, and, whether this is the result of metastatic spread or multifocal tumor development is not known. In that series, the median progression free and overall survival were 30 and 58 months, respectively, which were not affected by treatment type. According to this report [14], focal therapy, that is intra-ocular methotrexate or ocular radiotherapy, may minimize treatment toxicity without compromising disease control in PIOL patients. Conversely, there is some evidence that early systemic treatment for PIOL delays the onset of CNS disease, prolonging survival [83]. However, these studies failed to identify factors predicting CNS dissemination in patients presenting with lymphoma limited to the eyes, which makes it difficult to recommend focal versus systemic therapy for this group of patients.

An international retrospective study of 221 patients with PCNSL+IOL has been reported [67]. Patient characteristics were similar to those reported in other large series of patients with PCNSL, but without ocular involvement. Sixty-nine percent progressed at a median of 13 months; sites of progression included brain (52% of relapses), eyes (19%), brain and eyes (12%), meninges (23%), and systemic (2%). Median progression free survival and overall survival for the entire cohort were 18 and 31 months, suggesting a worse prognosis versus patients with PIOL [14]. In these patients, the addition of dedicated ocular therapy (ocular radiotherapy, intravitreal methotrexate or both) improved disease control, but did not affect overall survival.

Rare Forms of IOL

Choroidal Lymphoma

Primary choroidal lymphoma is an extremely rare condition, with an indolent clinical course, which has been previously termed "uveal or intraocular pseudotumor" or "reactive lymphoid hyperplasia" [84]. It can be subtyped according to the WHO classification as extranodal marginal zone B-cell lymphoma [85], displaying similar morphological and immunophenotypical features to extranodal marginal zone B-cell lymphomas arising in the gastrointestinal tract or ocular adnexa [86]. Lymphoid follicles with germinal centers are often present. Perforation of Bruch's membrane and infiltration of the adjacent retinal pigment epithelium can rarely occur, possibly representing the intraocular counterpart of "lymphoepithelial lesions" seen in extranodal marginal zone B-cell lymphomas elsewhere. Because of their rarity, few cases of primary choroidal marginal zone B-cell lymphoma have been studied for their genotype, showing some karyotypic alterations, including t(11;18)(q21;q21).

Primary choroidal lymphoma usually occurs unilaterally and is more common in men than women. Presentation characteristically occurs in the sixth and seventh decades of life. Typical presenting symptoms include recurrent, painless episodes of blurred vision and metamorphopsia caused by secondary serous retinal detachment involving the fovea [45]. The key, early signs of primary choroidal lymphoma include multifocal, yellow–pink choroidal swellings on fundus examination [87, 88]. These spots may resemble multifocal choroiditis or birdshot choroidopathy. Ultimately, a diffuse thickening of the uveal tract becomes obvious on funduscopy. This is often associated with serous retinal detachment. The appearance may mimic scleritis and sometimes ultrasonography shows fluid in subtenon's space; however, there is usually no pain. The vitreous remains clear. In some patients, subconjunctival or episcleral extensions may become apparent as "salmon patches" [87, 89]. Patients with large posterior lesions complain of proptosis and diplopia. Fluorescein angiography may show leopard spots secondary to effects on the overlying retinal pigment epithelium. Ultrasonography shows the tumor to have a low internal acoustic reflectivity (Fig. 12.4), and often reveals extraocular tumor extension near the optic nerve. Choroidal lymphoma must be differentiated from choroidal hemangioma, which, unlike lymphoma, has a high internal acoustic reflectivity. Metastasis and amelanotic melanoma should be considered in the differential diagnosis. If untreated, uveal lymphoma may cause glaucoma and retinal detachment, eventually rendering the eye blind and painful [90]. Treatment with low-dose radiotherapy induces complete tumor regression with few if any residual effects and good improvement in vision. The prognosis is usually good. An aggressive form of choroidal lymphoma exists, but is rare.

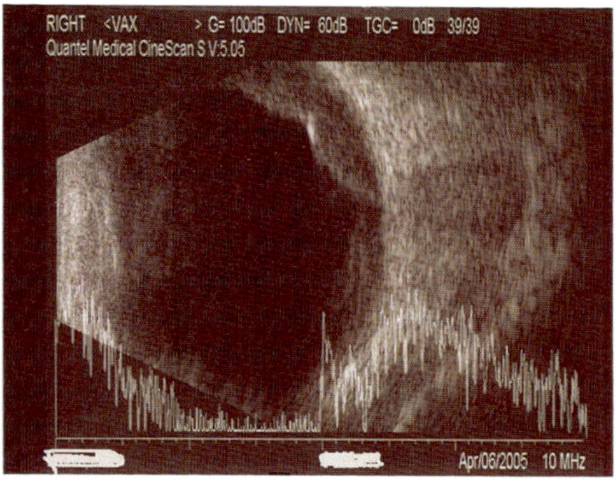

Fig. 12.4 Ultrasonographic examination of the eye in a patient affected by a choroidal lymphoma. Swelling of the choroid is observed

Iridal Lymphomas

Primary iris lymphomas are exceptionally rare forms of IOL of high-grade histotype, similar to those involving the retina [41, 51]. The few reported cases are equally divided between B- and T-cell lymphomas. No genotypic analysis of iris lymphomas has yet been reported. The typical presenting symptoms of primary iridal lymphoma include pain, redness, photophobia, and decreased vision. The clinical signs reported in the literature include uveitis of uncertain nature, nodular or diffuse iris precipitates, iris discoloration, anisocoria, hyphema, and pseudohypopyon. These appearances may resemble uveitis, metastases, and amelanotic iris melanoma. High-frequency echography shows ill-defined tumors of low internal reflectivity. Fine needle aspiration of anterior chamber cells and iris biopsy usually lead to a definitive diagnosis. Full ocular and systemic examination is indicated to exclude systemic dissemination, as well as choroidal and retinal lymphoma. Ocular treatment consisting of low-dose irradiation or systemic chemotherapy induces local tumor regression [91]; however, most patients with iridal lymphoma exhibit poor survival.

One case of primary ciliary body lymphoma has been reported. It presented, in an elderly woman, as an amelanotic tumor in the anterior chamber, which was confirmed by slit-lamp examination. There was a small hyphema. High-frequency ultrasonography demonstrated a small tumor involving the ciliary body, with a low internal acoustic reflectivity. The diagnosis was established by biopsy, which was performed with a 25-gauge vitreous cutter. Histopathological examination demonstrated a monoclonal population of small monomorphic B cells with chromatin-dense nuclei, aberrant immunophenotype (e.g., expression of CD43), and a growth fraction (Ki-67) of ~5%. The patient responded well to low-dose radiotherapy, but follow-up at the time of the report was still short.

Secondary Intraocular Lymphomas

Intraocular involvement of disseminated, systemic lymphomas is usually confined to the choroid [92]. Secondary involvement of the retina without uveal infiltration has been occasionally reported [93]. The morphology and immunophenotype of secondary choroidal lymphomas/leukemias correspond to the systemic lymphomas or leukemia. There are few reports on the details of genotypic features of secondary choroidal lymphomas [94]. Rarely, systemic lymphoma can present with anterior segment disease, such as pseudohypopyon or iris infiltration [90, 95]. Other unusual manifestations of SIOL include optic disc swelling [96] and serous macular detachment [97].

The most common systemic lymphoma subtype involving the choroid is diffuse large B-cell lymphoma, followed by multiple myeloma, extramedullary plasmacytoma, lymphoplasmacytic lymphoma, marginal zone B-cell lymphoma, and B-cell chronic lymphocytic leukemia [93]. Orbital Burkitt's lymphoma with direct ocular infiltration [98] and intravascular lymphoma with secondary involvement of the eye have been reported [99]. Definitive conclusions on therapeutic management can not be drawn, considering that the published experience is limited to a few case reports with short follow-up. However, no evidence in the literature suggests that these rare forms should be treated any differently than when these lymphoid malignancies present without ocular involvement.

References

1. Davis JW, Moriarty RP, Schlossberg SM et al (2001) Bilateral testicular lymphoma treated with chemotherapy and radiation without orchiectomy: complete response relapsed at 52 months in the vitreous humor. Urology 57:555
2. Choi JY, Kafkala C, Foster CS (2006) Primary intraocular lymphoma: a review. Semin Ophthalmol 21:125–133
3. Akpek EK, Ahmed I, Hochberg FH et al (1999) Intraocular-central nervous system lymphoma: clinical features, diagnosis, and outcomes. Ophthalmology 106:1805–1810
4. DeAngelis LM (2001) Primary central nervous system lymphomas. Curr Treat Options Oncol 2:309–318
5. Peterson K, Gordon KB, Heinemann MH et al (1993) The clinical spectrum of ocular lymphoma. Cancer 72:843–849
6. Chan CC (2003) Molecular pathology of primary intraocular lymphoma. Trans Am Ophthalmol Soc 101:275–292
7. Bardenstein DS (1998) Intraocular Lymphoma. Cancer Control 5:317–325
8. Herrlinger U, Schabet M, Brugger W et al (2001) Primary central nervous system lymphoma 1991–1997: outcome and late adverse effects after combined modality treatment. Cancer 91:130–135
9. Corn BW, Donahue BR, Rosenstock JG et al (1997) Palliation of AIDS-related primary lymphoma of the brain: observations from a multi-institutional database. Int J Radiat Oncol Biol Phys 38:601–605
10. Behin A, Hoang-Xuan K, Carpentier AF et al (2003) Primary brain tumours in adults. Lancet 361:323–331
11. Kadan-Lottick NS, Skluzacek MC, Gurney JG (2002) Decreasing incidence rates of primary central nervous system lymphoma. Cancer 95:193–202
12. Cote TR, Manns A, Hardy CR et al (1996) Epidemiology of brain lymphoma among people with or without acquired immunodeficiency syndrome. AIDS/Cancer Study Group. J Natl Cancer Inst 88:675–679
13. Hoffman PM, McKelvie P, Hall AJ et al (2003) Intraocular lymphoma: a series of 14 patients with clinicopathological features and treatment outcomes. Eye 17:513–521
14. Grimm SA, Pulido JS, Jahnke K et al (2007) Primary intraocular lymphoma: an International Primary Central Nervous System Lymphoma Collaborative Group Report. Ann Oncol 18:1851–1855
15. Wender A, Adar A, Maor E et al (1994) Primary B-cell lymphoma of the eyes and brain in a 3-year-old boy. Arch Ophthalmol 112:450–451
16. Cassoux N, Merle-Beral H, Leblond V et al (2000) Ocular and central nervous system lymphoma: clinical features and diagnosis. Ocul Immunol Inflamm 8:243–250
17. Surawicz TS, McCarthy BJ, Kupelian V et al (1999) Descriptive epidemiology of primary brain and CNS tumors: results from the Central Brain Tumor Registry of the United States, 1990–1994. Neuro Oncol 1:14–25
18. Pulido JS, Vierkant RA, Olson JE et al (2009) Racial differences in primary central nervous system lymphoma incidence and survival rates. Neuro Oncol 11:318–322

19. Bashir R, Luka J, Cheloha K et al (1993) Expression of Epstein-Barr virus proteins in primary CNS lymphoma in AIDS patients. Neurology 43:2358–2362
20. Martini F, Dolcetti R, Ferreri AJ et al (2004) No association between polyomaviruses and primary central nervous system lymphomas of HIV-seronegative and HIV-positive patients. Cancer Epidemiol Biomarkers Prev 13:1819–1820
21. Shen DF, Herbort CP, Tuaillon N et al (2001) Detection of Toxoplasma gondii DNA in primary intraocular B-cell lymphoma. Mod Pathol 14:995–999
22. Corboy JR, Garl PJ, Kleinschmidt-DeMasters BK (1998) Human herpesvirus 8 DNA in CNS lymphomas from patients with and without AIDS. Neurology 50:335–340
23. Levy-Clarke GA, Chan CC, Nussenblatt RB (2005) Diagnosis and management of primary intraocular lymphoma. Hematol Oncol Clin North Am 19:739–749
24. Coupland SE, Heimann H, Bechrakis NE (2004) Primary intraocular lymphoma: a review of the clinical, histopathological and molecular biological features. Graefes Arch Clin Exp Ophthalmol 242:901–913
25. Minckler DS, Font RL, Zimmerman LE (1975) Uveitis and reticulum cell sarcoma of brain with bilateral neoplastic seeding of vitreous without retinal or uveal involvement. Am J Ophthalmol 80:433–439
26. Fardeau C, Lee CP, Merle-Beral H et al (2009) Retinal fluorescein, indocyanine green angiography, and optic coherence tomography in non-Hodgkin primary intraocular lymphoma. Am J Ophthalmol 147:886–894
27. Ferreri AJ, Blay JY, Reni M et al (2002) Relevance of intraocular involvement in the management of primary central nervous system lymphomas. Ann Oncol 13:531–538
28. Chan CC, Buggage RR, Nussenblatt RB (2002) Intraocular lymphoma. Curr Opin Ophthalmol 13:411–418
29. Read RW, Zamir E, Rao NA (2002) Neoplastic masquerade syndromes. Surv Ophthalmol 47:81–124
30. Velez G, Chan CC, Csaky KG (2002) Fluorescein angiographic findings in primary intraocular lymphoma. Retina 22:37–43
31. Rothova A, Ooijman F, Kerkhoff F et al (2001) Uveitis masquerade syndromes. Ophthalmology 108:386–399
32. Ferreri AJ, Reni M, Pasini F et al (2002b) A multicenter study of treatment of primary CNS lymphoma. Neurology 58:1513–1520
33. van der Sanden GA, Schouten LJ, van Dijck JA et al (2002) Primary central nervous system lymphomas: incidence and survival in the Southern and Eastern Netherlands. Cancer 94:1548–1556
34. Whitcup SM, de Smet MD, Rubin BI et al (1993) Intraocular lymphoma. Clinical and histopathologic diagnosis. Ophthalmology 100:1399–1406
35. Zamiri P, Boyd S, Lightman S (1997) Uveitis in the elderly–is it easy to identify the masquerade? Br J Ophthalmol 81:827–831
36. Matsuo T, Yamaoka A, Shiraga F et al (1998) Two types of initial ocular manifestations in intraocular-central nervous system lymphoma. Retina 18:301–307
37. Gass JD, Sever RJ, Grizzard WS et al (1984) Multifocal pigment epithelial detachments by reticulum cell sarcoma. A characteristic funduscopic picture. Retina 4:135–143
38. Behbehani RS, Vacarezza N, Sergott RC et al (2005) Isolated optic nerve lymphoma diagnosed by optic nerve biopsy. Am J Ophthalmol 139:1128–1130
39. Merchant A, Foster CS (1997) Primary intraocular lymphoma. Int Ophthalmol Clin 37: 101–115
40. Ridley ME, McDonald HR, Sternberg P Jr et al (1992) Retinal manifestations of ocular lymphoma (reticulum cell sarcoma). Ophthalmology 99:1153–1160
41. Velez G, de Smet MD, Whitcup SM et al (2000) Iris involvement in primary intraocular lymphoma: report of two cases and review of the literature. Surv Ophthalmol 44:518–526
42. Dean JM, Novak MA, Chan CC et al (1996) Tumor detachments of the retinal pigment epithelium in ocular/central nervous system lymphoma. Retina 16:47–56

43. Bernstein M, Parrent AG (1994) Complications of CT-guided stereotactic biopsy of intra-axial brain lesions. J Neurosurg 81:165–168
44. Coupland SE (2008a) Ocular adnexal lymphoid tumors: progress in need of clarification. Am J Ophthalmol 146:791–792
45. Coupland SE, Anastassiou G, Bornfeld N et al (2005) Primary intraocular lymphoma of T-cell type: report of a case and review of the literature. Graefes Arch Clin Exp Ophthalmol 243:189–197
46. Lobo A, Lightman S (2003) Vitreous aspiration needle tap in the diagnosis of intraocular inflammation. Ophthalmology 110:595–599
47. Davis JL, Solomon D, Nussenblatt RB et al (1992) Immunocytochemical staining of vitreous cells. Indications, techniques, and results. Ophthalmology 99:250–256
48. Coupland SE (2008b) The pathologist's perspective on vitreous opacities. Eye 22:1318–1329
49. Saenz AD, Amador A, Ruiz BM et al (2007) Cytofluorographic and molecular identification of a CD8-positive, TCR-alpha/beta-negative intraocular T cell lymphoma: a case report and review of the literature. J Med Case Reports 1:114
50. Gass JD, Weleber RG, Johnson DR (1987) Non-Hodgkin's lymphoma causing fundus picture simulating fundus flavimaculatus. Retina 7:209–214
51. Raju VK, Green WR (1982) Reticulum cell sarcoma of the uvea. Ann Ophthalmol 14:555–560
52. Zaldivar RA, Martin DF, Holden JT et al (2004) Primary intraocular lymphoma: clinical, cytologic, and flow cytometric analysis. Ophthalmology 111:1762–1767
53. Winiarska M, Bil J, Wilczek E et al (2008) Statins impair antitumor effects of rituximab by inducing conformational changes of CD20. PLoS Med 5:e64
54. Coupland SE, Bechrakis NE, Anastassiou G et al (2003) Evaluation of vitrectomy specimens and chorioretinal biopsies in the diagnosis of primary intraocular lymphoma in patients with Masquerade syndrome. Graefes Arch Clin Exp Ophthalmol 241:860–870
55. Davis JL (2004) Diagnosis of intraocular lymphoma. Ocul Immunol Inflamm 12:7–16
56. Nussenblatt RB, Chan CC, Wilson WH et al (2006) International Central Nervous System and Ocular Lymphoma Workshop: recommendations for the future. Ocul Immunol Inflamm 14:139–144
57. van Dongen JJ, Langerak AW, Bruggemann M et al (2003) Design and standardization of PCR primers and protocols for detection of clonal immunoglobulin and T-cell receptor gene recombinations in suspect lymphoproliferations: report of the BIOMED-2 Concerted Action BMH4-CT98-3936. Leukemia 17:2257–2317
58. Chen YT, Whitney KD, Chen Y (1994) Clonality analysis of B-cell lymphoma in fresh-frozen and paraffin-embedded tissues: the effects of variable polymerase chain reaction parameters. Mod Pathol 7:429–434
59. Shen DF, Zhuang Z, LeHoang P et al (1998) Utility of microdissection and polymerase chain reaction for the detection of immunoglobulin gene rearrangement and translocation in primary intraocular lymphoma. Ophthalmology 105:1664–1669
60. Yunis JJ, Oken MM, Kaplan ME et al (1982) Distinctive chromosomal abnormalities in histologic subtypes of non-Hodgkin's lymphoma. N Engl J Med 307:1231–1236
61. Robinson MR, Lee SS, Sneller MC et al (2003) Tarsal-conjunctival disease associated with Wegener's granulomatosis. Ophthalmology 110:1770–1780
62. Chan CC, Whitcup SM, Solomon D et al (1995) Interleukin-10 in the vitreous of patients with primary intraocular lymphoma. Am J Ophthalmol 120:671–673
63. Whitcup SM, Stark-Vancs V, Wittes RE et al (1997) Association of interleukin 10 in the vitreous and cerebrospinal fluid and primary central nervous system lymphoma. Arch Ophthalmol 115:1157–1160
64. Cassoux N, Merle-Beral H, Lehoang P et al (2001) Interleukin-10 and intraocular-central nervous system lymphoma. Ophthalmology 108:426–427
65. Abrey LE, Batchelor TT, Ferreri AJ et al (2005) Report of an international workshop to standardize baseline evaluation and response criteria for primary CNS lymphoma. J Clin Oncol 23:5034–5043

66. Ferreri AJ, Reni M, Zoldan MC et al (1996) Importance of complete staging in non-Hodgkin's lymphoma presenting as a cerebral mass lesion. Cancer 77:827–833
67. Grimm SA, McCannel CA, Omuro AM et al (2008) Primary CNS lymphoma with intraocular involvement: International PCNSL Collaborative Group Report. Neurology 71:1355–1360
68. Kuker W, Herrlinger U, Gronewaller E et al (2002) Ocular manifestation of primary nervous system lymphoma: what can be expected from imaging? J Neurol 249:1713–1716
69. Baumann MA, Ritch PS, Hande KR et al (1986) Treatment of intraocular lymphoma with high-dose Ara-C. Cancer 57:1273–1275
70. Cunha-Vaz J (1979) The blood-ocular barriers. Surv Ophthalmol 23:279–296
71. Batchelor TT, Kolak G, Ciordia R et al (2003) High-dose methotrexate for intraocular lymphoma. Clin Cancer Res 9:711–715
72. Soussain C, Suzan F, Hoang-Xuan K et al (2001) Results of intensive chemotherapy followed by hematopoietic stem-cell rescue in 22 patients with refractory or recurrent primary CNS lymphoma or intraocular lymphoma. J Clin Oncol 19:742–749
73. Smith JR, Rosenbaum JT, Wilson DJ et al (2002) Role of intravitreal methotrexate in the management of primary central nervous system lymphoma with ocular involvement. Ophthalmology 109:1709–1716
74. de Smet MD, Vancs VS, Kohler D et al (1999) Intravitreal chemotherapy for the treatment of recurrent intraocular lymphoma. Br J Ophthalmol 83:448–451
75. Berenbom A, Davila RM, Lin HS et al (2007) Treatment outcomes for primary intraocular lymphoma: implications for external beam radiotherapy. Eye 21:1198–1201
76. Pulido JS, Bakri SJ, Valyi-Nagy T et al (2007) Rituximab penetrates full-thickness retina in contrast to tissue plasminogen activator control. Retina 27:1071–1073
77. Ohguro N, Hashida N, Tano Y (2008) Effect of intravitreous rituximab injections in patients with recurrent ocular lesions associated with central nervous system lymphoma. Arch Ophthalmol 126:1002–1003
78. Rubenstein JL, Fridlyand J, Shen A et al (2006) Gene expression and angiotropism in primary CNS lymphoma. Blood 107:3716–3723
79. Margolis L, Fraser R, Lichter A et al (1980) The role of radiation therapy in the management of ocular reticulum cell sarcoma. Cancer 45:688–692
80. Helbig H, Cerny T, de Smet MD (2003) Intravitreal chemotherapy for intraocular lymphoma. Ophthalmology 100:145–149
81. Kitzmann AS, Pulido JS, Mohney BG et al (2007) Intraocular use of rituximab. Eye 21: 1524–1527
82. Doolittle ND, Anderson CP, Bleyer WA et al (2001) Importance of dose intensity in neuro-oncology clinical trials: summary report of the Sixth Annual Meeting of the Blood-Brain Barrier Disruption Consortium. Neuro Oncol 3:46–54
83. Hormigo A, Abrey L, Heinemann MH et al (2004) Ocular presentation of primary central nervous system lymphoma: diagnosis and treatment. Br J Haematol 126:202–208
84. Cockerham GC, Hidayat AA, Bijwaard KE et al (2000) Re-evaluation of "reactive lymphoid hyperplasia of the uvea": an immunohistochemical and molecular analysis of 10 cases. Ophthalmology 107:151–158
85. Coupland SE, Foss HD, Hidayat AA et al (2002) Extranodal marginal zone B cell lymphomas of the uvea: an analysis of 13 cases. J Pathol 197:333–340
86. Coupland SE, Damato B (2006) Lymphomas involving the eye and the ocular adnexa. Curr Opin Ophthalmol 17:523–531
87. Ciulla TA, Bains RA, Jakobiec FA et al (1997) Uveal lymphoid neoplasia: a clinical-pathologic correlation and review of the early form. Surv Ophthalmol 41:467–476
88. Jakobiec FA, Sacks E, Kronish JW et al (1987) Multifocal static creamy choroidal infiltrates. An early sign of lymphoid neoplasia. Ophthalmology 94:397–406
89. Chang TS, Byrne SF, Gass JD et al (1996) Echographic findings in benign reactive lymphoid hyperplasia of the choroid. Arch Ophthalmol 114:669–675

90. Duker JS, Shields JA, Ross M (1987) Intraocular large cell lymphoma presenting as massive thickening of the uveal tract. Retina 7:41–45
91. Lobo A, Larkin G, Clark BJ et al (2003) Pseudo-hypopyon as the presenting feature in B-cell and T-cell intraocular lymphoma. Clin Experiment Ophthalmol 31:155–158
92. Verbraeken HE, Hanssens M, Priem H et al (1997) Ocular non-Hodgkin's lymphoma: a clinical study of nine cases. Br J Ophthalmol 81:31–36
93. Parikh AH, Khan SH, Wright JD Jr et al (2005) Systemic non-Hodgkin's lymphoma simulating primary intraocular lymphoma. Am J Ophthalmol 139:573–574
94. Coupland SE, Foss HD, Bechrakis NE et al (2001) Secondary ocular involvement in systemic "memory" B-cell lymphocytic leukemia. Ophthalmology 108:1289–1295
95. Tranos PG, Andreou PS, Wickremasinghe SS, Brazier JD (2002) Pseudohypopyon as a feature of multiple myeloma. Arch Ophthalmol 120:87–88
96. Pinna A, Dore S, Dore F et al (2003) Bilateral optic disc swelling as the presenting sign of Waldenstrom's macroglobulinaemia. Acta Ophthalmol Scand 81:413–415
97. Pilon AF, Rhee PS, Messner LV (2005) Bilateral, persistent serous macular detachments with Waldenstrom's macroglobulinemia. Optom Vis Sci 82:573–578
98. Wysenbeek YS, Nissenkorn I, Cohen S et al (1987) Intraocular involvement of Burkitt's lymphoma in a Bedouin child. Pediatr Hematol Oncol 4:309–314
99. Elner VM, Hidayat AA, Charles NC et al (1986) Neoplastic angioendotheliomatosis. A variant of malignant lymphoma immunohistochemical and ultrastructural observations of three cases. Ophthalmology 93:1237–1245

Chapter 13
Neurolymphomatosis

Tali Siegal, Sigal Grisariu, Batia Avni, and Joachim M. Baehring

Introduction

Neurolymphomatosis (NL) is defined as a clinical neuropathy induced by infiltration of peripheral nerves, nerve roots, plexus, or cranial nerves by malignant lymphocytes. The term NL encompasses nerve infiltration by nerve-seeking neoplastic cells in the setting of an unknown or a known hematologic malignancy. The majority of the patients described in the literature (Table 13.1) suffered from non-Hodgkin lymphoma (NHL), and in that setting NL represents a unique subtype of extranodal disease. However, nerve-seeking disease may occur rarely in leukemias [1, 2] and therefore, this chapter includes description of neuropathy, which is induced by malignant lymphocytic infiltration in both NHL and leukemias under the common term of NL.

NL is usually identified when the clinical neuropathy affects nerve structures outside the thecal sac, in contrast to the infiltration of nerve roots from leptomeningeal seeding or neural compression by epidural lymphoma. The malignant lymphocytes of NL distinguish it from the benign infiltrates, observed in paraneoplastic or inflammatory neuropathies, such as chronic inflammatory demyelinating polyneuropathy (CIDP) or paraproteinemias, and from the acellular neuropathic complications of chemotherapeutic agents, such as vinca alkaloids or bortezomib. Successful therapy is contingent upon the recognition of this unique neurological complication, yet the diagnosis is difficult. A high index of suspicion is essential in order to prove the diagnosis, but even with a careful search, definitive findings may sometimes be obtained only at autopsy [3].

T. Siegal (✉)
Gaffin Center for Neuro-Oncology, Hadassah Hebrew-University Medical Center, Jerusalem, Israel
e-mail: siegal@hadassah.org.il

T. Batchelor, L.M. DeAngelis (eds.), *Lymphoma and Leukemia of the Nervous System*, DOI 10.1007/978-1-4419-7668-0_13,

Table 13.1 Demographic and clinical features of neurolymphomatosis associated with lymphoproliferative malignancies

	Group A[a] Literature review with MGH case-series	Group B[b] Literature review	Group C[c] IPCG case series
Year period	1972–2000	2001–2008	1993–2008
Number of patients	72	43	50
Gender:			
Male	39 (54%)	25 (58%)	30 (60%)
Female	33 (46%)	16 (37%)	20 (40%)
Not reported		2 (4.6%)	
Median age (years)	63 (18–84)	56 (16–71)	55.5 (18–80)
NL as an extranodal site of systemic lymphoma	29 (40%)	27 (63%)	33 (66%)
NL as the presentation of malignancy	NA	13 (30%)	13 (26%)
Malignant cell type:			
B-cells	59 (82%)	29 (67%)	41 (82%)
T-cells	4 (5%)	11 (26%)	5 (10%)
NK cells		1 (2%)	
Not classified	9 (13%)	2 (4.6%)	4 (8%)
Parenchymal brain involvement	19 (26%)	NA	11 (22%)-PCNSL
Affected neural structures[d]:			
Peripheral nerves	46 (64%)	8 (17%)	30 (60%)
Spinal nerves	47 (65%)	14 (33%)	24 (48%)
Neural plexus	23 (32%)	15 (35%)	20 (40%)
Cranial nerves	37 (51%)	15 (35%)	23 (46%)
Painful neuropathy	34 (47%)	25 (58%)	38 (76%)
Type of neuropathy:			
Pure motor	NA	7 (16%)	11 (22%)
Pure sensory	NA	8 (17%)	1 (2%)
Sensorimotor	NA	22 (51%)	36 (72%)
Not reported		6 (14%)	2 (4%)

NA, not available; NL, neurolymphomatosis; PCNSL, primary central nervous system lymphoma.
[a]Group A consists of a retrospective case series of 25 patients diagnosed at the Massachusetts General Hospital (MGH) and a literature review of an additional 47 cases that were published together [3].
[b]Group B is based on literature review [5, 6, 12, 13, 26, 28–33, 35–59].
[c]Group C consists of a retrospective case series collected from 12 institutions in 5 countries as a part of the IPCG project [4].
[d]Involvement of multiple sites was common.

Epidemiology and Pathogenesis

NL is a very rare neurological manifestation of NHL and leukemias. Its true incidence is unknown. The most comprehensive review identified 72 cases reported during a 28 year period [3]; following this publication, we identified an additional 43 cases in the literature during the 8 year period from 2001 to 2008 (Table 13.1). Recently, the International Primary CNS Lymphoma Collaborative Group (IPCG) conducted a retrospective survey and identified 50 cases that were diagnosed in 12 centers from 5 countries during a 15 year period [4]. Judging from these 165 cases, it appears that the annual rate of diagnosis (across many centers) does not exceed 4 new cases per year. Still, this rate probably represents an underestimation as the majority of cases probably remain undiagnosed.

Pathogenesis

Most NL is due to diffuse large B-cell lymphoma (Table 13.1) and the causative cells stain for B-cell-associated surface antigens. NL in T-cell lymphoma accounts for about 10–20% of all cases (Table 13.1), and there are anecdotal reports of NK-cell types, or an association with Sezary syndrome [5, 6]. It is possible that on a molecular level, NL bears a resemblance to CNS lymphoma with cells similar to germinal center or post-germinal center B-cells, corroborating the theory that it is a systemic disease with unique proclivity to affect neural structures [7–10].

It has been claimed that NL patients have a higher than expected frequency of autoimmune disorders, such as recurrent chorioretinitis, hypothyroidism, Sjögren's syndrome, and lupus erythematosus [3]. Yet, the precise figures were not given, and population-based data to support this contention are lacking. Clinical similarities to Guillain-Barré syndrome and CIDP are obvious and a pathogenetic link might be supported by anecdotal reports [3, 11–13]. In these cases, years of exacerbations of painless polyradiculoneuropathy were observed. In one patient [13], a dramatic response to intravenous immunoglobulin therapy was documented years prior to the final episode of unremitting neurological worsening that led to the diagnosis of NL. Other descriptions include longstanding vasculitic neuropathy that preceded NL [14]. It is conceivable that lymphoma arises by malignant transformation of an autoreactive B-cell clone, targeting peripheral neural structures in patients with long-standing peripheral nervous system disorders.

Different trafficking pathways apply to lymphoid neoplasms of T- and B-cell lineage. T-lymphocytes accessing nonlymphoid tissues are equipped with a very different set of addressins and chemokine receptors than B-cells, which can act at a distance through secretion of antibodies. It has been suggested that B-cell migration to extralymphoid sites occurs almost exclusively in the context of chronic inflammation driven by various antigens. The reacting lymphoid tissue contains a specific expression pattern of vascular addressins and chemokine receptors [15]. Ectopic chemokine expression at sites of chronic inflammation is presumably responsible for selective homing of B cells to these sites.

Site-specificity in NL is presumed to be analogous to other antigen-driven extranodal NHLs, such as mucosa-associated lymphoid tissue (MALT) lymphomas and intravascular subtypes, and may share with these other lymphoid neoplasms, target-organ selection derived from tissue expression of a stimulating antigen. Putative antigens include autoantigens, bacterial, or viral antigens. As in normal lymphoid cells, adhesion receptors seem to determine the tissue-specific dissemination patterns of certain lymphoma subtypes [15–17]. The final distribution of neoplastic lymphocytes, like their physiologic counterparts, depends on the balance of entry, proliferation, and retention [15]. Several selectins, integrins, chemokines and adhesion molecules have been implicated in the pathogenesis of CNS and systemic NHL and they may play a role in the homing of lymphocytes to the CNS [18–23]. Still, specific adhesion molecules as the basis for organ selectivity of NL remain to be identified, if they exist.

NL has to be distinguished from other peripheral neuropathies occurring in the setting of hematologic malignancy (e.g. autoimmune, paraneoplastic, vasculitis, paraproteinemia, or chemotherapy-induced neuropathy). How difficult this distinction can be is exemplified by Marek's disease, a T-cell lymphoma in chicken induced by infection with oncogenic alphaherpes virus [24]. Marek's disease is characterized by four different forms: cutaneous, neural (nerve form), ocular, and visceral. When the disease was initially described, it was referred to as "neurolymphomatosis gallinarum" due to the associated rapidly progressive polyneuropathy. Histologic examination revealed thickened peripheral nerves infiltrated with mononuclear cells. The infiltrates affected both the sciatic nerves and areas of the spinal cord. Although the polyneuropathy is often neuritic and not neoplastic, some phenotypic studies demonstrated that nerve fibers were infiltrated by malignant T-cells [25].

Clinical Features

Symptoms and signs of NL may appear either in the setting of a known systemic lymphoproliferative malignancy or in a patient harboring the diagnosis of primary CNS lymphoma (PCNSL). It may, however, occur as the first relapse site of a previously treated lymphoma or as the first manifestation of the neoplastic disorder (Table 13.1). The latter is particularly challenging diagnostically. Primary NL (i.e. no previous evidence for malignancy) accounted for 26% of the cases collected retrospectively by the IPCG (Table 13.1). NL was due to lymphoma in 90% of patients and leukemia in 10% of cases in the IPCG series. PCNSL accounted for about 20% of the NL IPCG cases.

The most common clinical presentations of NL are a painful peripheral neuropathy or radiculopathy, followed by cranial neuropathy, painless polyneuropathy, and peripheral mononeuropathy (Table 13.1). The pain is usually severe, relentless, and dysesthetic. The neuropathy is most often characterized as a sensorimotor type, but pure motor neuropathy has been described in about 20% of patients, while pure sensory neuropathy is less frequent. Weakness often progresses, eventually resulting in symmetric paraparesis or quadriparesis with evolving muscle atrophy.

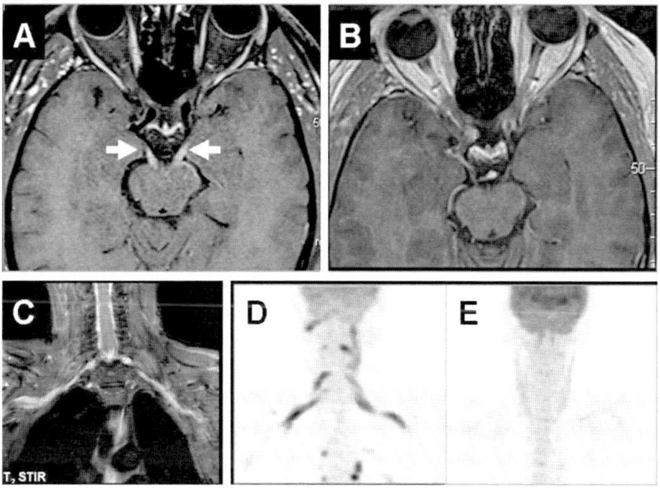

Fig. 13.1 Imaging in neurolymphomatosis. **a** Bilateral symmetric thickening and enhancement of the oculomotor nerves (arrows) demonstrated by MRI (axial, gadolinium enhanced T_1-weighted image) in a patient with neurolymphomatosis presenting as the first relapse site of systemic non-Hodgkin lymphoma (NHL). **b** Imaging of the same patients as in (**a**) following 2 months of treatment with high-dose methotrexate and intra-CSF cytarabine. The post-contrast MRI reveals normal oculomotor nerves without enhancement. **c** Bilateral involvement of the brachial plexus is demonstrated by MRI (coronal T_2 STIR) in a patient with a history of NHL who presented with asymmetric upper extremity weakness and muscle wasting associated with mild proximal pain. **d** FDG-PET scan of the same patient as shown in (**c**) demonstrating abnormal uptake of the tracer in cervical spinal nerve roots and along both brachial plexi suggesting infiltration of the neural structures by the lymphoma. **e** FDG-PET scan of the same patient as in (**d**) after treatment with high-dose methotrexate and procarbazine. The scan shows no abnormal uptake. The objective response was associated with marked clinical improvement

In some patients, the asymmetry of symptoms is similar to mononeuropathy multiplex. Plexopathies are frequent (30–40%) (Fig. 13.1c, d), but an isolated plexopathy is less common. The syndromes progress over weeks to months. Hyperacute variants reminiscent of Guillain-Barre syndrome are rare.

Mononeuropathies, secondary to malignant lymphocytic infiltration of nerves, occur in the sciatic, median, radial, ulnar, and intercostal nerves, or may manifest as cranial mononeuropathy [26–32]. Motor and sensory deficits are more common than pain syndromes and may precede diagnosis of NL by months to years.

A painless neuropathy occurs in 25–30% of cases. Paresthesias, numbness, and loss of deep tendon reflexes precede weakness. Examples of painless asymmetric or patchy numbness, as well as early painless proximal limb weakness reflecting plexus invasion are rare.

Involvement of cranial nerves has been described in about 50% of patients with NL during the course of the disease, but a single cranial neuropathy may herald diagnosis in approximately 20% [3]. The cranial neuropathies are usually painless, but painful trigeminal neuropathies have been reported [26, 27, 29, 33].

The majority of the patients are known to have a history of systemic or CNS lymphoma at the time of presentation with a clinical syndrome compatible with NL. In about 25–30% of cases, NL is the first manifestation of the malignancy (Table 13.1), but it is likely that systemic involvement will also be discovered after diagnostic evaluation at NL presentation. However, in some patients, no dissemination, either systemically or in the CNS, is recognized and this rare variant, isolated NL, may be diagnosed only at the time of autopsy [1–3, 34]. The majority of patients with NL have a B-cell malignancy, but the proportion of reported T-cell neoplasms is higher than anticipated (Table 13.1). Yet, as the source of data is largely based on published case reports, this may reflect a reporting bias.

Diagnosis

Diagnosis of NL requires integration of information from the clinical presentation (symptoms/signs), imaging findings, and morphological data obtained from neural or nonneural tissue and the CSF. A high index of suspicion and familiarity with the clinical manifestations of NL is necessary. As it is a rare expression of a hematologic malignancy, diagnosis is often delayed. Clinically, NL mimics nonneoplastic or paraneoplastic neuropathies. Clinical findings that suggest NL, as opposed to a remote effect of cancer or an inflammatory process, includes severe pain, asymmetric distribution, and rapid evolution. Still, the diagnosis is often elusive and 46% of patients identified up to the year 2000 [3] were diagnosed only at autopsy. With increasing awareness of this entity, NL is identified *ante mortem* more frequently, and diagnosis at autopsy was reported in only 8% of the 50 patients in the most recent IPCG series (Table 13.2); these four patients had an extensive evaluation prior to death for suspected NL, but no definite diagnosis could be established.

Imaging studies are of greatest utility. Magnetic resonance imaging (MRI) reveals nerve or nerve root enlargement or enhancement, and sometimes involvement of a neural plexus, which is more difficult to detect [3, 29, 35–41] (Fig. 13.1a, c). MRI findings are not specific for NL and might sometimes be seen in acute or chronic inflammatory radiculoneuropathies, in neurofibromatosis, in inflammatory pseudotumor, and in malignant tumors of the peripheral nerve sheath. Interpretation of imaging studies in the context of the clinical manifestations and laboratory tests is necessary. MRI yields abnormal findings in approximately 80% of patients (Table 13.2), and facilitates the diagnosis particularly when there is a history of hematologic malignancy.

In lymphomas, fusion ^{18}F-fluoro-2-deoxy-D-glucose (FDG) PET-CT is a standard diagnostic tool, which is used for staging and monitoring of therapeutic response. It seems to be a highly sensitive test in NL and although the total number of reported cases is still small, it may indicate the diagnosis and suggest which nerve is the best target for biopsy (Fig. 13.1d). Table 13.2 shows that FDG-PET yielded positive findings in up to 90% of patients studied. Yet, FDG-PET is not specific for NL and it may be positive when other malignancies affect peripheral or

Table 13.2 Diagnostic modalities and response to treatment of neurolymphomatosis associated with lymphoproliferative malignancies

	Group A[a] Literature review with MGH case-series 1972–2000 N = 72	Group B[b] Literature review 2001–2008 N = 43	Group C[c] IPCG case series 1993–2008 N = 50
Diagnostic/treatment modality	No. positive/No. of tests	No. positive/No. of tests	No. positive/No. of tests
Imaging:			
CT	NA	3/11 (27%)	7/11 (64%)
MRI	28/40 (70%)	27/34 (79%)	36/47 (77%)
FDG-PET	NA	18/20 (90%)	16/19 (84%)
CSF cytology	21/52 (40%)	9/23 (39%)	18/45 (40%)
CSF PCR gene rearrangement	NA	2/2 (100%)	3/11 (27%)
Biopsy of affected nerve	24/30 (80%)	19/21 (90%)	23/26 (88%)
Diagnosis established only by autopsy	33 (46%)	2 (5%)	4 (8%)
No. pts treated for NL[d]	43 (60%)	33 (77%)	47 (94%)
IV HD-MTX	5/43 (12%)	7/33 (21%)	23/47 (49%)
Intra CSF chemoTx.	15/43 (35%)	13/33 (39%)	23/47 (49%)
Radiotherapy	10/43 (23%)	16/33 (48%)	16/47 (34%)
Response rate[e]	31/43 (72%)	19/33 (58%)	16/35 (46%)

ChemoTx., chemotherapy; CSF, cerebrospinal fluid; HD-MTX, high dose methotrexate; IV, intravenous; NA, not available; NL, neurolymphomatosis; No., number; PCR, polymerase chain reaction; pts, patients.

[a]Group A consists of a retrospective case series of 25 patients diagnosed in Massachusetts General Hospital (MGH) and literature review of additional 47 cases that were published together [3].

[b]Group B is based on literature review (for references see Table 13.1).

[c]Group C consists of a retrospective case series collected from 12 institutions in 5 countries as a part of the IPCG project [4].

[d]Some patients were treated by chemotherapy other than high dose methotrexate.

[e]Includes complete and partial response by clinical improvement or by post treatment imaging.

cranial nerves. However, in the setting of known lymphoma, with clinical findings compatible with NL, it may be diagnostic.

Identification of malignant cells in the CSF is a confirmatory diagnostic test for NL. However, both cytologic evaluation and flow cytometry have modest sensitivity and positive findings are reported in only about 40% of patients (Table 13.2). Tests that suggest monoclonality of cells within the CSF (e.g. flow cytometry and PCR-based gene rearrangement of either the immunoglobulin heavy-chain in B-cells or of the T-cell receptor) have been applied sporadically (Table 13.2). These tests may confirm that malignant cells entered the CSF when the morphology is in doubt.

Although most of the reported cases were evaluated by multiple diagnostic modalities, a biopsy of an affected nerve was still indicated and has been performed in more than 40% of NL patients. The diagnostic yield of a biopsy is high and infiltration of a peripheral or cranial nerve by malignant cells is demonstrated histopathologically in 80–90% of biopsy samples (Table 13.2). The majority of cases are classified by immunohistochemistry as a B-cell malignancy (Table 13.1).

Treatment and Outcome

Treatment of NL consists of either chemotherapy alone or chemotherapy combined with radiotherapy. In order to select the appropriate treatment, knowledge of the systemic and neurological extent of involvement is essential. Staging with FDG-PET is effective for delineation of systemic disease, as well as the involved nerves (Fig. 13.1d). Contrast-enhanced MR images of brain and the complete spine should be obtained as well. NL involves roots within, as well as beyond, the borders of the subarachnoid space and thus, intrathecal drugs and standard craniospinal radiation fields will not treat all of the involved areas.

Chemotherapy is critical to address the multiple sites of involvement. Overall, 70% of patients who received treatment for NL in the IPCG series were managed by chemotherapy (Table 13.2). The most effective regimen is unknown and the selection is often based on protocols used to treat CNS involvement by malignant lymphoma. Many centers employed intravenous, high-dose methotrexate, either alone or in combination with other drugs and particularly with high-dose cytarabine. Doses of methotrexate ranged between 3 and 8 g/m^2. Methotrexate is effective against lymphoma, affecting the nervous system and when given in high doses, can penetrate the blood-brain and blood-nerve barrier. Any other choice of chemotherapy must also meet those criteria. However, in the IPCG series approximately 30% of treated patients did not receive systemic chemotherapy due to the fact that NL represented relapse of a chemoresistant disease. Intrathecal chemotherapy (methotrexate, cytarabine, rituximab) has been used in 35–50% of patients to treat either overt leptomeningeal seeding or to prevent its occurrence.

Radiotherapy has a limited role in the treatment of NL due to involvement of multiple sites, affecting both the CNS and the peripheral nervous system. Extensive radiation fields are poorly tolerated in most patients, but focal radiotherapy can be very effective in relieving unremitting neuropathic pain attributed to a particular nerve, plexus, or nerve root.

Clinical improvement (functional recovery, reduction of pain), as well as radiographic resolution (improvement of nerve root enlargement and enhancement or normalization of FDG-PET uptake) have been observed in 50–70% of treated patients (Table 13.2) (Fig. 13.1a, b, d, e). Standardized criteria to measure response are not available. There is limited data available on overall survival data. The median survival from diagnosis of NL in the IPCG series was 10 months, with 12 and

36 month survival rates of 46 and 24%, respectively. These data indicate that an aggressive multimodality therapeutic approach can achieve long term survival in some patients.

References

1. Grisold W, Jellinger K et al (1990) Human neurolymphomatosis in a patient with chronic lymphatic leukemia. Clin Neuropathol 9(5):224–230
2. Kuroda Y, Nakata H et al (1989) Human neurolymphomatosis by adult T-cell leukemia. Neurology 39(1):144–146
3. Baehring JM, Damek D et al (2003) Neurolymphomatosis. Neuro Oncol 5(2):104–115
4. Grisariu S, Avni B et al (2010) Neurolymphomatosis: An international primary CNS lymphoma collaborative group report. Blood 115(24):5005–5011
5. Bezier M, Reguiai Z et al (2009) Neurolymphomatosis associated with Sezary syndrome. Arch Dermatol 145(3):294–296
6. Odabasi Z, Parrott JH et al (2001) Neurolymphomatosis associated with muscle and cerebral involvement caused by natural killer cell lymphoma: a case report and review of literature. J Peripher Nerv Syst 6(4):197–203
7. Julien S, Radosavljevic M et al (1999) AIDS primary central nervous system lymphoma: molecular analysis of the expressed VH genes and possible implications for lymphomagenesis. J Immunol 162(3):1551–1558
8. Larocca LM, Capello D et al (1998) The molecular and phenotypic profile of primary central nervous system lymphoma identifies distinct categories of the disease and is consistent with histogenetic derivation from germinal center-related B cells. Blood 92(3): 1011–1019
9. McCann KJ, Ashton-Key M et al (2009) Primary central nervous system lymphoma: tumor-related clones exist in the blood and bone marrow with evidence for separate development. Blood 113(19):4677–4680
10. Montesinos-Rongen M, Kuppers R et al (1999) Primary central nervous system lymphomas are derived from germinal-center B cells and show a preferential usage of the V4-34 gene segment. Am J Pathol 155(6):2077–2086
11. Borit A, Altrocchi PH (1971) Recurrent polyneuropathy and neurolymphomatosis. Arch Neurol 24(1):40–49
12. Pages M, Marty-Double C et al (2004) Sensory neuropathy as revealing symptom of neurolymphomatosis: report of a case with a 15-year duration. Eur Neurol 52(1):57–58
13. Tajima Y, Sudo K et al (2007) Malignant lymphoma originating in the cauda equina mimicking the inflammatory polyradiculoneuropathy. Intern Med 46(13):1029–1032
14. Kuntzer T, Lobrinus JA et al (2000) Clinicopathological and molecular biological studies in a patient with neurolymphomatosis. Muscle Nerve 23(10):1604–1609
15. Pals ST, de Gorter DJ et al (2007) Lymphoma dissemination: the other face of lymphocyte homing. Blood 110(9):3102–3111
16. Drillenburg P, Pals ST (2000) Cell adhesion receptors in lymphoma dissemination. Blood 95(6):1900–1910
17. Pals ST, Drillenburg P et al (1997) Adhesion molecules in the dissemination of non-Hodgkin's lymphomas. Acta Haematol 97(1-2):73–80
18. Aho R, Ekfors T et al (1993) Pathogenesis of primary central nervous system lymphoma: invasion of malignant lymphoid cells into and within the brain parenchyma. Acta Neuropathol 86(1):71–76
19. Aho R, Kalimo H et al (1997) Binding of malignant lymphoid cells to the white matter of the human central nervous system: role of different CD44 isoforms, beta 1, beta 2 and beta 7 integrins, and L-selectin. J Neuropathol Exp Neurol 56(5):557–568

20. Albelda SM (1993) Role of integrins and other cell adhesion molecules in tumor progression and metastasis. Lab Invest 68(1):4–17
21. Bashir R, Coakham H et al (1992) Expression of LFA-1/ICAM-1 in CNS lymphomas: possible mechanism for lymphoma homing into the brain. J Neurooncol 12(2):103–110
22. Kern WF, Spier CM et al (1992) Neural cell adhesion molecule-positive peripheral T-cell lymphoma: a rare variant with a propensity for unusual sites of involvement. Blood 79(9):2432–2437
23. Matsumura Y, Tarin D (1992) Significance of CD44 gene products for cancer diagnosis and disease evaluation. Lancet 340(8827):1053–1058
24. Osterrieder N, Kamil JP et al (2006) Marek's disease virus: from miasma to model. Nat Rev Microbiol 4(4):283–294
25. Okada K, Tanaka Y et al (1997) Phenotype analysis of lymphoid cells in Marek's disease of CD4(+) or CD8(+) T-cell-deficient chickens: occurrence of double negative T-cell tumour. Avian Pathol 26(3):525–534
26. Bulsara KR, Kadri PA et al (2005) Malignant lymphoma of the trigeminal region. Case illustration. J Neurooncol 73(3):279–280
27. Czepczynski R, Guzikowska-Ruszkowska I et al (2008) Neurolymphomatosis detected by (18)F-FDG PET/CT scan – a case report. Nucl Med Rev Cent East Eur 11(2):73–75
28. Dakwar E, Teja S et al (2004) Sciatic neurolymphomatosis. Neurology 63(9):1751
29. Iplikcioglu AC, Dinc C et al (2006) Primary lymphoma of the trigeminal nerve. Br J Neurosurg 20(2):103–105
30. Karadag D, Karagulle AT et al (2002) Trigeminal nerve involvement in T-cell acute lymphoblastic leukemia: value of MR imaging. Eur J Radiol 44(1):16–18
31. Kitzmann AS, Pulido JS et al (2008) Histologic findings in T-cell lymphoma infiltration of the optic nerve. Ophthalmology 115(5):e1–e6
32. Strobel K, Fischer K et al (2007) Sciatic nerve neurolymphomatosis – extent and therapy response assessment with PET/CT. Clin Nucl Med 32(8):646–648
33. Kinoshita M, Izumoto S et al (2003) Primary malignant lymphoma of the trigeminal region treated with rapid infusion of high-dose MTX and radiation: case report and review of the literature. Surg Neurol 60(4):343–348; discussion 348
34. Diaz-Arrastia R, Younger DS et al (1992) Neurolymphomatosis: a clinicopathologic syndrome re-emerges. Neurology 42(6):1136–1141
35. Baehring J, Cooper D (2004) Neurolymphomatosis. J Neurooncol 68(3):243–244
36. Dong Q, Wong KK et al (2008) Sacral nerve root neurolymphomatosis diagnosed on FDG-PET/CT and magnetic resonance imaging. Clin Nucl Med 33(1):30–31
37. Khong P, Pitham T et al (2008) Isolated neurolymphomatosis of the cauda equina and filum terminale: case report. Spine 33(21):E807–E811
38. Kim JH, Jang JH et al (2006) A case of neurolymphomatosis involving cranial nerves: MRI and fusion PET-CT findings. J Neurooncol 80(2):209–210
39. Levin N, Soffer D et al (2008) Primary T-cell CNS lymphoma presenting with leptomeningeal spread and neurolymphomatosis. J Neurooncol 90(1):77–83
40. Matano S, Shirasaki H et al (2006) Thickening of multiple cranial nerves in a patient with extranodal peripheral T-cell lymphoma. J Neuroimaging 16(2):167–169
41. Moore KR, Blumenthal DT et al (2001) Neurolymphomatosis of the lumbar plexus: high-resolution MR neurography findings. Neurology 57(4):740–742
42. Shibata-Hamaguchi A, Samuraki M et al (2007) B-cell neurolymphomatosis confined to the peripheral nervous system. J Neurol Sci 260(1–2):249–252
43. Boes M, Pels H et al (2008) High-grade B-cell NHL of the brachial plexus followed by infiltration of the spinal cord. J Neurol 255(1):135–137
44. Bokstein F, Goor O et al (2005) Assessment of neurolymphomatosis by brachial plexus biopsy and PET/CT. Report of a case. J Neurooncol 72(2):163–167
45. Ghobrial IM, Buadi F et al (2004) High-dose intravenous methotrexate followed by autologous stem cell transplantation as a potentially effective therapy for neurolymphomatosis. Cancer 100(11):2403–2407

46. Grisold W, Klimpfinger M et al (2007) Peripheral nerve involvement in lymphoma: the meninges as the crucial barrier between meningoradicular spread and neurolymphomatosis. J Peripher Nerv Syst 12(1):58–60
47. Kanter P, Zeidman A et al (2005) PET-CT imaging of combined brachial and lumbosacral neurolymphomatosis. Eur J Haematol 74(1):66–69
48. Koerbel A, Roser F et al (2005) Primary non-Hodgkin lymphoma of the cranial nerves mimicking neurofibromatosis Type 2. Case illustration. J Neurosurg 102(6):1166
49. Kosa SC, Peller PJ et al (2009) T-cell neurolymphomatosis involving cauda equina and sciatic nerves. Neurology 72(1):98
50. Lin M, Kilanowska J et al (2008) Neurolymphomatosis–diagnosis and assessment of treatment response by FDG PET-CT. Hematol Oncol 26(1):43–45
51. Ohta H (2002) A case of non-Hodgkin's lymphoma infiltrating the brachial plexus detected by Ga-67 scintigraphy. Ann Nucl Med 16(4):297–298
52. Ozturk E, Arpaci F et al (2006) Detection of widespread neurolymphomatosis with 18F-FDG PET. Eur J Nucl Med Mol Imaging 33(8):975–976
53. Peruzzi P, Ray-Chaudhuri A et al (2009) Reversal of neurological deficit after chemotherapy in BCL-6-positive neurolymphomatosis. J Neurosurg 111(2):247–251
54. Pietrangeli A, Milella M et al (2000) Brachial plexus neuropathy as unusual onset of diffuse neurolymphomatosis. Neurol Sci 21(4):241–245
55. Rosso SM, de Bruin HG et al (2006) Diagnosis of neurolymphomatosis with FDG PET. Neurology 67(4):722–723
56. Seror P (2001) Brachial plexus neoplastic lesions assessed by conduction study of medial antebrachial cutaneous nerve. Muscle Nerve 24(8):1068–1070
57. Shima K, Ishida C et al (2008) A linear lesion along the brachial plexus on FDG-PET in neurolymphomatosis. Intern Med 47(12):1159–1160
58. Trojan A, Jermann M et al (2002) Fusion PET-CT imaging of neurolymphomatosis. Ann Oncol 13(5):802–805
59. Yazawa S, Ohi T et al (2007) Brachial plexus neurolymphomatosis: a discrepancy between electrophysiological and radiological findings. Intern Med 46(8):533–534

Chapter 14
Intravascular Lymphoma of the CNS

Maurilio Ponzoni, Jon Glass, and Emanuele Zucca

Introduction

By virtue of its distinctive, almost selective growth within vessel lumina, intravascular large B-cell lymphoma (IVLBCL) represents perhaps the best *in vivo* model for the evaluation of lymphocytic migration, trafficking and invasiveness of lymphoma cells [1].

IVLBCL, previously described as "angiotropic lymphoma" refers to a disease described in 1959 by Pfeger and Tappeneimer as an endothelial neoplasia with vascular dissemination [2]. This disease was recognized as "lymphoid" more recently [3] and is designated as a distinct clinicopathological entity in the 2008 edition of the WHO classification of lymphoid neoplasms [4]. Accordingly, IVLBCL is currently defined as "a rare type of extranodal large B-cell lymphoma characterized by selective growth of lymphoma cells within the lumina of vessels, particularly capillaries, with exception of larger arteries and veins" [4]. Rare cases with T-cell or NK-cell phenotype have been reported, but they are considered to represent a different entity [4].

Pathology and Biology

Tissue biopsy is essential for the diagnosis of IVLBCL. The tumor cells must be visualized as contained within blood vessels to establish the diagnosis of IVLBCL. In those patients with suspected CNS involvement by IVLBCL, a random skin [6], gastric [7], or even a bone marrow biopsy [8] may establish the diagnosis as IVLBCL is always a systemic disease, even if systemic involvement is not immediately apparent clinically. The main challenge is to determine which target tissue should be subjected to biopsy. Sometimes multiple random biopsies might

---

M. Ponzoni (✉)
Pathology Unit, Unit of Lymphoid Malignancies, Scientific Institute, San Raffaele Hospital, Milan, Italy
e-mail: ponzoni.maurilio@hsr.it

T. Batchelor, L.M. DeAngelis (eds.), *Lymphoma and Leukemia of the Nervous System*, DOI 10.1007/978-1-4419-7668-0_14,

be required to achieve the diagnosis [9]. Lymph node biopsy is discouraged, as IVLBCL rarely affects these structures.

Histopathology

IVLBCL cells are usually large, with enlarged nuclei and scant cytoplasm; only rarely are these cells a medium-to-large size. The nuclear outline is smooth, sometimes with irregular contour. The nucleolus may be single or multiple. These cells share intermediate features between centroblasts and immunoblasts. Importantly, mitotic figures are present, suggesting that the blood vessel lumen could be the site of active replication for IVLBCL cells [1, 4].

The degree and growth patterns within blood vessel lumina vary from case to case, or more than one pattern may occur in the same patient. Basically, four patterns are recognized: (1) “dyscohesive”, in which neoplastic lymphocytes are free-floating in the lumen; (2) “cohesive”, where the cells form aggregates completely filling the lumen, sometimes disrupting the blood vessel structure; (3) “adhesive”, when IVLBCL cells are selectively close to the endothelia and the lumen is almost devoid of neoplastic cells; (4) “tumor associated”, when IVLBCL selectively colonizes vessels contained within an associated benign or malignant neoplasm [10]. When IVLBCL occurs in the CNS, the first two patterns predominate (Fig. 14.1).

Aside from the above-mentioned features, which could be defined collectively as the “classic variant” of IVL, a so-called “hemophagocytosis related” variant (formerly called the “Asian variant”) of IVLBCL has also been described [11, 12]. In this variant, the neoplastic lymphocytes do not show substantial morphologic differences compared to the classic patterns, but are accompanied by a striking array

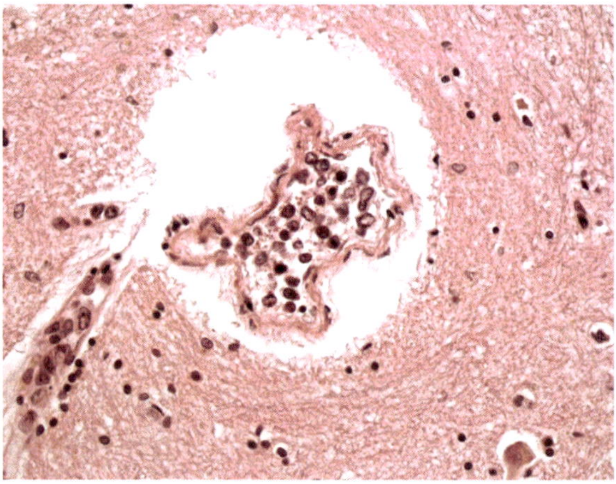

Fig. 14.1 Intravascular lymphomatosis: neoplastic large lymphocytes are “free floating” in a brain parenchymal vessel (Hematoxylin and Eosin, 40X)

of non-neoplastic elements, among which hemophagocytic histiocytes predominate [11]. In non-IVLBCL cases, a case of IVL with "anaplastic" morphology has also been reported [13].

Immunophenotype and Molecular Biology

IVLBCL cells display the immunophenotype of a "mature" (i.e. not precursor) lymphocyte. More than 90% of the reported cases show a B-cell phenotype and with few exceptions, are CD20 positive [11]. Few studies have focused on the immunophenotypic characterization of IVLBCL. In a series of cases diagnosed in Western countries, only one fifth displayed a so-called "germinal center phenotype" in terms of either CD10 or BCL-6 immunoreactivity [14] and, unexpectedly, half of these patients were also CD5 positive. In addition, a study from Japan demonstrated that the majority of IVLBCL express the late/post-germinal center-associated molecule, MUM-1, as well as BCL-2 protein [15]. Taken together, these data demonstrate marked immunophenotypic heterogeneity of IVL.

Few exceptions to B-cell lineage occur in IVL, and these have either a T-cell immunophenotype [13, 16], which are sometimes associated with HIV infection [17], or an NK immunophenotype [18].

There are anecdotal reports that describe immunoreactivity for the myeloid-lineage associated molecule myeloperoxidase [19] and prostatic acid phosphatase [20] in IVLBCL. The significance of these phenotypic features is unknown and confirmatory studies are necessary.

The clonal nature of IVLBCL has been demonstrated by Southern blot technique [21] or, more recently, by PCR [22], using immunoglobulin heavy chain rearrangement or T-cell receptor rearrangement to identify the B-cell or T-cell phenotype, respectively. Furthermore, identification of somatic hypermutation of the immunoglobulin heavy chain in five of six cases of IVLBCL [23] suggests that these cells arise from the germinal center. Interestingly, t(14;18) rearrangement is rare in IVLBCL [24]. Cytogenetic abnormalities in IVLBCL have not been investigated thoroughly; these abnormalities are relatively frequent, albeit not characteristic; the most frequent abnormalities in a series of 6 patients were structural aberrations in chromosomes 1(especially 1p), 6, and 18, and trisomy 18 [25].

Adhesion Molecules

The most distinctive property of IVL cells is their propensity to grow within blood vessel lumina without substantial extravasation. Neoplastic B-cells in IVLBCL may be able to adhere, at least in part, to endothelial cells, but the cells seem to lack molecules, such as CD29 (β1 integrin subunit), which are critical for extravasation [10, 26, 27]. It is likely that adhesion/extravasation defects at multiple levels may be implicated in the pathogenesis of these lymphomas.

Table 14.1 Most frequent presenting symptoms in IVLBCL

Systemic symptoms	55%
Fever	18%
Fever + weight loss ± night sweats	23%
Fever + night sweats	3%
Weight loss	10%
Cutaneous lesions	40%
Neurological symptoms	35%
Pain	20%
Fatigue	16%

Relationship with Infectious Agents

Although IVLBCL has not been linked to any particular infectious agent, some microorganisms have been demonstrated in patients with these lymphomas. Infectious agents include some helminths, as suggested by the detection of serum antibodies to *Fasciola* and *Anisakis* in these patients [28]. The human T-cell lymphotropic virus type-1 (HTLV-1) has been associated with T-cell intravascular lymphoma [29], mostly in Japanese patients. EBV infection is usually not observed in IVLBCL [18, 30, 31], while there are reports of EBV detection in IVL with NK-cell and T-cell immunophenotype [18, 31–33] or associated with HIV infection [34]. Therefore, in IVLBCL it is important to assess whether the non-neoplastic bystander lymphocytes versus the tumor cells are positive for EBV. An association between IVLBCL and CMV, as well as other infectious agents, such as herpes simplex, herpes zoster, or human herpes virus-6 has not been detected [35]. However, a case of IVLBCL associated with human herpes virus-8 has been reported [36].

Clinical Presentation

The median age at diagnosis of IVL is 70 years, but there is a wide age range (34–90 years), and there is a similar prevalence in men and women. IVLBCL can involve any organ, thus accounting for the widely variable clinical presentation. Fever, pain, or organ-specific local symptoms may occur in combination with B symptoms and rapidly progressive manifestations, resulting from multiorgan failure. Frequently patients complain of non-specific symptoms accompanied by global deterioration in performance status (PS). This presentation, although non-specific, has led to an *in vivo* diagnosis in almost 80% of patients. In the past 10–20 years, the majority of diagnoses were made on post-mortem.

The most common presenting signs and symptoms of IVLBCL are summarized in Table 14.1. More than half of the cases are accompanied by systemic symptoms, which are the sole manifestation of disease in approximately 25% of subjects. Fever accounts for the most common systemic symptom (45%), a figure which is much more common with respect to other aggressive extranodal lymphomas (≤25%).

Neurological manifestations at presentation are seen in approximately one third of patients, and neurological symptoms may occur subsequently in an additional one third [37]. The majority of patients with neurological disease have one or more of four clinical syndromes: progressive, multifocal cerebrovascular events; spinal cord and nerve root vascular syndromes; a subacute progressive encephalopathy; or peripheral or cranial neuropathies [38].

The most common form of neurological presentation is characterized by acute episodes of neurological impairment. These events, resulting in either transient or permanent neurological deficits, are due to occlusion of small arteries by neoplastic lymphocytes with resulting ischemia [39–41]. Brain-imaging characteristics reflect that of stroke. CT scanning reveals decreased attenuation in the distribution of large vessels or penetrating vessels [42]. MRI reveals increased intensity on T2 and FLAIR sequences, and restricted diffusion on diffusion-weighted images [5]. These areas do not typically enhance after contrast administration, although focal areas of enhancement in patchy, punctate, or linear patterns have been described. These radiographic findings may be present even if the patient has not had classical cerebrovascular symptoms [43]. Discrete, diffusely enhancing mass lesions with surrounding edema have also been described [44].

Cerebral angiography is commonly non-diagnostic, but may reveal multiple occlusions or stenoses of medium or small vessels [40]. An initially normal angiogram may later reveal multiple areas of stenosis or occlusion [44].

Venous occlusive disease has also been described. Kenéz et al. described a patient with a left frontal venous infarction accompanied by a defect on MR venography in the posterior third of the superior sagittal sinus and internal cerebral vein. Involvement of smaller arterioles and venules, large veins, and the superior sagittal sinus was observed at autopsy [45].

A subacute encephalopathy with a decline in the level of consciousness without focal cerebral signs may occur in up to 25% of patients. Other neurological syndromes, particularly paraparesis, may accompany this subacute encephalopathy. Encephalopathy may be initially attributed to a metabolic cause, delaying diagnosis [38, 48]. Seizures occur late in the course of the disease and accompany either encephalopathy or focal vascular events. Ocular manifestations include visual loss or blurring, reflecting occlusion of the retinal artery or its branches, ischemic optic neuropathy, papilledema, uveitis, vitiritis, and iridocyclitis [38].

Less commonly, patients will develop a syndrome of progressive paraparesis, localized or radicular back pain, urinary retention and incontinence, attributable to involvement of the vessels supplying the spinal cord, nerve roots, or peripheral nerves. Symptoms are initially referable to lower spinal segments and progress to involve higher levels. Although paraparesis is usually flaccid, it can also be spastic. Involvement in the upper extremities is less common and less severe [38, 39]. Radiographic findings are usually non-specific. Areas of abnormal T2 signal may be found within the spinal cord, particularly the conus medullaris. Myelography is usually described as negative, though swelling of nerve roots has been described on post-myelographic CT scanning [38, 47]. Electromyography and nerve conduction testing (EMG/NCV) often reveals evidence of acute denervation in the distribution of both nerve roots and peripheral nerves. Nerve conduction velocities may be normal or decreased. Electrophysiological findings consistent with myopathy have also been described [46]. Peripheral distal polyneuropathies, mononeuropathies, mononeuropathy multiplex, and cranial neuropathies and myopathy have also been described [38].

Approximately 25% of IVLBCL patients have only cutaneous involvement; termed the "cutaneous variant" of IVLBCL [8]. Single or multiple lesions of the skin in combination with negative systemic staging are consistent with this clinical presentation of IVLBCL. Patients with this variant display distinctive clinical characteristics and prognosis. Almost all patients with the "cutaneous variant" are women with normal leukocyte and platelet counts, ECOG-PS usually ≤ 1, younger age (59 years), and a lower rate of systemic symptoms than "classic" IVLBCL. Patients with the "cutaneous variant" survive longer than other patients, even after controlling for the International Prognostic Index (IPI) score and all other known prognostic variables. Therapeutic outcome is remarkably better in patients with single cutaneous lesions compared to patients with multiple lesions [8].

In the remaining 75% of cases, cutaneous involvement may variably occur; in these situations, however, cutaneous lesions are associated with other manifestations, mostly represented by neurological or B symptoms, and standard lymphoma staging procedures often detect additional sites of disease, mostly in the liver, CNS, and bone marrow.

Stage and Sites of Disease

Forty percent of patients have stage I_E disease at diagnosis, according to the Ann Arbor staging system. A portion of these cases have disease limited to the skin ("cutaneous variant"). However, 60% of IVLBCL patients have stage IV disease at diagnosis, and disseminated disease is reported in all autopsied cases (Table 14.2). The most commonly involved organs are skin, CNS, bone marrow, liver, and spleen, with 60–80% of patients having skin or CNS involvement.

In rare cases of IVL, the bone marrow or lymphatic system is involved and complete staging evaluation should include a bone marrow biopsy in all patients [1]. Peripheral blood involvement is rare (5% of cases), in contrast to the distinct propensity of lymphoma cells to grow within blood vessel lumen [49]. It should be emphasized, however, that a systematic search for neoplastic cells is not routinely performed; therefore, a more systematic morphologic evaluation or a cytogenetic

Table 14.2 Main sites of IVLBCL localization

Skin	single lesion	11%
	multiple lesions	30%
CNS		40%
Liver		26%
Spleen		26%
Bone marrow		32%
Peripheral blood smear		5%
Lymph nodes		11%

analysis of peripheral blood smears, may increase the identification of peripheral blood involvement by IVLBCL [1].

Association with Other Tumors

Approximately 15% of IVL patients have a history of prior or concomitant malignancies, with an interval between tumor occurrences of approximately 4–5 years. The non-IVLBCL tumor may be either a hematopoietic or non-hematopoietic malignancy. Among hematopoietic tumors, non-Hodgkin lymphomas are the most commonly associated malignancies, since they occur in approximately one third of cases [50]. NHLs may occur before, concomitantly, or after the IVLBCL diagnosis; the most represented histiotype is diffuse large B-cell lymphoma, but other histiotypes may occur as well [1]. This is a relevant issue considering that extravascular infiltration, which is observed in 11% of IVL cases, does not exclude the diagnosis of IVL, because the coexistence of both components has been described previously. In the CNS, some IVLBCL may be associated, at diagnosis or during the course of disease, with macroscopic lymphomatous brain masses [51].

Associated non-hematopoietic tumors include benign or malignant neoplasms. IVLBCL cells can be detected either in epithelial [52], mesenchymal [53] or vascular [10, 35] benign tumors. In the malignant non-hematopoietic category, epithelial tumors, such as renal cell carcinoma, have been reported [10]; in these patients, the IVLBCL cells were present preferentially within tumor-associated vessels (see "pathologic findings"); this finding suggests that the cancer-associated endothelia express particular molecules that attract or induce IVLBCL.

Laboratory Findings

The peripheral blood count is usually abnormal in IVLBCL patients. Anemia is the most frequent cytopenia (63%); leukopenia, or thrombocytopenia, usually does not occur without anemia. Cytopenias (particularly thrombocytopenia) are associated with bone marrow infiltration and hepatosplenic involvement. Increased serum lactic dehydrogenase and β_2-microglobulin levels are observed in more than 80% of IVLBCL patients. An elevated erythrocyte sedimentation rate is present in approximately one-half of cases, and a monoclonal serum spike is reported in 14% of patients. Altered hepatic, renal, or thyroid function tests are observed in approximately 15% of cases and are invariably associated with organ involvement by lymphoma cells.

The "Hemophagocytosis-Associated" Variant

Clinical features in IVLBCL cases diagnosed in Western countries are remarkably different than those reported in Japanese series [12, 54]. In Japanese patients, IVL is associated with hemophagocytic syndrome, bone marrow involvement, fever, hepatosplenomegaly, and thrombocytopenia in 73–100% of cases, while CNS and cutaneous involvement are uncommon. These features have been defined as diagnostic for hemophagocytic syndrome-associated IVLBCL (formerly the "Asian variant"). In this variant, IVLBCL has a rapidly aggressive course, with a median survival of 2–8 months. Since "classic IVLBCL" occurs in many Asian countries outside Japan, and some cases of hemophagocytic syndrome-associated IVLBCL may be present in Western countries, it is perhaps better to describe the classic and the hemophagocytosis-associated variants, without reference to geographical areas [12].

Treatment

IVLBCL usually displays a rapidly progressive and, ultimately, fatal course. However, there are exceptions with some patients achieving durable remission after chemotherapy, and rare reports of long-term survivors. Prompt diagnosis is critical as delayed diagnosis is often associated with rapid and progressive multiorgan failure and impairment of performance status. The latter complications may prevent the administration of aggressive chemotherapy. Since it is widely accepted that IVLBCL is a disseminated disease, with the exception of the cutaneous variant, polychemotherapy is advisable [7, 37]. Historically, encouraging results in these lymphomas have been achieved with anthracycline-containing regimens [55]; with these drugs, the response rate is approximately 60%, although an optimal evaluation of response is challenging due to the diffuse nature of IVLBCL, and the inability to fully define the sites of measurable disease (i.e., lymphadenopathy and tumor masses). A 53% complete remission rate and a 2-year OS of 32% was observed in Japanese patients with hemophagocytic syndrome-associated IVLBCL, which is comparable to response rates reported for classic IVLBCL in Western countries.

Relapses occur in half of patients treated with anthracycline-based chemotherapy, with a median time to progression of 8 months, and death within 18 months from diagnosis, with 3-year event-free survival of 27%. These relapses, in which the CNS is involved in one third of cases, invariably involve extranodal organs, mostly represented by the primary site of disease. The 3-year OS is approximately 30% and, interestingly enough, relapses after 5 years are rare. Predictors of durable remission after anthracycline-based chemotherapy are the cutaneous variant, good PS and small tumor burden. Despite initial responses, most patients with CNS involvement treated with anthracycline-based chemotherapy die early due to lymphoma progression or septic complications.

An important achievement in IVLBCL has been the introduction of rituximab to the therapeutic regimen. In studies both from Japan [56, 57] and Western countries [58, 59], complete remission rates are reported in more than 80% of IVLBCL patients at a median follow-up of 2 years. Interestingly, 5/6 relapses occurring within this period involved the CNS [59]. This suggests that more intensive combinations including drugs with higher CNS bioavailability, such as methotrexate or cytarabine, are needed in cases with CNS involvement [59].

The observations above support the view that IVLBCL represents an oncologic emergency and, if this lymphoma is promptly and successfully treated, patients may experience a more favorable prognosis.

Additional/alternative therapeutic strategies are based on anecdotal evidence. For example, some cases treated with methotrexate-containing chemotherapy followed by consolidation with high-dose chemotherapy supported by autologous stem cell transplantation (ASCT) have achieved good outcomes [7, 37], but this therapy appears feasible for only a small proportion of patients with IVLBCL, given the advanced median age (i.e. >70 years), and compromised performance status in many at diagnosis. However, the impact of early consolidation with high-dose chemotherapy supported by ASCT may hold some promise and deserves to be investigated further, mostly in young patients with unfavorable features.

Finally, radiotherapy may be considered the sole treatment for IVL in elderly patients with a single cutaneous lesion; however, it has yet to be evaluated in patients with CNS involvement.

Future Perspectives

In the last 20 years, significant improvements have been achieved in this rare disease with a dismal prognosis, in terms of better knowledge of the histopathologic features and improved therapy. Notwithstanding these advances, many questions remain unanswered in IVLBCL. These issues involve biological aspects, such as: the need for better immunophenotypic characterization; recognition of the putative normal cellular counterpart; the possible immunophenotypic/molecular differences between the "classic" and the "cutaneous" variants, as well as between the Western and Asian variants; a better understanding of the relationship of IVLBCL to NHL; improved knowledge of immunoglobulin V_H family recruitment; a better characterization of cytogenetic abnormalities; and a more detailed characterization of the cytokine/adhesion molecules involved in IVLBCL. In addition, urgent clinical questions, such as the future role of drugs with good CNS bioavailability in the treatment of IVLBCL are equally important and likely will represent the forthcoming research strategies in this rare disease.

References

1. Ponzoni M, Ferreri AJ, Campo E et al (2007) Definition, diagnosis, and management of intravascular large B-cell lymphoma: proposals and perspectives from an international consensus meeting. J Clin Oncol 25:3168–3173
2. Pfleger L, Tappeiner J (1959) On the recognition of systematized endotheliomatosis of the cutaneous blood vessels (reticuloendotheliosis?). Hautarzt 10:359–363
3. Sheibani K, Battifora H, Winberg CD et al (1986) Further evidence that "malignant angioendotheliomatosis" is an angiotropic large-cell lymphoma. N Engl J Med 314:943–948
4. Nakamura S, Ponzoni M, Campo E (2008) Intravascular large B-cell lymphoma. In: Swerdlow S, Campo E, Harris NL et al (eds) WHO Classification of Tumours of Haematopoietic and Lymphoid Tissues. IARC, Lyon, pp 252–253

5. Baehring JM, Henchcliffe C, Ledezma CJ et al (2005) Intravascular lymphoma: magnetic resonance imaging correlates of disease dynamics within the central nervous system. J Neurol Neurosurg Psychiatry 76:540–544
6. Gill S, Melosky B, Haley L, ChanYan C (2003) Use of random skin biopsy to diagnose intravascular lymphoma presenting as fever of unknown origin. Am J Med 114:56–58
7. Ponzoni M, Ferreri AJ (2006) Intravascular lymphoma: a neoplasm of "homeless" lymphocytes? Hematol Oncol 24:105–112
8. Ferreri AJ, Campo E, Seymour JF et al (2004) Intravascular lymphoma: clinical presentation, natural history, management and prognostic factors in a series of 38 cases, with special emphasis on the "cutaneous variant". Br J Haematol 127:173–183
9. Kiyohara T, Kumakiri M, Kobayashi H et al (2000) A case of intravascular large B-cell lymphoma mimicking erythema nodosum: the importance of multiple skin biopsies. J Cutan Pathol 27:413–418
10. Ponzoni M, Arrigoni G, Gould VE et al (2000) Lack of CD 29 (beta1 integrin) and CD 54 (ICAM-1) adhesion molecules in intravascular lymphomatosis. Hum Pathol 31:220–226
11. Murase T, Nakamura S, Kawauchi K et al (2000) An Asian variant of intravascular large B-cell lymphoma: clinical, pathological and cytogenetic approaches to diffuse large B-cell lymphoma associated with haemophagocytic syndrome. Br J Haematol 111:826–834
12. Ferreri AJ, Dognini GP, Campo E et al (2007) Variations in clinical presentation, frequency of hemophagocytosis and clinical behavior of intravascular lymphoma diagnosed in different geographical regions. Haematologica 92:486–492
13. Takahashi E, Kajimoto K, Fukatsu T et al (2005) Intravascular large T-cell lymphoma: a case report of CD30-positive and ALK-negative anaplastic type with cytotoxic molecule expression. Virchows Arch 447:1000–1006
14. Yegappan S, Coupland R, Arber DA et al (2001) Angiotropic lymphoma: an immunophenotypically and clinically heterogeneous lymphoma. Mod Pathol 14:1147–1156
15. Murase T, Yamaguchi M, Suzuki R et al (2007) Intravascular large B-cell lymphoma (IVLBCL): a clinicopathologic study of 96 cases with special reference to the immunophenotypic heterogeneity of CD5. Blood 109:478–485
16. Williams G, Foyle A, White D et al (2005) Intravascular T-cell lymphoma with bowel involvement: case report and literature review. Am J Hematol 78:207–211
17. Malicki DM, Suh YK, Fuller GN, Shin SS (1999) Angiotropic (intravascular) large cell lymphoma of T-cell phenotype presenting as acute appendicitis in a patient with acquired immunodeficiency syndrome. Arch Pathol Lab Med 123:335–337
18. Nakamichi N, Fukuhara S, Aozasa K, Morii E (2008) NK-cell intravascular lymphomatosis–a mini-review. Eur J Haematol 81:1–7
19. Conlin PA, Orden MB, Hough TR, Morgan DL (2001) Myeloperoxidase-positive intravascular large B-cell lymphoma. Arch Pathol Lab Med 125:948–950
20. Seki K, Miyakoshi S, Lee GH et al (2004) Prostatic acid phosphatase is a possible tumor marker for intravascular large B-cell lymphoma. Am J Surg Pathol 28:1384–1388
21. Otrakji CL, Voigt W, Amador A et al (1988) Malignant angioendotheliomatosis–a true lymphoma: a case of intravascular malignant lymphomatosis studied by southern blot hybridization analysis. Hum Pathol 19:475–478
22. Sleater JP, Segal GH, Scott MD, Masih AS (1994) Intravascular (angiotropic) large cell lymphoma: determination of monoclonality by polymerase chain reaction on paraffin-embedded tissues. Mod Pathol 7:593–598
23. Kanda M, Suzumiya J, Ohshima K et al (2001) Analysis of the immunoglobulin heavy chain gene variable region of intravascular large B-cell lymphoma. Virchows Arch 439:540–546
24. Vieites B, Fraga M, Lopez-Presas E et al (2005) Detection of t(14;18) translocation in a case of intravascular large B-cell lymphoma: a germinal centre cell origin in a subset of these lymphomas? Histopathology 46:466–468
25. Tsukadaira A, Okubo Y, Ogasawara H et al (2002) Chromosomal aberrations in intravascular lymphomatosis. Am J Clin Oncol 25:178–181

26. Kinoshita M, Izumoto S, Hashimoto N et al (2008) Immunohistochemical analysis of adhesion molecules and matrix metalloproteinases in malignant CNS lymphomas: a study comparing primary CNS malignant and CNS intravascular lymphomas. Brain Tumor Pathol 25:73–78
27. Ferry JA, Harris NL, Picker LJ et al (1988) Intravascular lymphomatosis (malignant angioendotheliomatosis). A B-cell neoplasm expressing surface homing receptors. Mod Pathol 1:444–452
28. Murase T, Tashiro K, Suzuki T et al (1998) Detection of antibodies to Fasciola and Anisakis in Japanese patients with intravascular lymphomatosis. Blood 92:2182–2183
29. Shimokawa I, Higami Y, Sakai H et al (1991) Intravascular malignant lymphomatosis: a case of T-cell lymphoma probably associated with human T-cell lymphotropic virus. Hum Pathol 22:200–202
30. Bergmann M, Terzija-Wessel U, Blasius S et al (1994) Intravascular lymphomatosis of the CNS: clinicopathologic study and search for expression of oncoproteins and Epstein-Barr virus. Clin Neurol Neurosurg 96:236–243
31. Au WY, Shek WH, Nicholls J et al (1997) T-cell intravascular lymphomatosis (angiotropic large cell lymphoma): association with Epstein-Barr viral infection. Histopathology 31:563–567
32. Song DE, Lee M-W, Ryu M-H et al (2007) Intravascular Large Cell Lymphoma of the Natural Killer Cell Type. J Clin Oncol 25:1279–1282
33. Cerroni L, Massone C, Kutzner H et al (2008) Intravascular large T-cell or NK-cell lymphoma: a rare variant of intravascular large cell lymphoma with frequent cytotoxic phenotype and association with Epstein-Barr virus infection. Am J Surg Pathol 32:891–898
34. Hsiao CH, Su IJ, Hsieh SW et al (1999) Epstein-Barr virus-associated intravascular lymphomatosis within Kaposi's sarcoma in an AIDS patient. Am J Surg Pathol 23:482–487
35. Nixon BK, Kussick SJ, Carlon MJ, Rubin BP (2005) Intravascular large B-cell lymphoma involving hemangiomas: an unusual presentation of a rare neoplasm. Mod Pathol 18: 1121–1126
36. Ferry JA, Sohani AR, Longtine JA et al (2009) HHV8-positive, EBV-positive Hodgkin lymphoma-like large B-cell lymphoma and HHV8-positive intravascular large B-cell lymphoma. Mod Pathol 22:618–626
37. Shimada K, Kinoshita T, Naoe T, Nakamura S (2009) Presentation and management of intravascular large B-cell lymphoma. Lancet Oncol 10:895–902
38. Glass J, Hochberg FH, Miller DC (1993) Intravascular lymphomatosis. A systemic disease with neurologic manifestations. Cancer 15(71):3156–3164
39. Beristain X, Azzarelli B (2002) The neurological masquerade of intravascular lymphomatosis. Arch Neurol 59:439–443
40. Calamia KT, Miller A, Shuster EA et al (1999) Intravascular lymphomatosis. A report of ten patients with central nervous system involvement and a review of the disease process. Adv Exp Med Biol 455:249–265
41. Sienknecht CW, Whetsell WO Jr, Pollock P (1995) Intravascular malignant lymphoma ("malignant angioendotheliomatosis") mimicking primary angiitis of the central nervous system. J Rheumatol 22:1769–1770
42. Song DK, Boulis NM, McKeever PE, Quint DJ (2002) Angiotropic large cell lymphoma with imaging characteristics of CNS vasculitis. AJNR Am J Neuroradiol 23:239–242
43. Hashimoto H, Naritomi H, Kazui S et al (1998) Presymptomatic brain lesions on MRI in a patient with intravascular malignant lymphomatosis. J Neuroimaging 8:110–113
44. Schonfeld SM, Pinto RS, Aleksic S, Pearson J (1985 May) Cerebral angioendotheliomatosis: a report of two cases and review of the literature. AJNR Am J Neuroradiol 6:437–441
45. Kenéz J, Barsi P, Majtényi K et al (2000) Can intravascular lymphomatosis mimic sinus thrombosis? A case report with 8 months" follow-up and fatal outcome. Neuroradiology 42:436–440
46. Oei ME, Kraft GH, Sarnat HB (2002) Intravascular lymphomatosis. Muscle Nerve 25: 742–746

47. Levin KH, Lutz G (1996) Angiotropic large-cell lymphoma with peripheral nerve and skeletal muscle involvement: early diagnosis and treatment. Neurology 47:1009–1011
48. Lacomis D, Smith TW, Long RR (1992) Angiotropic lymphoma (intravascular large cell lymphoma) presenting with cauda equina syndrome. Clin Neurol Neurosurg 94:311–315
49. Van Droogenbroeck J, Altintas S, Polleflíet C et al (2001) Intravascular large B-cell lymphoma or intravascular lymphomatosis: report of a case diagnosed by testicle biopsy. Ann Hematol 80:316–318
50. Kayano H, Katayama I (1990) Primary hepatic lymphoma presenting as intravascular lymphomatosis. Arch Pathol Lab Med 114:580–584
51. Imai H, Kajimoto K, Taniwaki M et al (2004) Intravascular large B-cell lymphoma presenting with mass lesions in the central nervous system: a report of five cases. Pathol Int 54: 231–236
52. O'Connor SR, Tan JH, Walewska R et al (2002) Angiotropic lymphoma occurring in a lacrimal sac oncocytoma. J Clin Pathol 55:787–788
53. Yamada N, Uchida R, Fuchida S et al (2005) CD5+ Epstein-Barr virus-positive intravascular large B-cell lymphoma in the uterus co-existing with huge myoma. Am J Hematol 78: 221–224
54. Nakamura S, Murase T, Kinoshita T (2007) Intravascular large B-cell lymphoma: the heterogeneous clinical manifestations of its classical and hemophagocytosis-related forms. Haematologica 92:434–436
55. Ferreri AJ, Campo E, Ambrosetti A et al (2004) Anthracycline-based chemotherapy as primary treatment for intravascular lymphoma. Ann Oncol 15:1215–1221
56. Shimada K, Kosugi H, Narimatsu H et al (2008) Sustained remission after rituximab-containing chemotherapy for intravascular large B-cell lymphoma. J Clin Exp Hematop 48:25–28
57. Shimada K, Matsue K, Yamamoto K et al (2008) Retrospective analysis of intravascular large B-cell lymphoma treated with rituximab-containing chemotherapy as reported by the IVL study group in Japan. J Clin Oncol 26:3189–3195
58. Ferreri AJ, Dognini GP, Bairey O et al (2008) The addition of rituximab to anthracycline-based chemotherapy significantly improves outcome in "Western" patients with intravascular large B-cell lymphoma. Br J Haematol 143:253–257
59. Ferreri AJ, Dognini GP, Govi S et al (2008) Can rituximab change the usually dismal prognosis of patients with intravascular large B-cell lymphoma? J Clin Oncol 26:5134–5136; author reply 5136–5137

Chapter 15
Rare Variants of Primary CNS Lymphoma

Kristoph Jahnke, Tamara N. Shenkier, and Oussama Abla

Low-Grade Primary Central Nervous System Lymphoma

Introduction

Almost all primary central nervous system lymphomas (PCNSL) are aggressive neoplasms of the diffuse large B-cell lymphoma (DLBCL) type, according to the World Health Organization (WHO) classification (referred to as classic PCNSL in this chapter) [1], usually having growth fractions of 50% or greater. As opposed to classic PCNSL, the limited data on low-grade PCNSL derive from a few case reports and series, most of them focusing on pathological aspects and including human immunodeficiency virus (HIV)-positive patients. Thus, little is known about the characteristics of this entity.

The precise incidence of low-grade PCNSL is unknown. In published pathological series, the percentage of low-grade histology ranges from zero, in more recent publications, to 75 in older ones [2, 3]. This is probably due not only to the lack of an exact histological definition, but also to the application of different histological classification systems, the inclusion of immunosuppressed patients in some series, and the classification of small-cell and T-cell-rich B-cell subtypes of high-grade PCNSL as low-grade lymphomas [4]. Low-grade histology, defined by both morphological and immunological criteria, was observed in 3% of 332 immunocompetent patients screened for inclusion in three multicenter prospective studies [5, 6], and in 4% of patients in a retrospective series [7]. The majority of available data on low-grade PCNSL stem from a retrospective series compiled by the International Primary Central Nervous System Lymphoma Collaborative Group (IPCG) that included 40 patients [8]. In that report, the clinical picture, course, and outcome of low-grade PCNSL patients were characterized for the first time in a larger cohort. There have been detailed reports on only two patients with low-grade PCNSL not included in the IPCG study [9, 10].

K. Jahnke (✉)
Department of Hematology and Oncology, Charité-Universitätsmedizin Berlin, D-12200 Berlin, Germany
e-mail: kristoph.jahnke@charite.de

T. Batchelor, L.M. DeAngelis (eds.), *Lymphoma and Leukemia of the Nervous System*, DOI 10.1007/978-1-4419-7668-0_15,

Pathology

There is no generally accepted pathological definition for low-grade PCNSL. In the largest available detailed report on low-grade PCNSL [8], the inclusion criteria were histological/cytological diagnosis of low-grade or, if this term was not mentioned in the original pathology report, small lymphocytic lymphoma; disease restricted to the central nervous system with no signs of systemic involvement; and no evidence of HIV infection. The diagnosis of low-grade/small lymphocytic PCNSL made by local pathologists was based always on the morphological tumor cell appearance and, if performed, on immunophenotyping, including the proliferation index and the detection of rearranged immunoglobulin heavy-chain genes by polymerase chain reaction. The proliferation index (Ki-67, MIB-1 antibody), if determined, had to be 20% or less. Central pathology review could be performed by a referral pathologist in 19 cases. However, the application of older lymphoma classification systems and the paucity of available biopsy material prevented further subclassification of many B-cell lymphoma cases in that study. Thirty-two patients (80%) had a B-cell and eight had a T-cell lymphoma. B-cell histology included lymphoplasmacytic lymphoma (n = 11), follicular grade 1 lymphoma (n = 1), and lymphomas not further classified but described as "small lymphocytic, low-grade," "small lymphocytic," or "poorly differentiated lymphocytic, low-grade" (n = 20). The diagnosis was confirmed by immunophenotyping in 21 patients and by polymerase chain reaction in 3 patients. The T-cell cases were described as "angiocentric" (n = 3) and "small lymphocytic, low-grade" (n = 5) and were ultimately diagnosed by the presence of T-cell markers and the absence of B-cell markers in immunophenotyping. The proliferative index was documented in 11 cases. It was specified with a median of 4.5% (range, 1–20%) in 8 patients and was estimated as being less than 5% in 3 cases. Low-grade PCNSL appears to share some of the histopathological features of classic PCNSL, including diffuse and predominantly perivascular lymphocytic infiltrates [4, 11] and frequent (lympho)plasmacellular differentiation [11]. In the low-grade PCNSL IPCG study [8], an apparent difference from classic PCNSL was the relatively high percentage of T-cell cases. T-cell histology has been reported in less than 4% of PCNSL patients from Western countries [12, 13], and in 8.5% of patients from Japan [14]. It has been reported that low-grade histology appears to be more frequent in T-cell PCNSL [15]. The low-grade features observed in a significant proportion of T-PCNSL cases appeared to suggest that a more favorable prognosis could be expected [16]. However, the largest study on T-PCNSL thus far, reported an outcome similar to that of B-cell PCNSL [15].

Clinical Presentation and Diagnosis

Some clinical characteristics of low-grade PCNSL appear to be comparable with those of classic PCNSL [8]. For example, the median age of 60 years and the absence of B symptoms have often been reported for PCNSL [13, 17–19]. Supratentorial tumor localization was as common as in a large case series on classic PCNSL compiled by the International Extranodal Lymphoma Study Group (IELSG) [13], and positive cerebrospinal fluid (CSF) cytology was similarly infrequent [13, 20]). Compared with the IELSG data, more patients (65% versus 31%) seem to present with an Eastern Cooperative Oncology Group performance status of 0–1, and no male preponderance was observed. Moreover, serum lactate dehydrogenase elevation was infrequent (5% versus 35%), and ocular involvement was not diagnosed. Seizures were the most frequent symptom at presentation (44%) in the series compiled by the IPCG [8], whereas mental changes were relatively rare (24%). Mental changes were reported as the major initial symptom in classic PCNSL, with epilepsy being less frequent [19]. The mean time from symptom presentation to diagnosis of 14.8 months in low-grade PCNSL appears to be relatively long compared with the 2.8 months reported for PCNSL in general [19], most probably due to the relatively indolent clinical course of the disease.

Some low-grade PCNSL seem to have distinct brain magnetic resonance imaging (MRI) features. In the IPCG study [8], frequent MRI features usually not seen in high-grade PCNSL (Fig. 15.1) were: (1) hyperintensity on T2-weighted images (n = 16); (2) inhomogeneous contrast enhancement (n = 11); (3) moderate (n = 11) or absent (n = 1) contrast enhancement; and (4) lack of periventricular localization (n = 10). Six patients had four of these features, whereas four had three, another

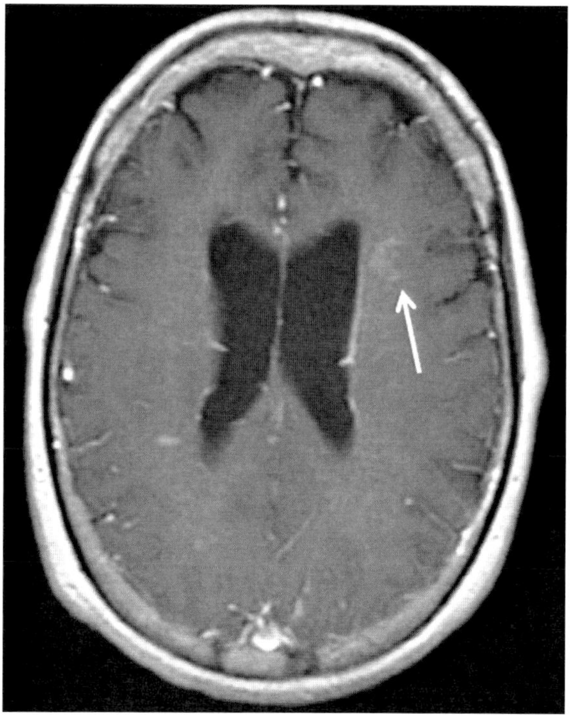

Fig. 15.1 T1-weighted MRI of a patient with low-grade PCNSL in the *left* hemisphere (*arrow*), demonstrating moderate and inhomogeneous contrast enhancement

four had two of them, and three had one feature. In contrast, characteristic MRI features of classic PCNSL are supratentorial localization, intensive and homogeneous contrast enhancement, slight or moderate edema, the absence of necrosis, and proximity to the ventricles [21, 22].

Treatment and Prognosis

The limited data on low-grade PCNSL preclude definitive treatment recommendations. Classic PCNSL is usually an aggressive tumor with a median survival of a few months after local therapy alone (i.e., surgery or local radiotherapy), up to 18 months after whole-brain radiation therapy (WBRT), and up to 50 months after high-dose methotrexate (HDMTX)-based chemotherapy with or without WBRT [7, 20, 23–25]. In Table 15.1, response and survival data of the IPCG study on low-grade PCNSL [8] are compared to data from treatment studies, in which classic PCNSL comprised the vast majority of patients. Low-grade PCNSL appears to have a longer median survival than classic PCNSL in general, even though many patients only received local or no therapy or did not achieve a treatment response, thus suggesting a better prognosis for low-grade PCNSL. For example, two patients were alive without evidence of disease 40 and 20.5 months after tumor resection alone, and three non-responders were alive and progression-free without further therapy after 85.5, 63 and 39.5 months. The relatively indolent clinical course, the possibility of disease control by local therapy alone or even no treatment, and the long survival compared with classic PCNSL suggest that treatment of low-grade PCNSL should be less aggressive than in classic PCNSL. In the IPCG publication [8], age $\geq$ 60 years was associated with shorter progression-free ($p = 0.009$), disease-specific ($p = 0.015$), and overall survival ($p = 0.001$) in multivariate analysis.

T-Cell Primary Central Nervous System Lymphoma

Mature T-cell lymphomas are heterogeneous and refer to a group of nodal and extranodal lymphoid neoplasms that comprise approximately 12–15% of all non-Hodgkin lymphomas (NHL), with a higher proportion in South-East Asia [26]. While T-cell lymphomas make up a significant minority of systemic lymphomas, these tumors represent a small proportion of all PCNSL cases in both the immunocompetent and immunosuppressed host, the vast majority of which are diffuse large B-cell lymphomas.

Epidemiology and Etiology

T-cell PCNSL appears to be infrequent in all reported series regardless of region. A review of 64 cases of PCNSL from Duke University identified only two cases which were phenotypic T-cell neoplasms [27]. Another case series of 100 patients

Table 15.1 Patient characteristics and treatment outcomes of clinical studies for PCNSL using chemotherapy alone or in conjunction with whole-brain radiotherapy, compared to data from a retrospective study on low-grade PCNSL [8], in bold type)

First author	Treatment	No. of patients	Median age (years)	Median Karnofsky performance status	Overall response rate (%)	Median overall survival (months)	Five-year overall survival (%)
Abrey et al. [72]	CHT+WBRT	31	59	Not reported	87.1[a]	40.3[b]	22.3
Blay et al. [7]	CHT, WBRT	226	61	Not reported	Not reported	16	19
McAllister et al. [60]	CHT	74	Not reported[c]	Not reported[c]	65[a]	40.7	42
DeAngelis et al. [24]	CHT+WBRT	102	56.5	80	94	36.9	32
Batchelor et al. [94]	CHT	25	60	80	74	22.8+	Not reported
Pels et al. [25]	CHT	65	62	70	71	50	43
Poortmans et al. [95]	CHT+WBRT	52	51	70	81	46	58
Hoang-Xuan et al. [96]	CHT	50	72	50	48	14.3	Not reported
Illerhaus et al. [97]	CHT+WBRT	30[d]	54	70	100[e]	Not reported	69[f]

Table 15.1 (continued)

First author	Treatment	No. of patients	Median age (years)	Median Karnofsky performance status	Overall response rate (%)	Median overall survival (months)	Five-year overall survival (%)
Jahnke et al. [8]	**Diverse**	**40**	**60**	**1**[g]	**77**	**79**	**67**
Omuro et al. [98]	CHT	23[h]	68	60	55	35	Not reported
Illerhaus et al. [99]	CHT[i]	30[h]	70	60	70.3	15.4	33
Angelov et al. [100]	CHT	149	54.5[j]	69.4[j]	81.9	37.2	41

[a]Complete remissions only.
[b]Median disease-free survival.
[c]In this cohort, 36 patients (49%) were <60, and 38 (51%) were $\geq$60 years of age. The Karnofsky performance was >70 in 46 patients (62%), and $\leq$70 in 26 patients (35%).
[d]Only patients <65 years were included.
[e]After high-dose chemotherapy with autologous stem cell transplantation and whole-brain radiation therapy.
[f]87% for patients that received high-dose chemotherapy with autologous stem cell transplantation.
[g]Eastern Cooperative Oncology Group (ECOG) performance status.
[h]Only patients >60 years were included.
[i]Whole-brain radiation therapy was administered to patients refractory to primary chemotherapy.
[j]Mean values.
CHT, chemotherapy; WBRT, whole-brain radiation therapy.

from Italy described 96 DLBCL, two Burkitt-like lymphomas, one anaplastic large T-cell lymphoma, and one unclassified B-cell lymphoma [28]. A prospective study in Germany accrued 14 cases, one of which was of T-cell origin [29]. Three of 14 patients from Melbourne with intraocular lymphoma had T-cell phenotype [30]. Since 1981, the Lymphoma Tumour Group at the British Columbia Cancer Agency (BCCA) has gathered demographic, clinical, pathologic, treatment, and follow-up information on all referred patients with lymphoid malignancies in the BCCA Lymphoid Database. This group has confirmed 5 cases of T-cell immunophenotype out of 179 patients with PCNSL.

In a 19-year study period, one Indian center reported only one case of CD3 positive T-cell lymphoma out of 56 patients with PCNSL [31]. Another series of 100 cases of PCNSL in Israel contained 5 cases of T-cell origin, all of whom presented with leptomeningeal involvement (with or without neurolymphomatosis) and no parenchymal lesion [32].

In South-East Asia, T-cell lymphomas appear to make up a larger proportion of these neoplasms. A 1999 survey of 466 cases of PCNSL over a decade in Japan demonstrated that 20 of 214 cases with available immunophenotyping expressed T-cell markers (8.5%) [14]. Seven of 45 Korean cases (16.7%) of PCNSL had molecularly confirmed clonal T-cell origin [33].

There is a higher incidence of PCNSL in immunosuppressed populations. Viral infectious agents such as HIV, human T-cell leukemia/lymphoma virus-1 (HTLV-1), and Epstein-Barr virus (EBV) are permissive and/or etiologic. As in immunocompetent hosts with PCNSL, the T-cell phenotype is also rare in immunosuppressed patients. In one series of 23 patients (20 HIV positive), the predominant immunophenotype was B-cell (19), although T-cell (2) and biphenotypic (1) cases were also identified. EBV RNA was detected in the malignant cells in 19 of 23 cases (83%) [34]. Another report of two HIV positive individuals with T-cell CNS lymphoma described one confirmed and one suspected case of co-infection with HTLV-1 [35].

The IPCG assembled 221 cases of PCNSL with ocular involvement from 16 centers in seven countries. Of the 166 cases in which immunophenotyping was available, five had T-cell disease [36]. In a separate publication, 83 patients with intraocular disease as the exclusive site of disease were described. Five of 60 lymphomas with available information were of T-cell origin [37].

In summary, T-cell lymphoid neoplasms presenting as primary CNS lesions in immunocompetent or immunosuppressed hosts, occur infrequently. They show significant regional variation comprising between 1 and 17% of all PCNSL.

Pathology

The diagnosis of CNS T-cell lymphoma is challenging. Stereotactic biopsy tissue yields small amounts of material, there are no immunohistochemical markers for

T-cell monoclonality, and intermixed inflammatory cells are often present in the specimen. Molecular genetic testing has proven indispensable in establishing the diagnosis [38].

A group from Stanford recently cautioned that T-cell lymphomas may be under-recognized due to a high degree of overlap between non-specific inflammatory and neoplastic lesions. Histologically, the malignant T-cell infiltrate can be composed of small, mature lymphocytes within a heterogeneous background infiltrate, which can be impossible to distinguish from a reactive infiltrate [39]. In addition, neither immunohistochemistry nor the proliferation index appeared sufficiently discriminating to distinguish reactive from neoplastic lesions. In five of the six reported cases, genotypic analysis for clonal T-cell receptor-gamma gene rearrangement was required to establish the diagnosis of T-cell PCNSL.

T-cell lymphoma itself is a heterogeneous entity. Of the 27 mature T-cell neoplasms in the new WHO classification [40], the following subtypes have been reported to involve the CNS as a primary phenomenon: peripheral T-cell lymphoma, not otherwise specified (PTCL), anaplastic large cell lymphoma (ALCL), adult T-cell leukemia/lymphoma, and extranodal NK/T-cell lymphoma (nasal type) [41–44]. Four out of the five BCCA patients had PTCL and the other had a T-cell intravascular lymphoma, exclusively involving the brain.

Within each subtype, unique observations have been made. PTCL most commonly exhibits a CD4+/CD8- phenotype. One reported case described a T-cell lymphoma with an unusual cytotoxic/suppressor T-cell immunophenotype; positive for CD3, CD8, CD57 and negative for CD4 and CD56. The case strongly resembled T-cell large granular lymphocytic leukemia with cytoplasmic granule-associated proteins and morphologically bland cells [43]. The seven cases described in the Korean study also displayed a preponderance of CD8 expression [33].

Most ALCLs exhibit a characteristic translocation which encodes a novel protein by fusing the anaplastic lymphoma kinase gene (ALK) of chromosome 2 and the nucleophosmin gene (NPM) of chromosome 5. Detectable expression with the ALK-1 antibody is highly sensitive and specific for ALK gene translocation. In the current WHO classification, ALK positive and ALK negative ALCLs are considered separate entities [40]. A series of nine cases of ALCL, involving the CNS was comprised of both T and null immunophenotype (seven and two, respectively), and five of these were ALK positive [42].

Isolated cases of retrovirus mediated adult T-cell lymphoma/leukemia with primary CNS involvement are reported in both immunocompetent and immunosuppressed patients [35, 41]. One case of extranodal NK/T-cell lymphoma (nasal type) in the CNS developed in an immunosuppressed renal transplant patient and was associated with EBV [44]. Another renal transplant recipient developed a monomorphic T-cell lymphoma [45].

In summary, T-cell PCNSL can be challenging to distinguish from reactive lesions. The application of molecular genetic techniques to verify clonal T-cell receptor rearrangements is an indispensable tool to establish the diagnosis. There is a spectrum of mature T-cell neoplasms represented in the CNS with the majority of reported cases being PTCL and ALCL.

Clinical Features

Most descriptions of T-cell PCNSL involve case reports or small series from which it is difficult to draw conclusions. A few papers have assembled larger series which have helped characterize this entity [15].

Diagnosis

In the series of 45 T-cell PCNSL cases from the IPCG, presenting complaints included headache, seizures, focal motor and sensory deficits, cranial neuropathies, gait disorders, and confusion. The symptoms preceded the identification of the lymphoma by 0–6 months. Stereotactic biopsy (80%) and resection (16%) established the diagnosis in most cases [15].

Imaging

There is little information regarding diagnostic imaging findings specific to T-cell PCNSL. In the one paper in which this was detailed, seven T-cell cases presented with distinct radiologic features compared to the 35 B-cell ones. Radiologically, T-cell PCNSL was correlated with superficial location, solitary lesions, presence of rim enhancement, and peritumoral edema [33].

In another series describing the MRI findings of seven cases, T-PCNSL showed a predilection for a subcortical location, tumor-associated hemorrhage in three of seven cases, rim enhancement in five cases, and cystic areas consistent with necrosis in three [46]. There was no evidence of leptomeningeal enhancement in any of the cases.

Patient and Disease Characteristics

The series from the IPCG only included centers from North America and Europe. The demographic and tumor characteristics are shown in Table 15.2 and did not appear to differ from patients with B-cell PCNSL [15]. The study from Israel described 100 patients with PCNSL. Five of them had T-cell PCNSL, and in an unusual finding, all presented with leptomeningeal involvement as the sole manifestation of disease. In addition, four of these cases also had features consistent with neurolymphomatosis. Neither MRI nor examination of the CSF was conclusive and diagnosis had to be made with meningeal or nerve biopsy. In contrast, the reports from Japan and Korea do not corroborate this observation. Overall, 15% of the Japanese patients with PCNSL (56 of 366 with available data) presented with meningeal dissemination, but none of the seven T-cell PCNSL cases from the Korean series involved the CSF [14, 33].

The report from the Mayo Clinic described 13 cases of confirmed CNS ALCL [42]. The cases had a bimodal age distribution: ALK-positive tumors occurred in younger individuals than the ALK negative tumors. Like the series reported by Levin, CNS ALCL affected the dura or leptomeninges in nine of 13 cases, but

Table 15.2 Patient and disease characteristics for 45 T-cell PCNSL cases

	Number of patients	%
Age Median	59 years	
Range	3–84 years	
≥70 yr	6	
Male	35	78
B symptoms	5	11
ECOG Performance Status		
0–1	20/41	48
2–3	20/41	48
4	1/41	2
LDH >normal	7/22	32
Ocular disease	1/26	4
Positive CSF cytology	6/32	19
Multiple lesions	13	29
Involvement of deep structures[a]	16	36
Sites of disease[b]		
Cerebral hemisphere	29	64
Basal ganglia	5	11
Corpus callosum	6	13
Brain stem	4	9
Cerebellum	3	7
Meninges[c]	1	2
Spinal cord	2	4

Not all data available for all patients. PCNSL, primary central nervous system lymphoma; ECOG, Eastern Cooperative Oncology Group; LDH, lactate dehydrogenase; CSF, cerebrospinal fluid.
[a]Deep structures of the brain include: basal ganglia, brain stem, corpus callosum, cerebellum.
[b]Some patients had involvement of multiple sites.
[c]As exclusive site of disease.

unlike the exclusive involvement of the meninges in those five patients, there was simultaneous brain involvement in seven of the nine.

The diagnosis of T-cell PCNSL is so rare that no typical or common pattern emerges, either clinically, radiologically, or pathologically, and firm conclusions cannot be reached [39].

Treatment and Outcome

Compared to systemic DLBCL, the clinical outcome for patients with aggressive T-cell lymphoma is poor with standard therapies [47]. In contrast, based on the available limited information, the prognosis for T-cell PCNSL does not appear to differ significantly from that of B-cell PCNSL, suggesting that the site of disease and other standard factors, such as age and performance status exert the dominant effect on prognosis and not immunophenotype [15].

The 13 patients with ALCL of the CNS were treated heterogeneously with chemotherapy, irradiation, or both. Eight patients succumbed of disease less than 6 months after diagnosis, but the five others are long-term survivors 2–6 years after treatment. Multifocal tumors, extensive necrosis, older age, and ALK-1 negativity were negative prognostic factors, with the latter two factors exerting similar negative prognosis when ALCL is diagnosed outside the nervous system [42].

The 45 patients in the IPCG series were assembled retrospectively and treated heterogeneously. Twenty-four of these patients received chemotherapy followed by irradiation, eleven patients had irradiation alone, seven had chemotherapy alone, and two patients were treated with blood brain barrier disruption and intra-arterial chemotherapy. The median overall survival and disease specific survival for all patients was 25 months (95% CI 11–38 months). These results are comparable to retrospectively assembled population-based series reported in the literature [48, 49] The IPCG series noted that performance status <2 was a good prognostic feature (odds ration for death 0.2) and that inclusion of intravenous HDMTX in the treatment regimen also reduced the risk of death substantially (odds ratio 0.4) [15]. Despite the bias inherent in such an assembled cohort, this observation is congruent with our recommendation for the treatment of classic PCNSL. Based on the current evidence, T-cell PCNSL should be treated like its B-cell counterpart.

Pediatric Primary Central Nervous System Lymphoma

Introduction

Brain tumors represent the second most common pediatric cancer after leukemias, while NHL occupies third place. However, PCNSL is extremely rare in childhood, thus the incidence and optimal therapy have not been defined. Among 596 cases of PCNSL reported to the Brain Tumor registry of Japan (1969–1990), only nine pediatric cases (1.5%) were documented [50]. In the United States (US), the Surveillance, Epidemiology, and End Results (SEER) program (1973–1998) only 1% of all PCNSL occurred in patients less than 19 years of age, giving an estimated incidence of 15–20 cases per year in North America [51]. Patients with congenital or acquired immune deficiencies are at increased risk for developing PCNSL, although it was diagnosed in only two of 350 HIV-infected children in the pediatric branch of the National Cancer Institute (US) [52–54]. Nevertheless, more than 50 pediatric patients with PCNSL have been reported during the last decade and most of them were immunocompetent. PCNSL tends to be more common in males than in females and the median age at diagnosis during childhood is 9 years (range 2–18) [55], although it has been reported in infants as young as 1 month of age [50].

Clinical Presentation and Diagnosis

Clinical features in children with PCNSL include increased intracranial pressure symptoms, facial nerve palsy, diplopia, dysarthria, ataxia, bulbar palsy, quadriparesis, and obtundation. Less common findings include seizures, acute blindness, optic neuritis, proptosis, lower and upper limb muscle weakness, nystagmus, paresthesias, personality change, lethargy, and somnolence. Children with PCNSL may also present with isolated diabetes insipidus and panhypopituitarism due to pituitary and hypothalamic involvement [55]. The clinical findings of children with primary CNS ALCL can often mimic those of an infectious, immunologic, or rheumatologic etiology (i.e. fever, seizures, emesis and neck stiffness), thus making the diagnosis challenging. Also, 77% of CNS ALCL had simultaneous brain and leptomeningeal involvement [56]. Since PCNSL can occur in the brain, leptomeninges, spinal cord, and the eyes, diagnostic evaluation should include assessment of these regions, as well as screening for occult systemic disease. Also, acquired and congenital immune deficiencies need to be ruled out in children.

On neuroimaging, pediatric PCNSL may present as a solitary mass or as a multifocal tumor [57]. While most adult PCNSL commonly involve the periventricular region, basal ganglia, corpus callosum, and the deep white matter [58], the most frequent tumor locations in children are the parietal and frontal lobes followed by the cerebellum, pituitary stalk, and hypothalamus [57].

In children with PCNSL, contrast-enhanced CT usually shows a heterogeneous, often ring-like pattern of enhancement, marked edema, and prominent mass effect [59]. Heterogeneous and ring-like enhancement are less common in adults. Furthermore, at least 18% of pediatric cases have predominant leptomeningeal involvement without any intracranial mass [55].

Pathology

A recent review of 43 pediatric PCNSL cases showed that the most frequent histological subtype is DLBCL (30%) followed by ALCL (21%; 7 T-cell and 2 null), lymphoblastic lymphoma (16%; 5 precursor-B and 2 T-cell), Burkitts (12%), histiocytic (5%), and other (6%). The most common immunophenotype was mature B-cell (43%) followed by T-cell (21%), precursor-B cell (12%), null-type (10%), and histiocytic (5%) subtypes. The diagnosis was established in most cases either by a stereotactic biopsy or by immunocytochemical/PCR analysis of the CSF [55].

Prognosis and Biology: Differences Between Children and Adults

A previous review of pediatric PCNSL cases treated between 1975 and 1991 demonstrated a mean survival time of 17 months with cranial radiotherapy (CRT) alone or combined with moderate chemotherapy [50]. However, a more recent pediatric retrospective series demonstrated improved survival with a 5-year event-free survival (EFS) of 70% in patients treated with chemotherapy alone without CRT [57], as opposed to 25–40% in most adult series [60]. The use of intensive CNS-directed chemotherapy, including HDMTX and high-dose cytarabine (HD-Ara-C) with intensive intrathecal therapy may have contributed to this improvement. The improved outcome may also be accounted for by different biological and molecular characteristics of pediatric PCNSL, as well as to the ability of younger patients to tolerate more intensive therapy.

In adult systemic DLBCL, the germinal center (GC) phenotype (CD10+, Bcl-6+) had a significantly better prognosis, and most adult PCNSL are either late GC or post-GC stage [61]. Braaten et al. demonstrated a median survival of 101 months for PCNSL patients with Bcl-6 expression compared to 14.7 months in patients whose tumors were Bcl-6 negative [62]. Pediatric DLBCL has an increased frequency of the GC phenotype (75%) and decreased Bcl-2 expression (28%), which may contribute to the excellent prognosis of children with DLBCL [63]. If this is true for all patients with PCNSL, it may partially explain the better prognosis in childhood. Among the patients diagnosed with ALCL-PCNSL, a relatively better outcome was associated with ALK-1 positivity, lack of necrosis and unifocal tumor [42]. The three children with ALCL-PCNSL from our previous series were alive and in CR at 79, 98, and 122 months, respectively, at the time of report [57]. However, the majority of ALCL involving primarily the CNS (adults and children) have had a rapidly fatal course with death occurring in 8 out of the 14 cases reported in the literature [56].

The lymphoblastic PCNSL subtype was previously thought to have a worse prognosis, with a high relapse rate and a tendency to leukemic transformation [50]. In a recent review, however, pediatric patients with precursor B-lymphoblastic PCNSL were alive at 22+ to 77+ months after treatment with intensive chemo-radiotherapy combinations [55]. The histiocytic subtype is the most aggressive among published pediatric PCNSL, with an overall survival of only 3–4 months [64, 65], thus confirming the correlation between histology and prognosis.

Treatment

The most appropriate therapeutic approach for pediatric PCNSL has not yet been determined because of the rarity of the disease and the lack of large prospective studies. Surgical resection has been shown to worsen the neurological deficits in adults with PCNSL and resection confers no survival benefit (overall survival (OS) 3–5 months) [66]. Thus, tumor debulking should be reserved for the rare patient with increased intracranial pressure and brain herniation. The utility of surgery in both pediatric and adult PCNSL is limited to a stereotactic biopsy, which should be performed only if the CSF is negative [55].

Cranial radiotherapy alone is insufficient with a 5-year OS of 4% and an 80% relapse rate over 10–14 months in adult PCNSL; furthermore, it is associated with a high risk of severe neurotoxicity in elderly patients [67].

Among the very few pediatric cases reported in the last decade, 4 were treated with CRT alone: 3 were alive and in remission at 4.5, 5 and 14 years, respectively, at the time of report; the fourth relapsed at 12 months [42, 50, 58, 68]. These numbers are too small for any reliable assessment of efficacy, however, due to the high risk of secondary brain tumors [69], and the risk of severe neurocognitive deficit [70] associated with the use of CRT in young children, first-line treatment of pediatric PCNSL with CRT alone is not routinely recommended, except in the palliative setting [55].

Due to the inability of vincristine and doxorubicin to cross the blood-brain-barrier (BBB), the addition of the cyclophosphamide/doxorubicin/vincristin/prednisone (CHOP) regimen to CRT has failed to improve survival rates in adult PCNSL [71]. The combination of CRT and HDMTX gave better survival rates (30–60 months), although neurotoxicity was significantly worse in patients older than 60 years [72]. Abla and Weitzman reviewed 43 pediatric cases published between 1996 and 2006. Twelve children received chemo-radiotherapy and 8 of them (66%) were alive at the time of report (22–98 months from diagnosis). Cranial irradiation doses ranged from 12 to 50 Gy, whereas chemotherapy regimens consisted mainly of HDMTX combined with HD-Ara-C and steroids. Long-term neurotoxicity has not been evaluated in these reports [55].

It is evident from the adult literature that by using chemotherapy alone, with drugs that cross the BBB, survival is comparable to that of regimens with chemotherapy combined with CRT, but with significantly less cognitive dysfunction [25, 73–75]. The largest pediatric PCNSL case series included 12 patients from six cancer centers in four countries, and suggested that most children with PCNSL can achieve long-term remissions with chemotherapy alone without CRT. In this series, 2 children received chemotherapy and CRT; one relapsed and died from his disease while the other remained in complete remission at 98+ months from diagnosis. Ten children received first-line therapy with chemotherapy regimens consisting mainly of HDMTX and HD-Ara-C combinations. The 5-year EFS of this group was 70% with a median follow-up time of 79 months (range 31–122) [57]. These results are almost equivalent to the international FAB/LMB-96 study results in children and adolescents with CNS positive B-NHL, where the deletion of CRT and an additional course of HDMTX (8 g/m^2) plus extra intrathecal therapy resulted in 75% 4-year EFS [76], which was not significantly different from the 4-year EFS of 79% in historical controls with CNS positive B-NHL treated on the LMB-89 with cranial irradiation.

Twenty-three of the 43 pediatric PCNSL cases reported in the last decade were treated with chemotherapy alone; 18 (78%) were alive at the time of report [55]. Two of the patients who relapsed without prior radiation therapy were salvaged with autologous stem cell transplantation (ASCT) combined with CRT [57], and with EBV-cytotoxic immunotherapy followed by allogeneic stem cell transplant [77], respectively.

It is well established that HDMTX is the most important agent in the treatment of PCNSL. Although the optimal dose of this drug in PCNSL has not yet been defined, intensifying the MTX dose to 8 g/m^2, a dose commonly used in pediatric systemic NHL was found to be beneficial in one study [78]. HDMTX is associated with response rates of 52–88% when given as single agent, and 70–94% when combined with other drugs and CRT [24]. Single-agent MTX therapy, however, even with very high doses (8 g/m^2), can lead to higher risk of relapse, at least in adults with PCNSL [79]. Accordingly, one HIV-positive child with PCNSL who was treated with HDMTX monotherapy relapsed and died at 4 months after diagnosis [57]. The combination of HD-Ara-C with HDMTX has a synergistic action, and was shown to improve survival rates in adult PCNSL when compared to HDMTX alone (2-year OS 64% versus 18%) [13]. This benefit was confirmed by one adult prospective study that used HDMTX at 5 g/m^2 combined with HD-Ara-C at 3 g/m^2 [25]. Furthermore, the LMB and BFM studies have confirmed the benefit from introducing HD-Ara-C to regimens containing increased doses of MTX (8 g/m^2) in CNS-positive childhood systemic B-cell lymphomas [80]. In our last pediatric review, 16 children with PCNSL who received HD-Ara-C, combined with other agents, achieved long-term remissions [55].

Due to their good CNS penetration, etoposide and ifosfamide were used in combination with cytarabine as salvage regimen in relapsed PCNSL with a 1-year OS of 41% [81]. Etoposide was given also in the intensification phase of the LMB-89 protocol [82], a therapy which was used successfully in some pediatric PCNSL cases [55].

Blood-brain-barrier disruption (BBBD) can enhance chemotherapy delivery to microscopic tumoral areas. Intraarterial MTX in conjunction with BBBD, and without CRT, produced a survival rate of 42% when used as first-line therapy in adult PCNSL, without causing any cognitive impairment [60]. These results are inferior to the results found in pediatric PCNSL cases treated with systemic chemotherapy alone. One of these cases was treated with BBBD-enhanced MTX chemotherapy and remained well at 104 months without any cognitive dysfunction [83]. With the current state of knowledge, however, there is no evidence that BBBD is superior to systemic HDMTX therapy, at least in children, particularly when considering the toxicity associated with its use, such as seizures, stroke, thromboembolic events, and edema [84].

Primary leptomeningeal lymphoma without parenchymal CNS disease was identified in 8 of 43 (18%) pediatric cases reviewed, five of them are long-term survivors [55]. The role of intrathecal and intraventricular therapy in PCNSL is still controversial, especially when used in combination with high doses of systemic MTX (>3 g/m^2) [85]. Twenty-six of the 43 pediatric patients received intrathecal chemotherapy, and due to the retrospective nature of the review and because of diversity in treatment strategies, the impact of intrathecal therapy on the outcome of childhood PCNSL cannot be evaluated. Intraventricular administration of the anti-CD20 monoclonal antibody rituximab, combined with systemic rituximab, has been used with success for refractory B-cell PCNSL in a child [86]. However, the safety and feasibility of intrathecal rituximab in children needs to be tested in phase I trials prior to the introduction in front-line therapies.

Due to the beneficial effect on survival of high-dose therapy and ASCT in adults with relapsed PCNSL [87], several studies have examined the role of ASCT as front-line therapy for PCNSL with survival rates between 50 and 69% at 5 years [88, 89]. Abla et al. reported on 2 children with PCNSL who underwent ASCT; one had stem cell rescue as part of her front-line therapy and remained in complete remission at 91+ months from diagnosis, while the second child had ASCT followed by CRT after relapse and was still in CCR at 55+ months at the time of report [57]. Wynn et al. reported a case of a refractory PCNSL in a child who was treated with allogeneic stem cell transplant and was alive at 17 months [77]. Although high-dose therapy with rescue appears to be a reasonable alternative for slowly responding or refractory disease, the role of stem cell transplant as first-line therapy in pediatric PCNSL is still unclear. Due to the high incidence of neurotoxicity, SCT may not be the perfect option in patients who have received prior cranial irradiation [87, 88].

Immunocompromised Children

Eight of the 43 children with PCNSL in the pediatric review were immune-deficient. Three children with congenital immune deficiencies and PCNSL were in CCR at 17+, 90+ and 122+ months from initial diagnosis, following multiagent chemotherapy protocols [55]. One patient with EBV-positive-CNS post-transplant lymphoproliferative disorder remained in complete remission at 26+ months after withdrawal of immunosuppression and intravenous acyclovir [90].

Four children were diagnosed with HIV-related PCNSL; 2 were not treated, while the other 2 patients were treated with single-agent therapies (HDMTX and hydroxyurea, respectively). All patients died at 2–26 months from diagnosis. Eleven other pediatric cases of HIV-associated PCNSL have been reported since 1986, and all have died [55, 57, 91]. Highly active anti-retroviral therapy (HAART) combined with CRT ($\geq$ 30 Gy) improved survival in adults with HIV-related PCNSL [92]. Due to the coexistence of AIDS encephalopathy in most of these cases, however, this therapy cannot be recommended for pediatric HIV patients and CRT should be reserved for palliation purposes [93]. Furthermore, the utility of HAART in combination with intensive chemotherapy in childhood HIV-PCNSL has not been proven.

The true incidence of pediatric PCNSL is unknown, and it is very likely that many cases are not being reported. Except for HIV-associated PCNSL, a review of the published pediatric cases suggests that the prognosis is better in childhood PCNSL patients than in their adult counterparts. The role of intrathecal rituximab and of high-dose therapy followed by stem cell rescue is yet to be defined. The majority of pediatric patients can be cured with high-dose multiagent chemotherapy, which should include HDMTX and HD-Ara-C, while CRT can be reserved for refractory or recurrent disease. The IPCG is currently conducting a large retrospective series in children and adolescents with PCNSL, with the goal of confirming these results. However, a true assessment can only derive from prospective international studies, which are very difficult to conduct in such a rare disease. Improved collaboration among the international pediatric lymphoma groups might give an answer to all these issues.

References

1. Jaffe ES, Harris NL, Stein H et al (2001) World Health Organization classification of tumours. Pathology and genetics of tumours of haematopoietic and lymphoid tissues. IARC Press, Lyon
2. Jellinger K, Radaskiewicz TH, Slowik F (1975) Primary malignant lymphomas of the central nervous system in man. Acta Neuropathol Suppl (Berl) suppl 6:95–102
3. Lanfermann H, Heindel W, Schaper J et al (1997) CT and MR imaging in primary cerebral non-Hodgkin's lymphoma. Acta Radiol 38:259–267
4. Bergmann M, Kuchelmeister K, Edel G (1993) Primary non-Hodgkin lymphomas of the CNS. Classification, tissue reaction and proliferative activity. Zentralbl Pathol 139:37–44
5. Jahnke K, Schilling A, Heidenreich J et al (2005a) Radiological morphology of low-grade primary central nervous system lymphoma in immunocompetent patients. AJNR Am J Neuroradiol 26:2446–2454
6. Jahnke K, Thiel E, Schilling A et al (2005b) Low-grade primary central nervous system lymphoma in immunocompetent patients. Br J Haematol 128:616–624
7. Blay JY, Conroy T, Chevreau C et al (1998) High-dose methotrexate for the treatment of primary cerebral lymphomas: analysis of survival and late neurologic toxicity in a retrospective series. J Clin Oncol 16:864–871
8. Jahnke K, Korfel A, O'Neill BP et al (2006) International study on low-grade primary central nervous system lymphoma. Ann Neurol 59:755–762
9. King A, Wilson H, Penney C et al (1998) An unusual case of primary leptomeningeal marginal zone B-cell lymphoma. Clin Neuropathol 17:326–329
10. Mikol J, Wassef M, Galian A et al (1987) Primary malignant non-Hodgkin's lymphomas of the central nervous system. Report of two cases with a predominant callosal localization. In: Chatel M, Darcel F, Pecker J (eds) Brain oncology. Martinus Nijhoff Publishers, Dordrecht, pp 257–266
11. Kanavaros P, Mikol J, Nemeth J et al (1990) Stereotactic biopsy diagnosis of primary non-Hodgkin's lymphoma of the central nervous system. A histological and immunohistochemical study. Pathol Res Pract 186:459–466
12. Bataille B, Delwail V, Menet E et al (2000) Primary intracerebral malignant lymphoma: report of 248 cases. J Neurosurg 92:261–266
13. Ferreri AJ, Reni M, Pasini F et al (2002) A multicenter study of treatment of primary CNS lymphoma. Neurology 58:1513–1520
14. Hayabuchi N, Shibamoto Y, Onizuka Y (1999) Primary central nervous system lymphoma in Japan: a nationwide survey. Int J Radiat Oncol Biol Phys 44:265–272
15. Shenkier TN, Blay JY, O'Neill BP et al (2005) Primary CNS lymphoma of T-cell origin: a descriptive analysis from the international primary CNS lymphoma collaborative group. J Clin Oncol 23:2233–2239
16. Gijtenbeek JM, Rosenblum MK, DeAngelis LM (2001) Primary central nervous system T-cell lymphoma. Neurology 57:716–718
17. DeAngelis LM (2001) Primary central nervous system lymphomas. Curr Treat Options Oncol 2:309–318
18. Fine HA, Mayer RJ (1993) Primary central nervous system lymphoma. Ann Intern Med 119:1093–1104

19. Hochberg FH, Miller DC (1988) Primary central nervous system lymphoma. J Neurosurg 168:835–853
20. Ferreri AJ, Blay JY, Reni M et al (2003) Prognostic scoring system for primary CNS lymphomas: the International Extranodal Lymphoma Study Group experience. J Clin Oncol 21:266–272
21. Bühring U, Herrlinger U, Krings T et al (2001) MRI features of primary central nervous system lymphomas at presentation. Neurology 57:393–396
22. Roman-Goldstein SM, Goldman DL, Howieson J et al (1992) MR of primary CNS lymphoma in immunologically normal patients. AJNR Am J Neuroradiol 13:1207–1213
23. DeAngelis LM, Hormigo A (2004) Treatment of primary central nervous system lymphoma. Semin Oncol 31:684–692
24. DeAngelis LM, Seiferheld W, Schold SC et al; Radiation Therapy Oncology Group Study 93-10 (2002) Combination chemotherapy and radiotherapy for primary central nervous system lymphoma: radiation therapy oncology group study 93-10. J Clin Oncol 20:4643–4648
25. Pels H, Schmidt-Wolf IG, Glasmacher A et al (2003) Primary central nervous system lymphoma: results of a pilot and phase II study of systemic and intraventricular chemotherapy with deferred radiotherapy. J Clin Oncol 15:4489–4495
26. No authors listed (1997) A clinical evaluation of the International Lymphoma Study Group classification of non-Hodgkin's lymphoma. The Non-Hodgkin's Lymphoma Classification Project. Blood 89(11):3909–3918
27. Nuckols JD, Liu K et al (1999) Primary central nervous system lymphomas: a 30-year experience at a single institution. Mod Pathol 12(12):1167–1173
28. Ponzoni M, Berger F et al (2007) Reactive perivascular T-cell infiltrate predicts survival in primary central nervous system B-cell lymphomas. Br J Haematol 138(3):316–323
29. Pottgen C, Stuschke M et al (2003) Long-term survival following radiotherapy and cytarabine chemotherapy for sporadic primary central nervous system lymphoma. Strahlenther Onkol 179(9):626–632
30. Hoffman PM, McKelvie P et al (2003) Intraocular lymphoma: a series of 14 patients with clinicopathological features and treatment outcomes. Eye 17(4):513–521
31. Paul T, Challa S et al (2008) Primary central nervous system lymphomas: Indian experience, and review of literature. Indian J Cancer 45(3):112–118
32. Levin N, Soffer D et al (2008) Primary T-cell CNS lymphoma presenting with leptomeningeal spread and neurolymphomatosis. J Neuro Oncol 90(1):77–83
33. Choi JS, Nam D-H et al (2003) Primary central nervous system lymphoma in Korea: comparison of B- and T-cell lymphomas. Am J Surg Pathol 27(7):919–928
34. Yu GH, Montone KT et al (1996) Cytomorphology of primary CNS lymphoma: review of 23 cases and evidence for the role of EBV. Diagn Cytopathol 14(2):114–120
35. Calderon EJ, Japon MA et al (2002) Primary lymphoma of the central nervous system and HTLV-I infection. Haematologia (Budap) 31(4):365–367
36. Grimm SA, McCannel CA et al (2008) Primary CNS lymphoma with intraocular involvement: International PCNSL Collaborative Group Report. Neurology 71(17):1355–1360
37. Grimm SA, Pulido JS et al (2007) Primary intraocular lymphoma: an International Primary Central Nervous System Lymphoma Collaborative Group Report. Ann Oncol 18(11): 1851–1855
38. Harder A, Dudel C et al (2003) Molecular genetic diagnosis of a primary central nervous system T cell lymphoma. Acta Neuropathol 105(1):65–68
39. Dulai MS, Park CY et al (2008) CNS T-cell lymphoma: an under-recognized entity? Acta Neuropathol 115(3):345–356
40. Jaffe ES, Harris NL et al (2008) Classification of lymphoid neoplasms: the microscope as a tool for disease discovery. Blood 112(12):4384–4399
41. Dungerwalla M, Osuji N et al (2005) Isolated central nervous system involvement in adult T-cell lymphoma/leukemia. Br J Haematol 130(4):511–515

42. George DH, Scheithauer BW, Aker FV et al (2003) Primary anaplastic large cell lymphoma of the central nervous system: prognostic effect of ALK-1 expression. Am J Surg Pathol 27(4):487–493
43. Liu D, Schelper RL et al (2003) Primary central nervous system cytotoxic/suppressor T-cell lymphoma: report of a unique case and review of the literature. Am J Surg Pathol 27(5): 682–688
44. Omori N, Narai H et al (2008) Epstein-Barr virus-associated T/NK cell-type central nervous system lymphoma which manifested as a post-transplantation lymphoproliferative disorder in a renal transplant recipient. J Neurooncol 87(2):189–191
45. Su IC, Lien HC et al (2006) Primary brain T-cell lymphoma after kidney transplantation: a case report. Surg Neurol 66(Suppl 2):S60–S63
46. Kim EY, Kim SS (2005) Magnetic resonance findings of primary central nervous system T-cell lymphoma in immunocompetent patients. Acta Radiol 46(2):187–192
47. Vose J, Armitage J et al (2008) International peripheral T-cell and natural killer/T-cell lymphoma study: pathology findings and clinical outcomes. J Clin Oncol 26(25):4124–4130
48. Quek R, Ty A et al (2006) Primary central nervous system lymphoma in an Asian population: a 15-year experience. Onkologie 29(10):455–459
49. Shenkier TN, Voss N et al (2005) The treatment of primary central nervous system lymphoma in 122 immunocompetent patients: a population-based study of successively treated cohorts from the British Colombia Cancer Agency. Cancer 103(5):1008–1017
50. Kai Y, Kuratsu J, Ushio Y (1998) Primary Malignant Lymphoma of the Brain in Childhood. Case report. Neurol Med Chir (Tokyo) 38:232–237
51. Kadan-Lottick NS, Skluzacek MC, Gurney JG (2002) Decreasing Incidence Rates of Primary central Nervous System Lymphoma. Cancer 95(1):193–202
52. Alderson L, Fetell MR, Sisti M et al (1996) Sentinel lesions of primary CNS lymphoma. J Neurol Neurosurg Psychiatry 60:102–105
53. Rodriguez M, Delgado P, Petito CK (1997) Epstein-Barr Virus-associated Primary Central Nervous System Lymphoma in a child With the Acquired Immunodeficiency Syndrome. Arch Pathol Lab Med 121:1287–1291
54. Schabet M (1999) Epidemiology of Primary CNS Lymphoma. J Neurooncol 43:199–201
55. Abla O, Sandlund JT, Sung L et al (2006a, Dec) A case series of Pediatric Primary Central nervous System Lymphoma- Favourable Outcome Without Cranial Irradiation. Pediatr Blood Cancer 47(7):880–885
56. Karikari IO, Thomas K, Lagoo A et al (2007) Primary Cerebral ALK-1-positive Anaplastic Large Cell Lymphoma in a Child. Pediatr Neurosurg 43:516–521
57. Abla O, Weitzman S (2006b, Nov 15) Primary CNS lymphoma in children. Neurosurg Focus 21(5):E8
58. Ciftci E, Erden I, Akyar S (1998) MR Findings of Primary Central Nervous System Lymphoma in a Child. Acta Radiol 39:727–729
59. Schulman H, Hertzanu Y, Maor E et al (1991) Primary lymphoma of brain in childhood. Pediatr Radiol 21:434–435
60. McAllister LD, Doolittle ND, Guastadisegni PE et al (2000) Cognitive outcomes and long-term follow-up results after enhanced chemotherapy delivery for primary central nervous system lymphoma. Neurosurgery 46:51–60
61. Coupland SE, Loddenkemper C, Smith JR et al (2005) Expression of Immunoglobulin Transcription Factors in Primary Intraocular Lymphoma and Primary Central Nervous System Lymphoma. Invest Ophthalmol Vis Sci 46(11):3957–3964
62. Braaten KM, Betensky RA, de Leval L et al (2003) BCL6 expression predicts improved survival in patients with primary central nervous system lymphoma. Clin Cancer Res 9:1063–1069
63. Miles R, Raphael M, McCarthy K et al (2008) Pediatric Diffuse Large B-Cell Lymphoma Demonstrates a High Proliferation Index, Frequent c-Myc Protein Expression, and a High Incidence of Germinal Center Subtype: report of the French-American-British (FAB) International Study Group. Pediatr Blood Cancer 51:369–374

64. Cheuk W, Walford N, Lou J et al (2001) Primary Histiocytic Lymphoma of the Central nervous System: a neoplasm Frequently Overshadowed by a Prominent Inflammatory Component. Am J Surg Pathol 25(11):372–1379
65. Torres CF, Korones DN, Powers JM et al (1996) Primary Leptomeningeal Histiocytic Lymphoma in a Young Child. Med Pediatr Oncol 27:547–550
66. Murray K, Kun L, Cox J (1986) Primary malignant lymphoma of the central nervous system. Results of treatment of 11 cases and review of the literature. J Neurosurg 65(5): 600–607
67. Blay JY, Ongolo-Zogo C, Sebban C et al (2000) Primary cerebral lymphomas: unsolved issues regarding first line treatment, follow-up, late neurological toxicity and treatment of relapses. Ann Oncol 11:39–44
68. Makino K, Nakamura H, Yano S et al (2007) Pediatric primary CNS lymphoma: long term survival after treatment with radiation monotherapy. Acta Neurochir 149:295–298
69. Loning L, Zimmermann M, Reiter A et al (2000) Secondary neoplasms subsequent to Berlin-Frankfurt-Munster therapy of acute lymphoblastic leukemia in childhood: significantly lower risk without cranial radiotherapy. Blood 95:2770–2775
70. Said JA, Waters BG, Cousens P et al (1989) Neuropsychological sequelae of central nervous system prophylaxis in survivors of childhood acute lymphoblastic leukemia. J Consult Clin Psychol 57:251–256
71. Mead GM, Bleehen NM, Gregor A et al (2000) A medical research council randomized trial in patients with primary cerebral non-Hodgkin lymphoma. Cancer 89:1359–1369
72. Abrey LE, DeAngelis LM, Yahalom J (1998) Long-term survival in primary CNS lymphoma. J Clin Oncol 16:859–863
73. Fliessbach K, Helmstedter C, Urbach H et al (2005) Neuropsychological outcome after chemotherapy for primary CNS lymphoma. A prospective study. Neurology 64: 1184–1188
74. Freilich RJ, Delattre J, Monjour A et al (1996) Chemotherapy without radiation therapy as initial treatment for primary CNS lymphoma in older patients. Neurology 46: 435–439
75. Sandor V, Stark-Vancs V, Pearson D et al (1998) Phase II trial of chemotherapy alone for primary CNS and intraocular lymphoma. J Clin Oncol 16:3000–3006
76. Cairo MS, Gerrard M, Sposto R et al (2007) Results of a randomized international study of high-risk central nervous system B non-Hodgkin lymphoma and B acute lymphoblastic leukemia in children and adolescents. Blood 109:2736–2743
77. Wynn R, Arkwright PD, Haque T et al (2005) Treatment of Epstein-Barr-virus-associated primary CNS B-cell lymphoma with allogeneic T-cell immunotherapy and stem-cell tranplantation. Lancet Oncol 6:344–346
78. Watanabe T, Katayama Y, Yoshino A et al (2003) Long-term remission of primary central nervous system lymphoma by intensified methotrexate chemotherapy. J Neurooncol 63: 87–95
79. Bessell EM, Lopez-Guillermo A, Villa S et al (2002) Importance of radiotherapy in the outcome of patients with primary CNS lymphoma: an analysis of the CHOD/BVAM regimen followed by two different radiotherapy treatments. J Clin Oncol 20:231–236
80. Patte C (2006) Treatment Strategies and Outcome in childhood B-Cell Lymphoma. Proc Second International Symposium on Childhood, Adolescent And Young Adult Non-Hodgkin Lymphoma, New York, NY, May 18–20 Abstract 2, p 834
81. Arellano-Rodrigo E, Lopez-Guillermo A, Bessell EM et al (2003) Salvage treatment with etoposide (VP-16), ifosfamide and cytarabine (Ara-C) for patients with recurrent primary central nervous system lymphoma. Eur J Haematol 70:219–224
82. Patte C, Auperin A, Michon J et al (2001) The Societe Francaise d'Oncologie Pediatrique LMB 89 protocol: highly effective multiagent chemotherapy tailored to the tumor burden and initial response in 561 unselected children with B-cell lymphomas and L3 leukemia. Blood 97(11):3370–3379

83. Neuwelt EA, Guastadisegni PE, Varallyay P et al (2005) Imaging Changes and Cognitive Outcome in primary CNS Lymphoma after Enhanced Chemotherapy Delivery. Am J Neuroradiol 26:258–265
84. Kraemer DF, Fortin D, Doolittle ND et al (2001) Association of total dose intensity of chemotherapy in primary central nervous system lymphoma (human non-acquired immunodeficiency syndrome) and survival. Neurosurgery 48:1033–1041
85. Khan RB, Shi W, Thaler HT et al (2002) Is intrathecal methotrexate necessary in the treatment of primary CNS lymphoma? J Neurooncol 58:175–178
86. Akyuz C, Aydin GB, Cila A et al (2007) Successful use of intraventricular and intravenous rituximab therapy for refractory primary CNS lymphoma in a child. Leuk Lymphoma 48(6):1253–1255
87. Soussain C, Suzan F, Hoang-Xuan K et al (2001) Results of intensive chemotherapy followed by hematopoietic stem-cell rescue in 22 patients with refractory or recurrent primary CNS lymphoma or intraocular lymphoma. J Clin Oncol 19:742–749
88. Abrey LE, Moskowitz CH, Mason WP et al (2003) Intensive methotrexate and cytarabine followed by high-dose chemotherapy with autologous stem-cell rescue in patients with newly diagnosed primary CNS lymphoma. J Clin Oncol 21:4151–4156
89. Brevet M, Garidi R, Gruson B et al (2005) First-line autologous stem cell transplantation in primary CNS lymphoma. Eur J Haematol 75:288–292
90. Brennan KC, Lowe LH, Yeaney GA (2005) Pediatric Central Nervous System Posttransplant Lymphoproliferative Disorder. Am J Neuroradiol 26:1695–1697
91. Scrigni A, Nastri M, de Schiavi SR et al (2006) Leptomeningeal lymphoma in a child with Acquired Immune Deficiency Syndrome. Neuropediatrics 37:121–125
92. Newell ME, Hoy JF, Cooper SG et al (2004) Human immunodeficiency virus-related primary central nervous system lymphoma: Factors influencing survival in 111 patients. Cancer 100:2627–2636
93. Goldstein J, Dickson DW, Rubenstein A et al (1990) Primary central nervous system lymphoma in a pediatric patient with acquiured immunodeficiency syndrome. Cancer 66:2503–2508
94. Batchelor T, Carson K, O'Neill A et al (2003) Treatment of primary CNS lymphoma with methotrexate and deferred radiotherapy: a report of NABTT 96-07. J Clin Oncol 21: 1044–1049
95. Poortmans PM, Kluin-Nelemans HX, Haaxma-Reiche H et al (2003) High-dose methotrexate-based chemotherapy followed by consolidating radiotherapy in non-AIDS-related primary central nervous system lymphoma: European Organization for Research and Treatment of Cancer Lymphoma Group Phase II Trial 20962. J Clin Oncol 21:4483–4488
96. Hoang-Xuan K, Taillandier L, Chinot O et al; European Organization for Research and Treatment of Cancer Brain Tumor Group (2003) Chemotherapy alone as initial treatment for primary CNS lymphoma in patients older than 60 years: a multicenter phase II study (26952) of the European Organization for Research and Treatment of Cancer Brain Tumor Group. J Clin Oncol 21:2726–2731
97. Illerhaus G, Marks R, Ihorst G et al (2006) High-dose chemotherapy with autologous stem-cell transplantation and hyperfractionated radiotherapy as first-line treatment of primary CNS lymphoma. J Clin Oncol 24:3865–3870
98. Omuro AM, Taillandier L, Chinot O et al (2007) Temozolomide and methotrexate for primary central nervous system lymphoma in the elderly. J Neurooncol 85:207–211
99. Illerhaus G, Marks R, Müller F et al (2009) High-dose methotrexate combined with procarbazine and CCNU for primary CNS lymphoma in the elderly: results of a prospective pilot and phase II study. Ann Oncol 20:319–325
100. Angelov L, Doolittle ND, Kraemer DF et al (2009) Blood-brain barrier disruption and intra-arterial methotrexate-based therapy for newly diagnosed primary CNS lymphoma: a multi-institutional experience. J Clin Oncol 27:3503–3509

Part V
Neurological Complications of Lymphomas and Leukemias

Chapter 16
Neurological Complications of Non-Hodgkin Lymphoma

Mustafa Khasraw, Ariela Noy, Mark Gilbert, and Antonio Omuro

Introduction

Systemic non-Hodgkin lymphoma (NHL) may involve the nervous system at every level, including the neuromuscular junction, peripheral nerve, plexus, spinal nerve root, spinal cord, meninges, and brain. Such involvement may occur as a result of direct invasion or compression of these structures, as well as through non-invasive paraneoplastic effects of NHL. Typical central nervous system (CNS) manifestations include leptomeningeal metastasis, epidural extension with myelopathy, and brain parenchymal infiltration. Peripheral nervous system involvement is less frequent, and may present as radiculopathy, plexopathy, neuropathy, and myopathy. This chapter will focus on direct involvement of the nervous system by systemic NHL; paraneoplastic syndromes secondary to NHL are discussed in Chapter 19.

CNS Involvement in NHL

Incidence and Risk Factors

CNS involvement in NHL may be present at diagnosis, but most often occurs later in the course of disease, either as an isolated site of relapse or in combination with systemic relapse. CNS relapses tend to occur relatively early, at a median of 5–12 months from diagnosis. Approximately 70% of patients with CNS involvement will present with leptomeningeal metastasis and 30% will develop brain parenchymal involvement. The CNS will be the sole site of relapse in approximately one-half of patients with CNS involvement [1].

A number of studies have investigated the incidence and risk factors for the development of CNS involvement in NHL (Table 16.1), in an attempt to identify those patients who may benefit from CNS prophylaxis as part of initial treatment.

A. Omuro (✉)
Department of Neurology, Memorial Sloan-Kettering Cancer Center, New York, NY 10065, USA
e-mail: omuroa@mskcc.org

T. Batchelor, L.M. DeAngelis (eds.), *Lymphoma and Leukemia of the Nervous System*, DOI 10.1007/978-1-4419-7668-0_16,

Table 16.1 Reported risk factors for the development of CNS disease in Non-Hodgkin lymphoma

- *Advanced/ aggressive disease:*
  - Increased age-adjusted IPI
  - Albumin < 3.5 g/dL
  - LDH > 450
  - Age > 60
- *Disease location:*
  - Testicular
  - Paranasal sinuses/base of skull
  - Bone/bone marrow
  - Breast
  - Retroperitoneal
  - >1 extra-nodal site
- *Histologic subtypes*[a]:
  - Lymphoblastic
  - Burkitt's lymphoma
  - Mantle cell
  - Intravascular lymphoma
  - Mycosis fungoides with large-cell transformation

[a]Diffuse large-B cell lymphoma remains the most common histologic type.

However, interpreting these studies is difficult because of the various definitions of "CNS involvement", heterogeneous treatments and patient populations, and the retrospective nature of many of the reports. Overall, these studies have indicated a risk of CNS relapse of approximately 2–7% [2]. Most studies have shown that advanced and high risk disease, as determined by staging and the International Prognostic Index (IPI) ([3]), are important risk factors for CNS relapse. CNS relapse has been predicted by the presence of stage III/IV disease, neurological symptoms, bone marrow involvement, elevated serum lactate dehydrogenase (LDH), and high or high-intermediate IPI [4, 5]. A study involving 444 patients identified 29 (6.5%) with CNS disease after a median observation time of 115 months [6]. CNS occurrence was associated with testicular involvement, advanced clinical stage, and increased age-adjusted IPI. A retrospective Norwegian study of 2,514 patients with NHL, of whom 106 (4.2%) developed neuraxis involvement, identified the following independent risk factors: age >60 years, LDH >450 U/l, albumin <3.5 g/dL, retroperitoneal lymph node involvement, and involvement of >1 extranodal site [7]. Of note, if four or five of these risk factors were present, the risk of CNS recurrence was >25% at 5 years. A series of 1,693 patients with aggressive NHL treated on a variety of chemotherapy protocols reported a low incidence of CNS relapse (2.2%). On multivariate analysis, only elevated serum LDH and involvement of >1 extranodal site were independent risk factors for CNS involvement [8]. In a study of 399 elderly patients with diffuse large B-cell lymphoma (DLBCL) treated without CNS prophylaxis, 20 patients (5%) developed CNS involvement. Only the age-adjusted IPI predicted CNS recurrence [9]. In a study of 974 patients with aggressive NHL in complete response and treated with CNS prophylaxis, CNS recurrence developed in only 1.6%, and higher risk IPI was a strong predictor of isolated CNS recurrence [10]. Although DLBCL accounts for the majority of NHL patients with CNS involvement, nearly every lymphoma subtype has been reported to invade the nervous system [7, 11]. In a retrospective study of 498 patients with NHL, 26 of the 30 patients with CNS involvement had aggressive or highly aggressive disease. The risk of CNS recurrence was 23% for the highly aggressive variant lymphoblastic lymphoma and only 1.4% for those with indolent lymphoma [11]. The propensity for CNS involvement by Burkitt's lymphoma has also been well described, with an 8–10% incidence at diagnosis, and up to 30–50% throughout the course of disease [12]. Mantle cell lymphoma (MCL) has been reported to be associated with an unexpected high risk of CNS involvement, estimated at 4–6% [13]; Feugier et al. 2004; [14, 15]. However, such risks may be attributed to poor systemic control of disease, and CNS relapse in MCL is rare with modern therapies. Intravascular lymphoma is a rare DLBCL that frequently affects the CNS, although CNS manifestations are usually secondary to vascular occlusion and hypoxia (i.e., strokes) rather than direct brain infiltration [16].

Lymphomatous involvement of certain locations such as the testicles, paranasal sinuses/base of skull, retroperitoneum, bone and bone marrow has been associated with an increased risk of CNS involvement [17, 18]. The association of primary testicular lymphoma and CNS lymphoma is well known. One review found that 13 of 62 patients (21%) with testicular lymphoma experienced CNS relapse, with 8 of the 13 recurrences isolated to the CNS [19, 20]. Testicular involvement is an important predictor of CNS recurrence in elderly lymphoma patients as well [19, 20]. Base of skull and paranasal sinus involvement is frequently associated with intracranial disease through direct extension and seeding of the CSF. Cutaneous lymphoma has been associated with a high frequency of CNS involvement. An autopsy study reported up to 14% of patients with T-cell lymphoma mycosis fungoides (MF) had CNS involvement. However, this is rarely observed in clinical practice, and usually occurs in the setting of large-cell transformation [21]. Likewise, primary cutaneous B-cell lymphoma does not appear to be associated with a high frequency of CNS recurrence [22]. It is widely accepted that involvement of more than one extra-nodal site is associated with a significant increase in the risk of CNS relapses. Indications for CNS prophylaxis in these different clinical situations are discussed below.

Leptomeningeal Metastasis

Leptomeningeal metastasis (LM), also known as leptomeningeal disease or lymphomatous meningitis, is the most common nervous system complication of NHL. LM occurs in 6–8% of NHL patients [23, 24]; conversely, NHL patients represent one-quarter of all patients with LM [25].

Clinical Features

The most common presentation is cranial nerve palsies, observed in 42–80% of patients with LM. One or several nerves may be affected, with a predilection for cranial nerves II, III, V, VI, and VII. Other symptoms and signs include headaches, gait difficulty, altered mental status, radicular pain, vague back or neck pain, focal weakness or sensory loss. Dysfunction at multiple levels of the neuraxis is common; seizures may occasionally occur. Hydrocephalus and intracranial hypertension may cause headache, nausea, vomiting, and lethargy.

Imaging

Contrast-enhanced brain and spine MRI are the neuroimaging techniques of choice for the diagnosis of LM, although the diagnostic sensitivity in hematologic malignancies can be as low as 50%. Nevertheless, both brain and spine MRI are recommended in all patients with suspected LM to exclude parenchymal brain involvement, as well as hydrocephalus or bulky LM compressing the spinal cord, which require specific management. Optimally, MRI should be obtained prior to the lumbar puncture (LP) to exclude the presence of a large brain mass that would contraindicate the procedure. Moreover, an LP may cause pachymeningeal enhancement related to intracranial hypotension, which can mimic LM on spine and brain MRI and produce false-positive results. The presence of subarachnoid nodular enhancement along the neuraxis is diagnostic of LM, since other inflammatory processes, such as meningitis and Guillain-Barré syndrome are associated with linear, fine patterns of enhancement. Typical locations of leptomeningeal enhancement in LM include the cauda equina, basal cisterns, cerebellum, and cranial nerves; the contrast enhancement is frequently referred to as "sugar coating." Communicating hydrocephalus may occur, but is non-specific. Contrast-enhanced cranial CT can be used for the evaluation of LM, but is less sensitive and specific than MRI and should only be used when MRI is contraindicated. PET studies are inadequate for the characterization of LM due to low resolution.

Lumbar Puncture and Cerebrospinal Fluid (CSF) Analysis

In hematologic malignancies, LP and CSF analysis have a greater sensitivity and specificity than neuroimaging. CSF analysis has a lower sensitivity than specificity; i.e., false-negative results are more common than false-positive results. In addition, cellular atypia is common in immunosuppressed patients, increasing diagnostic confusion [26]. Fresh CSF, adequate preservation of cell structure and large CSF volume for analysis (5 ML or more) are required for adequate cytologic analysis. In the setting of high clinical suspicion and negative results, repeat LP is the standard of care.

The CSF protein level is usually increased in patients with LM. Low glucose levels in the CSF can also be present, as well as a lymphocytic pleocytosis. Elevation of CSF levels of beta 2-microglobulin and increased LDH isoenzymes have been reported in LM, but are non-specific findings and must be interpreted in conjunction with cytologic and clinical data [27, 28].

The identification of lymphoma cells in the CSF is the definitive diagnostic test for LM. Early studies reported positive cytology only 50% of the time with one sample, but in excess of 80% after three samples. As with other malignancies, repeated LPs may be necessary to make the diagnosis of LM. Occasionally, differentiating tumor cells from reactive lymphocytes can be challenging. Immunocytochemistry using disease-specific monoclonal antibodies selected according to the patient's previously known histologic type may be helpful to establish the diagnosis [29]. Additional techniques, such as flow cytometry and polymerase chain reaction (PCR) amplification of IgH_V genes or T-cell receptors, have been increasingly utilized and may improve the diagnostic accuracy of CSF analysis for the detection of LM.

Flow cytometry is a technique in which clonal populations of B-lymphocytes are separated from reactive cells on the basis of size, granularity, and surface antigen expression. Flow cytometry can detect populations of neoplastic cells comprising as few as 0.2% of CSF lymphocytes [30, 31]. In a study of flow cytometry in patients with aggressive B-cell lymphomas at risk for CNS involvement, 11 (22%) were found to have occult CSF involvement. All 11 were detected by flow cytometry and only 1 by cytology [30]. In clinical practice, technical issues (need for rapid processing, difficulties with multi-flow processing) have prevented universal adoption of such techniques.

PCR assay of the CDR3 encoding region of the immunoglobulin heavy chain locus on CSF lymphocytes has also been identified as a sensitive and rapid technique for distinguishing reactive B-cell populations from malignant ones [32]. PCR relies on the clonal rearrangement of immunoglobulin genes during B-cell development to identify malignant cells. In one study of patients with known CNS lymphoma, five of seven specimens suspicious but non-diagnostic by conventional cytology were positive by PCR. Of 13 specimens that were negative by cytology, five were positive by PCR [33]. T-cell receptor PCR can be used for patients with T-cell lymphomas. However, this technique is prone to both false-negative and false-positive results, due to the relative paucity of T-cell receptor genes and the occasional presence of oligoclonality in healthy individuals.

Treatment

Once the diagnosis of LM is confirmed, corticosteroids are often utilized for symptomatic relief. Corticosteroids should not be initiated until the diagnosis is confirmed because of their lympholytic activity, which decreases the sensitivity of diagnostic tests. Leptomeningeal dissemination from lymphoid malignancies tends to respond better to treatment than leptomeningeal involvement from solid tumors [34]. Control of meningeal disease is necessary to prevent neurological morbidity and preserve quality of life. However, optimal management for LM is unclear, and the prognosis remains poor [35, 36]. Reported median overall survival has been in the range of 2.2–19 months, but most often 4–5 months [35]. The available treatment options are discussed below.

Intrathecal Chemotherapy

Due to the poor penetration of most chemotherapy drugs through the blood-brain barrier, intrathecal (IT) chemotherapy remains a mainstay of treatment. Placement of an Ommaya reservoir for administration is preferred over repeat LPs for patient comfort, better drug distribution, and assurance of drug delivery into the CSF. Prior to the start of treatment, a radionuclide cisterno-scintigraphy is often performed to evaluate CSF flow, and IT chemotherapy should not be administered to patients with impaired CSF circulation.

Intrathecal MTX or cytarabine are the drugs of choice for LM. A limitation in the use of IT drugs is their rapid clearance from the CSF; frequent administrations are often necessary. Typical schedules are MTX 12 mg or cytarabine 50 mg, given twice a week. Leucovorin may be given orally to prevent mucositis and myelosuppression, but is usually not required given the low dose and limited systemic distribution.

Liposomal cytarabine (DepoCyt®) has been proposed as an alternative to MTX, given its longer half-life and more convenient schedule (every 2 weeks). In a randomized phase II trial comparing conventional IT cytarabine versus liposomal cytarabine, the liposomal formulation achieved a superior cytologic response rate (71% versus 15%) and a better quality of life [37]. The efficacy of IT liposomal cytarabine versus IT MTX has not been adequately evaluated in hematological malignancies. It must also be noted that in clinical practice, chemical arachnoiditis and aseptic meningitis are more common with the use of liposomal cytarabine than conventional therapy, particularly in patients on prolonged administration schedules. Corticosteroids with CNS penetration, specifically dexamethasone, must be administered for prophylaxis of arachnoiditis from liposomal cytarabine (e.g., dexamethasone 4 mg bid for 5 days beginning on the day of treatment).

Intrathecal use of the monoclonal anti-CD20 antibody rituximab has been proposed to overcome the lack of blood-brain barrier penetration after intravenous administration [38–40]. In a phase I dose-escalation study of 10 patients with recurrent CNS NHL [41], the maximal tolerated dose of IT rituximab was 25 mg twice weekly. This resulted in rapid craniospinal axis distribution and the achievement of intra-ventricular CSF concentrations similar to peak serum levels achieved after IV administration of standard doses (375 mg/m^2). Cytologic responses were observed in six of the eight patients who had LM. Interestingly, one patient exhibited resolution of a brain lesion after IT rituximab treatment. In a small retrospective study, IT rituximab was given in combination with liposomal cytarabine to patients with recurrent LM [42]. Modest palliative activity was observed, with 10/14 partial responses lasting a median time of 4 months; median overall survival was 5 months. Because of the paucity of data, to date, the IT use of rituximab with or without liposomal cytarabine should be considered experimental.

Intrathecal chemotherapy is generally well tolerated, but several complications may arise. Although new or worsening of existing symptoms that develop during IT chemotherapy are often due to disease progression, all patients should be promptly evaluated to rule out complications of treatment.

Aseptic or chemical meningitis/arachnoiditis may develop causing headache, neck stiffness, nausea, vomiting, CSF lymphocytic or neutrophilic pleocytosis, and occasionally fever. These symptoms often develop within hours in contrast to a septic meningitis or catheter infection, which typically develop $\geq$24 h following drug instillation and are rare. Aseptic meningitis responds well to steroids.

Hydrocephalus may develop as a result of treatment or as a complication of the LM, and needs to be recognized since further IT chemotherapy is contraindicated and a ventriculoperitoneal shunt must be considered.

Acute/subacute encephalopathy may also complicate IT chemotherapy, particularly in the setting of increased intracranial pressure and obstructed CSF flow. Patients usually present with mental status changes and gait difficulty; MRI demonstrates progressive leukoencephalopathy. Occasionally, the chemotherapy agent may track back along the ventricular catheter to produce a focal enhancing mass; this occurs in the setting of raised intracranial pressure or a damaged catheter. Discontinuation of IT chemotherapy and steroids are often sufficient for treatment and surgery is usually not required.

Systemic Chemotherapy

A critical aspect of LM management is control of extraneural systemic disease with chemotherapy, as a survival benefit from treatment of LM is unlikely unless this is achieved. Moreover, systemic chemotherapy can achieve uniform distribution throughout the CSF compartment and can penetrate bulky sites of disease that will not be adequately treated by IT chemotherapy. The choice of systemic drugs for patients with LM is dictated by the histologic type and previous chemotherapies used; whenever possible, the regimen should include drugs with CNS penetration, particularly high-dose MTX (>3 g/m^2) and cytarabine; nitrosoureas, thiotepa, and other lipophilic agents may also be used. Most often, systemic chemotherapy is used in combination with IT chemotherapy, and the role of systemic chemotherapy with drugs such as high-dose IV methotrexate and cytarabine, without IT chemotherapy has not been established.

High-Dose Chemotherapy (HDCT) with Autologous Stem-Cell Transplant (ASCT)

HDCT-ASCT is an emerging option for consolidation treatment in patients with LM and chemosensitive disease. An early retrospective study of 1,464 patients with NHL undergoing HDCT-ASCT suggested that some patients with CNS disease may achieve durable remissions with HDCT. In that study, patients who achieved remission of CNS disease before transplantation fared better than those who had active CNS disease at the time of transplant [43].

In a retrospective review of 37 NHL patients with CNS involvement in remission before the high dose conditioning regimen, 24% had received IT chemotherapy alone, and 70% had received IT chemotherapy and CNS irradiation before HDCT. The main preparative regimens were cyclophosphamide/total body irradiation and busulfan/cyclophosphamide. Forty-one percent received an allogeneic transplant.

Lymphoma relapsed after hematopoietic stem cell transplant in 14 patients (38%), and at least five had documented or suspected CNS relapse. The 5-year event-free survival was 36%, and overall survival was 39% [44]. Taken together, these studies suggested that NHL patients with CNS involvement who achieve CNS remission should be offered HDCT, if it is otherwise not contraindicated. In another study of 481 patients undergoing HDCT-ASCT for NHL, 13 had secondary CNS NHL (seven with LM). Various treatments were utilized prior to HDCT-ASCT, including IT chemotherapy in all patients. At the time of transplantation, 8 patients had achieved a complete response. The preparative treatment consisted of carmustine, etoposide, and cyclophosphamide. The actuarial 5-year event-free survival was 46% and the overall survival was 41%, with a good quality of life in long-term survivors [45]. This study is limited by the low number of patients and retrospective nature. More robust results have been reported in recurrent primary CNS lymphoma. In a phase II prospective study, salvage chemotherapy with cytarabine and etoposide followed by high-dose thiotepa, busulfan and cyclophosphamide, and ASCT given to 43 patients achieved a 2-year survival of 45% [46]. Interestingly, 12 patients with chemoresistant disease that did not respond to the induction chemotherapy received HDCT-ASCT and experienced a complete response, suggesting that HDCT-ASCT may overcome chemoresistance mediated by poor drug CNS penetration. In fact, experience with primary CNS lymphoma also suggests that the HDCT regimens must be chosen carefully because milder regimens such as BCNU, etoposide, cytarabine, and melphalan (BEAM) may not be effective when applied to disease in the CNS [47], and more aggressive regimens may be required [46].

Radiotherapy

Whole brain radiotherapy (WBRT) has been used in the treatment of LM, both at the time of initial diagnosis (preceding and following IT chemotherapy) and as a salvage therapy after chemotherapy failure [43]. The upfront use of WBRT without chemotherapy is associated with higher risks of relapse, and is currently reserved for palliation in patients with terminal disease or in those who are not candidates for chemotherapy. Likewise, the upfront use of WBRT in combination with chemotherapy has been largely abandoned because of the high risk of radiotherapy-related neurotoxicity; HDCT-ASCT is increasingly preferred as a consolidation treatment. However, WBRT remains an option for palliation in patients who are refractory to chemotherapy. In some instances, focal radiotherapy is used when rapid decompression of neural structures is required, such as in patients with bulky LM compressing the optic nerves or the spinal cord. Concurrent use of IT chemotherapy is not recommended in patients receiving WBRT due to increased neurotoxicity. Craniospinal irradiation has been abandoned due to toxicity, lack of efficacy, and possible preclusion of further chemotherapy due to bone marrow suppression.

Attempts have been made to deliver radiation to the leptomeninges with radioactive IT elements, such as radiolabeled indium-111 and yttrium-90 ibritumomab tiuxetan in order to avoid neurotoxicity, but to date, such treatments remain experimental [48].

Brain Metastases

Clinical Presentation

Involvement of brain parenchyma is less common than leptomeningeal involvement in NHL. In a study of 592 patients, brain metastases were reported in 1.4% with NHL [49]. Depending on the number and location of the metastases, patients may present with mental status changes, gait abnormalities, focal motor or sensory deficits, cranial nerve deficits, or symptoms and signs of increased intracranial pressure.

Diagnosis

Contrast-enhanced cranial MRI provides an excellent definition of the location and number of metastatic lesions and associated edema, and constitutes the imaging modality of choice for diagnosis and evaluation of responses. Contrast-enhanced cranial CT scan can be helpful as a preliminary test in emergency situations or if MRI is contraindicated.

MRI findings are similar to those seen in PCNSL, and typically demonstrate one or more homogenously enhancing, intra-parenchymal lesions (Fig. 16.1), with an appearance often referred to as "cotton" or "snow ball" on T1 post-contrast sequences. T2 sequences may show hypointensity in the regions with contrast enhancement surrounded by hyperintensity corresponding to surrounding edema. This is a distinct feature compared to other types of brain tumors, in which enhancing cores are associated with T2 hyperintensity. In patients with a history of base

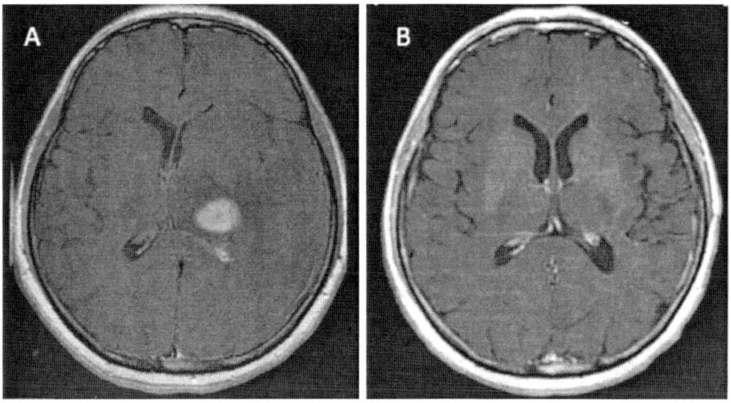

Fig. 16.1 Brain metastasis in a 61-year-old woman with a previous history of diffuse large B-cell lymphoma who presented with headaches. The T-1 post-contrast MRI sequence shows a typical parenchymal brain metastasis from NHL (**a**), consisting of a homogenously enhancing mass in the deep aspect of the left cerebral hemisphere. The diagnosis was confirmed by brain biopsy and the patient achieved a complete response (**b**) to high-dose methotrexate, procarbazine and vincristine, and received consolidation high-dose chemotherapy with thiotepa, busulfan and cyclophosphamide

of skull or paranasal disease, direct extension from the original lesion can be appreciated on the MRI.

Because brain metastases occur rarely in NHL, biopsy is required to confirm the diagnosis and to exclude the possibility of a second malignancy or other neurological diseases. Occasionally, the lesions are located in regions of difficult access (e.g., brainstem), and the risk of neurological injury from the biopsy outweighs the concern for misdiagnosis. As clinically indicated, such patients may be treated empirically, particularly if a remarkable response to steroids is observed, which favors the diagnosis of CNS lymphoma over other types of cancer. Additional non-invasive evaluation with MR spectroscopy, perfusion MRI or PET may be helpful when a biopsy is not an option. Although such modalities are not specific enough to confirm a diagnosis of CNS lymphoma, they may underscore the neoplastic nature of the lesion, and exclude inflammatory, infectious, or vascular diseases [50]. MR spectroscopy typically shows an increase in choline, indicating cell proliferation; the presence of a large lipid peak in the absence of necrosis is a suggestive, but non-diagnostic finding in CNS lymphomas. MR perfusion usually shows increased relative cerebral blood volumes (rCBVs), but occasionally the metastatic lesion can be hypoperfused, unlike most other malignant brain tumors. FDG-PET scan usually demonstrates hypermetabolism, but a dedicated brain PET is needed, as brain involvement is often missed on a full body PET scan.

Treatment

Because parenchymal brain relapse of NHL is rare, the optimal treatment has not been defined; these patients are often reported in conjunction with patients who have LM or recurrent primary CNS lymphoma. The most commonly utilized initial treatment is high-dose MTX-based chemotherapy. Other drugs are frequently used in combination with high-dose MTX, particularly in the setting of systemic recurrence. A retrospective series of 113 NHL patients presenting with isolated brain relapse after initial complete systemic remission suggested that MTX used as initial treatment is associated with significantly longer survival. Median overall survival from the date of brain relapse was 1.6 years, with a 3-year survival of 23%. Younger age (<60 years) at relapse, and MTX used as initial treatment for brain relapse, were associated with longer survival [51]. WBRT can be used for consolidation therapy following chemotherapy, but is most often reserved for recurrent or refractory disease due to the risks of neurotoxicity. HDCT-ASCT may be used as consolidation therapy in patients with chemosensitive disease, and is discussed above in conjunction with HDCT-ASCT for LM.

A challenging, but uncommon, situation is the synchronous presentation of parenchymal brain lymphoma and systemic NHL. Most of these patients will have DLBCL, and will require initial treatment for both systemic and brain disease. In a small retrospective study of nine patients, all but one patient received high-dose MTX in combination with other drugs and the median overall survival was 46 months [52]. In three of these patients, MTX could be combined safely with R-CHOP (MTX 3.5 g/m^2 on day 1 and R-CHOP starting on day 8 of 21 day cycles).

CNS Prophylaxis for NHL

The decision to incorporate CNS prophylaxis into the initial treatment regimen for a patient with NHL is influenced not only by the presence of risk factors, but also by the effectiveness and toxicity of the agents used for CNS prophylaxis. Because available studies have been unable to account for all these variables, results have been conflicting and little consensus exists on which patients should or should not receive CNS prophylaxis; clinical practice varies widely in terms of patient selection and type of CNS prophylaxis [1, 53–55].

In spite of this controversy, it is largely accepted that all patients with Burkitt's lymphoma and acute lymphoblastic leukemia/lymphoma should receive CNS prophylaxis, as the evidence, suggesting a reduction in CNS relapse and clinical benefit is strong. Most modern first-line regimens for these patients incorporate IT or high-dose MTX or cytarabine. Likewise, there is general acceptance that patients with indolent lymphoma, including MCL, do not require routine CSF prophylaxis.

The indications for CNS prophylaxis in DLBCL are more controversial, given the relatively low overall incidence of CNS relapse. A number of studies have suggested a role for CNS prophylaxis in selected and unselected populations of DLBCL patients. In an uncontrolled study, 51 patients with DLBCL involving sites associated with a high risk of CNS relapse received IT prophylaxis with MTX (plus cytarabine in some cases) [56]. The CNS relapse rate was 1.1%, which is substantially lower than the expected relapse rate based on other reports. A Japanese group analyzed 68 patients with aggressive NHL who had achieved CR after therapy with a MACOP-B like regimen and then received either IT MTX with hydrocortisone or no CNS prophylaxis [57]. CNS relapse did not occur in any of the 29 patients who received prophylaxis, compared with six of 39 patients (15%) who did not receive prophylaxis. Five-year overall survival (80% versus 58%) and recurrence-free survival (85% versus 51%) were significantly longer for the group that received prophylaxis. On multivariate analysis, lack of CNS prophylaxis was the strongest independent predictor of CNS recurrence. However, other studies have refuted a role for CNS prophylaxis in DLBCL. An Australian group retrospectively studied 27 patients who had received IT prophylaxis for B-cell malignancies. Six patients with DLBCL suffered secondary CNS relapse despite IT prophylaxis [58]. Taken together, these studies illustrate the difficulties in ascertaining the risks versus benefits of CNS prophylaxis, given the low number of patients and heterogeneous populations. In practical terms, CNS prophylaxis, particularly IT chemotherapy, is frequently utilized in patients with more than one extranodal site, elevated LDH or high/high-intermediate IPI. Many physicians have also systematically used CNS prophylaxis for patients with testicular, breast, epidural and nasopharynx/base of skull DLBCL; most often, IT MTX is used, although clear evidence of efficacy is lacking [1]. It is noteworthy that most studies of CNS prophylaxis in NHL date from the pre R-CHOP era, and newer studies are needed to evaluate the impact of rituximab in DLBCL. There is some evidence that rituximab may not decrease the risk of CNS relapse due to poor blood-brain barrier penetration [9], although other studies have found a decrease in CNS recurrence, perhaps reflecting better control of systemic disease [59].

In addition to the difficulty in defining clear criteria for patient selection, the choice of CNS prophylaxis also remains controversial. WBRT has been increasingly abandoned due to the risks of neurotoxicity and inability to address the entire CSF compartment. IT chemotherapy with MTX or cytarabine is used frequently, but can be associated with several complications and does not address parenchymal disease. High-dose MTX, at doses of at least 3 g/m^2, has been used increasingly for CNS prophylaxis, and has the advantage of better CNS drug distribution and addressing parenchymal disease. However, prospective studies directly comparing high-dose versus IT MTX are lacking. Cytarabine has also been used for CNS prophylaxis, both at doses of 1–3 g/m^2 intravenously, and 50 mg intrathecally, although the hematotoxicity with intravenous use is a concern for incorporation into first-line regimens. IT liposomal cytarabine may be an option for CNS prophylaxis, but efficacy data are lacking.

Spinal Cord Involvement

Clinical Presentation

A common neurological problem in NHL is epidural spinal cord or cauda equina compression (ESCC) from vertebral body involvement or direct invasion of the spinal canal through the intervertebral foramina. Back pain is the most common initial symptom. The pain is typically aggravated by the recumbent position and by Valsalva maneuver. As the spinal cord is compressed, patients develop symptoms of myelopathy with weakness, numbness, and bladder/bowel disturbances. In some cases, neurological deficits develop in a rapid manner; in others, symptoms and signs progress over days or weeks. Rapid onset and progression of clinical signs portend a poor prognosis. In either case, ESCC must be managed as a neurological emergency. Patients with severe weakness at presentation may have compromised functional recovery. Thus, prompt diagnosis and treatment of this condition has a significant impact on neurological outcome and the patient's quality of life.

Rarely, the spinal cord may also be involved by intramedullary metastases from NHL. The presentation typically includes weakness, sensory deficits, and urinary incontinence. Although pain may be present, it is usually less severe than in ESCC. Early signs indicating intramedullary disease include urinary and fecal incontinence, and a sensory level on examination.

Symptoms and signs of radiculopathy (radicular pain, sensory and motor abnormalities in the affected dermatome/myotome, sphincter abnormalities) may be observed in patients with vertebral or epidural disease (Fig. 16.2), with or without cord compression, but may also be observed in LM and neurolymphomatosis.

Diagnosis

Whole spine MRI, with and without gadolinium is the imaging modality of choice when ESCC, intramedullary metastases, or epidural disease are suspected. In

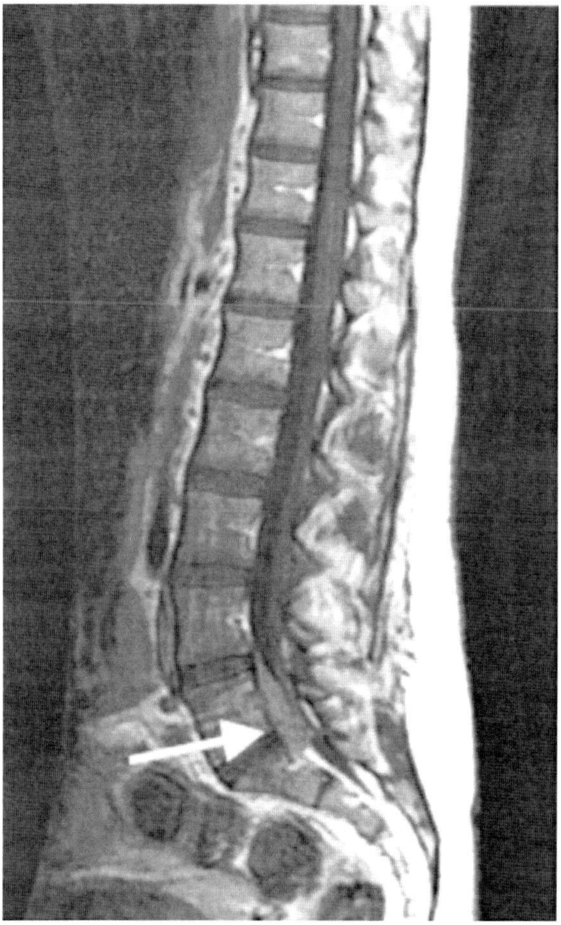

Fig. 16.2 Epidural lymphomatous involvement in a 32-year-old woman presenting with low back pain and lumbosacral radiculopathy. The saggital T1-weighted post contrast MRI shows a homogeneously enhancing epidural lesion (*arrow*) producing a complete effacement of the thecal sac. Biopsy of this lesion was consistent with follicular lymphoma

addition to defining the degree of compression, spinal MRI may also demonstrate disease at multiple levels. A sagittal T1-weighted "screening" image of the entire spine is ideal, with special attention to the level of involvement suggested by clinical evaluation. Gadolinium is not required to diagnose ESCC, but is essential to identify LM or an intramedullary lesion. Occasionally, the MRI may reveal concurrent LM, ESCC or a spinal cord metastasis. In a series of 21 autopsy-proven cases of LM, three patients presented clinically with spinal cord compression.

Treatment

Prompt diagnosis and treatment are critical when NHL causes spinal cord compression. High doses of corticosteroids should be promptly used, although the optimal corticosteroid dose has not been defined. Doses as high as 100 mg of dexamethasone or equivalent are usually administered, but there is no evidence that doses higher than 24 mg are more effective. Following the initial bolus, patients are usually given daily maintenance doses of corticosteroids. Once imaging has been obtained and the diagnosis confirmed, urgent radiotherapy is usually recommended. Some patients may also benefit from urgent decompressive surgery, particularly with bulky disease at one spinal level causing paraplegia. However, in practical terms, lymphomas are largely radiosensitive and radiation therapy is usually favored over surgery, if it can be rapidly initiated. Less frequently, NHL is diagnosed when patients without a cancer diagnosis present with spinal cord compression, and surgery is performed to establish the diagnosis. Anterior surgical decompression or synchronous vertebral decompression has also been advocated in ESCC cases that fail radiotherapy, although most of the experience with this approach has been with solid tumors, such as breast and lung cancer [60]. Bed rest is advocated only in patients with spinal instability, which usually requires surgical correction. Dedicated nursing care helps prevent skin complications in patients with weakness and sensory deficits. Bowel care with laxatives and bladder drainage (preferably with intermittent catheterization) are also essential for patients with sphincter disturbances. Chemotherapy is not usually employed in the urgent treatment of ESCC in NHL, since response to treatment is too slow to be effective. Nevertheless, successful chemotherapeutic treatment of ESCC in NHL has been reported [61], and may be considered in chemotherapy naive patients if neurological symptoms are mild. Because ESCC is typically associated with active systemic disease, chemotherapy is usually instituted once the patient's neurological condition is stabilized.

Patients with epidural disease or radiculopathy without ESCC may be managed with chemotherapy, as appropriate for their primary disease histology and stage [62]. Radiotherapy may be used for rapid relief of pain that cannot be controlled otherwise.

Patients with intramedullary NHL metastasis can be treated with focal radiotherapy, with or without chemotherapy. Chemotherapy should follow the same principles that guide treatment of brain metastasis from NHL. Although corticosteroids can often provide substantial symptom relief, management of pain, constipation and urinary dysfunction is also required.

Plexus and Peripheral Nerve Involvement

Lymphomatous Plexopathy

Plexopathies in NHL may occur as a result of direct compression or infiltration from a lymphomatous mass or from radiation-induced plexopathy. Since some patients with NHL have received prior radiation including the brachial or lumbosacral plexus, it can often be difficult to distinguish between malignant infiltration of the plexus by lymphoma cells versus radiation-induced neurotoxicity affecting the plexus (radiation plexopathy). Paraneoplastic plexopathy and idiopathic plexitis are other less common causes. Pain is a cardinal symptom in malignant plexopathy, and severe pain usually indicates malignant plexopathy rather than radiation injury [63]. Weakness and sensory loss occur in the distribution of the involved levels of the plexus. Diagnosis of plexopathy due to NHL is made by physical examination and appropriate imaging studies. Electrodiagnostic testing may reveal myokymia, spontaneous, fine fascicular contractions of muscle without muscular atrophy or weakness, which is pathognomonic for radiation injury, but still seen in only about 40% of patients with that diagnosis. Focal radiation therapy is useful for lymphomatous plexopathy and can relieve pain and preserve function; chemotherapy may be used if radiotherapy is not an option.

Peripheral Neuropathy

Peripheral nerve dysfunction is often seen in patients with NHL. Most commonly, the peripheral neuropathy is the result of chemotherapy-related polyneuropathy. These patients usually do not pose a diagnostic challenge, as a history of recent exposure to a known neurotoxic drug (e.g., vincristine) is usually clear and symptoms are typical: sensory symptoms (usually tingling and numbness or loss of sensation), loss of reflexes, and distal muscle weakness. Symptoms may persist for several months after the completion of chemotherapy. However, absence of exposure to a known neurotoxic agent or a significant delay between symptom onset and end of chemotherapy are indicators that other potential causes of polyneuropathy may be present: diabetes, nutritional deficits, paraproteinemia, paraneoplastic syndromes, and neurolymphomatosis should be considered.

Neurolymphomatosis (reviewed in Chapter 12) causes a progressive peripheral neuropathy, secondary to lymphomatous infiltration of nerve roots and peripheral nerves [64]. PET imaging may guide selection of a nerve for biopsy, which is required for diagnosis (Fig. 16.3).

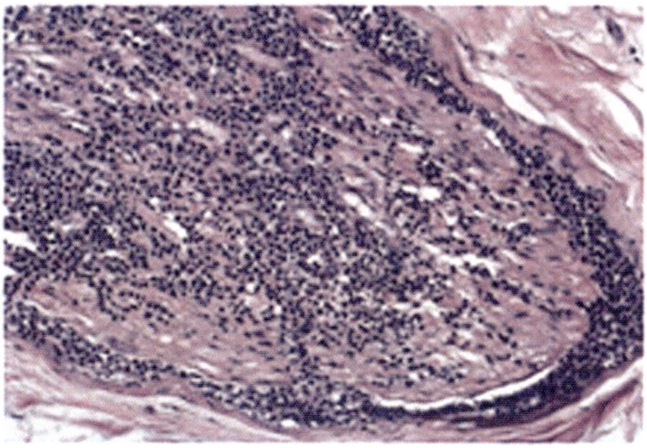

Fig. 16.3 Neurolymphomatosis: nerve biopsy (H/E) shows diffuse infiltration of the nerve by tumor and reactive cells

Individual nerves may be affected by direct compression by lymphoma, and usually present as a mononeuropathy. PET studies may disclose the affected region and dedicated imaging studies may be performed. Patients presenting with mononeuropathy multiplex (two or more individual nerves affected) should be evaluated for paraneoplastic syndromes, multiple compression sites, and neurolymphomatosis. Recognition of direct nerve compression and differentiation from root or plexus lesions is important as treatment must be directed to the lymphomatous mass and may result in marked clinical improvement [65].

Myopathies

The most common cause of myopathy in patients with NHL is corticosteroids. Lymphoma may occur rarely in skeletal muscle, and reports of such patients suggest that disease at this site portends a poor prognosis [66]. The quadriceps femoris is the most commonly reported site of involvement [67]. Presentation is usually with a painless enlarging mass in a muscle of the extremities, most commonly in the thigh. A Japanese study reported an association between NHL and dermatomyositis [68].

Neuromuscular junction disease (i.e., Lambert-Eaton and myasthenia gravis) may rarely be due to the paraneoplastic effects of NHL (reviewed in Chapter 19).

References

1. Hill QA, Owen RG (2006) CNS prophylaxis in lymphoma: who to target and what therapy to use. Blood Rev 20(6):319–332
2. van Besien K, Ha CS, Murphy S et al (1998) Risk factors, treatment, and outcome of central nervous system recurrence in adults with intermediate-grade and immunoblastic lymphoma. Blood 91(4):1178–1184
3. A predictive model for aggressive non-Hodgkin's lymphoma. The international non-Hodgkin's lymphoma prognostic factors project. N Engl J Med 329(14):987–994 (1993)
4. Tomita N, Kodama F, Sakai R et al (2000) Predictive factors for central nervous system involvement in non-Hodgkin's lymphoma: significance of very high serum LDH concentrations. Leuk Lymphoma 38(3–4):335–343
5. Zinzani PL, Magagnoli M, Frezza G et al (1999) Isolated central nervous system relapse in aggressive non-Hodgkin's lymphoma: the Bologna experience. Leuk Lymphoma 32(5–6):571–576
6. Bjorkholm M, Hagberg H, Holte H et al (2007) Central nervous system occurrence in elderly patients with aggressive lymphoma and a long-term follow-up. Ann Oncol 18(6):1085–1089
7. Hollender A, Kvaloy S, Nome O et al (2002) Central nervous system involvement following diagnosis of non-Hodgkin's lymphoma: a risk model. Ann Oncol 13(7):1099–1107
8. Boehme V, Zeynalova S, Kloess M et al (2007) Incidence and risk factors of central nervous system recurrence in aggressive lymphoma – a survey of 1693 patients treated in protocols of the German High-Grade Non-Hodgkin's Lymphoma Study Group (DSHNHL). Ann Oncol 18(1):149–157
9. Feugier P, Virion JM, Tilly H et al (2004) Incidence and risk factors for central nervous system occurrence in elderly patients with diffuse large-B-cell lymphoma: influence of rituximab. Ann Oncol 15(1):129–133

10. Haioun C, Besson C, Lepage E et al (2000) Incidence and risk factors of central nervous system relapse in histologically aggressive non-Hodgkin's lymphoma uniformly treated and receiving intrathecal central nervous system prophylaxis: a GELA study on 974 patients. Ann Oncol 11(6):685–690
11. Haernisimon G, Suchaud JP, Eghbali H et al (1987) Secondary involvement of the central-nervous-system in malignant Non-Hodgkins-lymphoma – a Study of 30 cases in a series of 498 Patients. Oncology 44(2):98–101
12. Salzburg J, Burkhardt B, Zimmermann M et al (2007) Prevalence, clinical pattern, and outcome of CNS involvement in childhood and adolescent non-Hodgkin's lymphoma differ by non-Hodgkin's lymphoma subtype: a Berlin-Frankfurt-Munster group report. J Clin Oncol 25(25):3915–3922
13. Oinonen R, Franssila K, Elonen E (1999) Central nervous system involvement in patients with mantle cell lymphoma. Ann Hematol 78(3):145–149
14. Ferrer A, Bosch F, Villamor N et al (2008) Central nervous system involvement in mantle cell lymphoma. Ann Oncol 19(1):135–141
15. Gill S, Prince HM, Wolf MM et al (2008) Mantle cell lymphoma with central nervous system involvement: frequency and clinical features. Ann Oncol 19:212–212
16. Ponzoni M, Ferreri AJ, Campo E et al (2007) Definition, diagnosis, and management of intravascular large B-cell lymphoma: proposals and perspectives from an international consensus meeting. J Clin Oncol 25(21):3168–3173
17. Liang R, Chiu E, Loke SL (1990) Secondary central-nervous-system involvement by Non-Hodgkins-lymphoma – the risk-factors. Hematol Oncol 8(3):141–145
18. McMillan A (2005) Central nervous system-directed preventative therapy in adults with lymphoma. Br J Haematol 131(1):13–21
19. Fonseca R, Habermann TM, Colgan JP et al (2000) Testicular lymphoma is associated with a high incidence of extranodal recurrence. Cancer 88(1):154–161
20. Fonseca R, Inwards DJ, Habermann TM et al (2000) Testicular lymphoma is associated with a high risk of extranodal recurrence – reply. Cancer 89(3):714–714
21. Vu BA, Duvic M (2008) Central nervous system involvement in patients with mycosis fungoides and cutaneous large-cell transformation. J Am Acad Dermatol 59(2 Suppl 1):S16–S22
22. Bekkenk MW, Postma TJ, Meijer CJ et al (2000) Frequency of central nervous system involvement in primary cutaneous B-cell lymphoma. Cancer 89(4):913–919
23. Mead GM, Kennedy P, Smith JL et al (1986) Involvement of the central nervous system by non-Hodgkin's lymphoma in adults. A review of 36 cases. Q J Med 60(231):699–714
24. Yoshida S, Morii K, Watanabe M et al (2000) Characteristic features of malignant lymphoma with central nervous system involvement. Surg Neurol 53(2):163–167
25. Kaplan JG, DeSouza TG, Farkash A et al (1990) Leptomeningeal metastases: comparison of clinical features and laboratory data of solid tumors, lymphomas and leukemias. J Neurooncol 9(3):225–229
26. Bigner SH (1992) Cerebrospinal fluid (CSF) cytology: current status and diagnostic applications. J Neuropathol Exp Neurol 51(3):235–245
27. Jeffery GM, Frampton CM, Legge HM et al (1990) Cerebrospinal fluid B2-microglobulin levels in meningeal involvement by malignancy. Pathology 22(1):20–23
28. Lossos IS, Breuer R, Intrator O et al (2000) Cerebrospinal fluid lactate dehydrogenase isoenzyme analysis for the diagnosis of central nervous system involvement in hematooncologic patients. Cancer 88(7):1599–1604
29. Zeiser R, Burger JA, Bley TA et al (2004) Clinical follow-up indicates differential accuracy of magnetic resonance imaging and immunocytology of the cerebral spinal fluid for the diagnosis of neoplastic meningitis – a single centre experience. Br J Haematol 124(6):762–768
30. Hegde U, Filie A, Little RF et al (2005) High incidence of occult leptomeningeal disease detected by flow cytometry in newly diagnosed aggressive B-cell lymphomas at risk for central nervous system involvement: the role of flow cytometry versus cytology. Blood 105(2):496–502

31. Quijano S, Lopez A, Manuel Sancho J et al (2009) Identification of leptomeningeal disease in aggressive B-cell non-Hodgkin's lymphoma: improved sensitivity of flow cytometry. J Clin Oncol 27(9):1462–1469
32. Storch-Hagenlocher B, Haas J, Vogt-Schaden ME et al (2000) Molecular analysis of the CDR3 encoding region of the immunoglobulin heavy chain locus in cerebrospinal fluid cells as a diagnostic tool in lymphomatous meningitis. Ann Neurol 47(2):211–217
33. Rhodes CH, Glantz MJ, Glantz L et al (1996) A comparison of polymerase chain reaction examination of cerebrospinal fluid and conventional cytology in the diagnosis of lymphomatous meningitis. Cancer 77(3):543–548
34. DeAngelis LM (1998) Current diagnosis and treatment of leptomeningeal metastasis. J Neurooncol 38(2-3):245–252
35. Ferreri AJ, Assanelli A, Crocchiolo R et al (2009) Central nervous system dissemination in immunocompetent patients with aggressive lymphomas: incidence, risk factors and therapeutic options. Hematol Oncol 27(2):61–70
36. Grier J, Batchelor T (2005) Metastatic neurologic complications of non-Hodgkin's lymphoma. Curr Oncol Rep 7(1):55–60
37. Glantz MJ, LaFollette S, Jaeckle KA et al (1999) Randomized trial of a slow-release versus a standard formulation of cytarabine for the intrathecal treatment of lymphomatous meningitis. J Clin Oncol 17(10):3110–3116
38. Rubenstein JL, Combs D, Rosenberg J et al (2003) Rituximab therapy for CNS lymphomas: targeting the leptomeningeal compartment. Blood 10:466–468
39. Schulz H, Pels H, Schmidt-Wolf I et al (2004) Intraventricular treatment of relapsed central nervous system lymphoma with the anti-CD20 antibody rituximab. Haematologica 89(6):753–754
40. Shah GD, Yahalom J, Correa D et al (2007) Combined immunochemotherapy with reduced whole-brain radiotherapy for newly diagnosed primary CNS lymphoma. J Clin Oncol 25(30):4730–4735
41. Rubenstein JL, Fridlyand J, Abrey L et al (2007) Phase I study of intraventricular administration of rituximab in patients with recurrent CNS and intraocular lymphoma. J Clin Oncol 25(11):1350–1356
42. Chamberlain MC, Johnston SK, Van Horn A et al (2009) Recurrent lymphomatous meningitis treated with intra-CSF rituximab and liposomal ara-C. J Neuro-oncol 91(3):271–277
43. Williams CD, Pearce R, Taghipour G et al (1994) Autologous bone marrow transplantation for patients with non-Hodgkin's lymphoma and CNS involvement: those transplanted with active CNS disease have a poor outcome – a report by the European bone marrow transplant lymphoma registry. J Clin Oncol 12(11):2415–2422
44. Kasamon YL, Jones RJ, Piantadosi S et al (2005) High-dose therapy and blood or marrow transplantation for non-Hodgkin lymphoma with central nervous system involvement. Biol Blood Marrow Transplant 11(2):93–100
45. Alvarnas JC, Negrin RS, Horning SJ et al (2000) High-dose therapy with hematopoietic cell transplantation for patients with central nervous system involvement by non-Hodgkin's lymphoma. Biol Blood Marrow Transplant 6(3A):352–358
46. Soussain C, Hoang-Xuan K, Taillandier L et al (2008) Intensive chemotherapy followed by hematopoietic stem-cell rescue for refractory and recurrent primary CNS and intraocular lymphoma: Societe Francaise de Greffe de Moelle Osseuse-Therapie Cellulaire. J Clin Oncol 26(15):2512–2518
47. Abrey LE, Moskowitz CH, Mason WP et al (2003) Intensive methotrexate and cytarabine followed by high-dose chemotherapy with autologous stem-cell rescue in patients with newly diagnosed primary CNS lymphoma: an intent-to-treat analysis. J Clin Oncol 21(22): 4151–4156
48. Hanssens PE, Lagerwaard FJ, Levendag PC (1998) Principles of radiotherapy of neoplastic meningosis. J Neuro-oncol 38(2-3):145–150
49. Levitt LJ, Dawson DM, Rosenthal DS et al (1980) CNS involvement in the non-Hodgkin's lymphomas. Cancer 45(3):545–552

50. Omuro AM, Leite CC, Mokhtari K et al (2006) Pitfalls in the diagnosis of brain tumours. Lancet Neurol 5(11):937–948
51. Doolittle ND, Abrey LE, Shenkier TN et al (2008) Brain parenchyma involvement as isolated central nervous system relapse of systemic non-Hodgkin lymphoma: an international primary CNS Lymphoma collaborative group report. Blood 111(3):1085–1093
52. Bazzoli E, Iwamoto FM, Zelenetz AD et al (2008) Synchronous presentation of systemic and brain non-Hodgkin lymphoma. Leuk Lymphoma 49(12):2370–2373
53. Buckstein R, Lim W, Franssen E et al (2003) CNS prophylaxis and treatment in non-Hodgkin's lymphoma: variation in practice and lessons from the literature. Leuk Lymphoma 44(6):955–962
54. Cheung CW, Burton C, Smith P et al (2005) Central nervous system chemoprophylaxis in non-Hodgkin lymphoma: current practice in the UK (vol 131, pg 193, 2005). Br J Haematol 131(5):673–673
55. Herrlinger U, Glantz M, Schlegel U et al (2009) Should intra-cerebrospinal fluid prophylaxis be part of initial therapy for patients with non-Hodgkin lymphoma: what we know, and how we can find out more. Semin Oncol 36(4 Suppl 2):S25–S34
56. Arkenau HT, Chong G, Cunningham D et al (2007) The role of intrathecal chemotherapy prophylaxis in patients with diffuse large B-cell lymphoma. Ann Oncol 18(3):541–545
57. Tomita N, Kodama F, Kanamori H et al (2002) Prophylactic intrathecal methotrexate and hydrocortisone reduces central nervous system recurrence and improves survival in aggressive non-Hodgkin lymphoma. Cancer 95(3):576–580
58. Chua SL, Seymour JF, Streater J et al (2002) Intrathecal chemotherapy alone is inadequate central nervous system prophylaxis in patients with intermediate-grade non-Hodgkin's lymphoma. Leuk Lymphoma 43(9):1783–1788
59. Boehme V, Schmitz N, Zeynalova S et al (2009) CNS events in elderly patients with aggressive lymphoma treated with modern chemotherapy (CHOP-14) with or without rituximab: an analysis of patients treated in the RICOVER-60 trial of the German High-Grade Non-Hodgkin Lymphoma Study Group (DSHNHL). Blood 113(17):3896–3902
60. Grant R, Papadopoulos SM, Greenberg HS (1991) Metastatic epidural spinal-cord compression. Neurol Clin 9(4):825–841
61. Oviatt DL, Kirshner HS, Stein RS (1982) Successful chemotherapeutic treatment of epidural compression in Non-Hodgkins lymphoma. Cancer 49(12):2446–2448
62. Wong ET, Portlock CS, O'Brien JP et al (1996) Chemosensitive epidural spinal cord disease in non-Hodgkins lymphoma. Neurology 46(6):1543–1547
63. Kori SH, Foley KM, Posner JB (1981) Brachial-plexus lesions in patients with cancer – 100 Cases. Neurology 31(1):45–50
64. Bezier M, Reguiai Z, Delaby P et al (2009) Neurolymphomatosis associated with Sezary syndrome. Arch Dermatol 145(3):294–296
65. Wulff EA, Simpson DM (2000) Peripheral neuropathy associated with acquired immunodeficiency syndrome (AIDS)-related Burkitt's lymphoma. Muscle Nerve 23(11): 1764–1766
66. Jeffery GM, Golding PF, Mead GM (1991) Non-Hodgkins-lymphoma arising in skeletal-muscle. Ann Oncol 2(7):501–504
67. Keung YK, Liang R (1996) Report of a case of primary skeletal muscle lymphoma and review of the literature. Acta Haematol-Basel 96(3):184–186
68. Anzai S, Katagiri K, Sato T et al (1997) Dermatomyositis associated with primary intramuscular B cell lymphoma. J Dermatol 24(10):649–653

Chapter 17
Neurological Complications of Hodgkin Lymphoma

Elizabeth R. Gerstner and Maciej M. Mrugala

Introduction

Hodgkin lymphoma (HL) is a cancer of the immune system that is typically characterized by the presence of Reed-Sternberg cells. Approximately 30% of all lymphomas are of Hodgkin type. Classical HL is the most common presentation (95% of all cases) and can be divided into four subtypes: lymphocyte predominance, nodular sclerosis, mixed cellularity, and lymphocyte depletion. Nodular lymphocyte-predominance HL is seen in the remaining 5% of cases and the malignant cell in this form of HL is the lymphocytic and histiocytic cell rather than the Reed Sternberg cell. The malignant cells in HL are derived from germinal-center B cells that have lost the B cell phenotype and are characterized by dysregulation of multiple signaling pathways [1].

The incidence of the disease is bimodal with a peak in young adulthood (ages 15–35), and a second peak in those older than 55. Patients with systemic HL can present with lymphadenopathy, fever, night sweats, or weight loss. Patients with early stage disease (stage IA or IIA) are typically treated with radiation, and have an excellent prognosis and a 10-year survival in excess of 80%. Patients with disseminated disease (stage IIIB or IV) have more variable outcome with 5-year survival rates in the range of 50–60% [2]. Older age and lymphocyte depletion or mixed cellularity histology are associated with a worse prognosis.

Central Nervous System Involvement

The first description of HL, involving the central nervous system (CNS), was by Murchison in 1870 who described lymphomatous meningeal infiltration [3]. Complications that result from direct involvement of the CNS by HL occur less

E.R. Gerstner (✉)
Department of Neurology, Massachusetts General Hospital and Harvard Medical School, Boston, MA, USA
e-mail: egerstner@partners.org

T. Batchelor, L.M. DeAngelis (eds.), *Lymphoma and Leukemia of the Nervous System*, DOI 10.1007/978-1-4419-7668-0_17,

Table 17.1 Neurological complications of Hodgkin lymphoma

Direct	Parenchymal lesions in the brain and spinal cord Epidural spinal cord compression Leptomeningeal involvement
Indirect	*Vascular*: Primary CNS angiitis
	Infectious: Meningitis/meningoencephalitis Encephalitis Brain abscess Progressive multifocal leukoencephalopathy
	Paraneoplastic: Subacute cerebellar degeneration Sensory and motor neuropathies Acquired neuromyotonia Limbic encephalitis Others
	Iatrogenic

Adapted from references [4, 58].

frequently than with other lymphomas and leukemias [4]. The reported incidence of CNS involvement is 0.02–0.5% [5–7]. Consequently, there is little information about neurological complications of HL, and minimal guidance for clinicians treating patients with CNS HL.

The CNS can be affected directly or indirectly (Table 17.1). Most cases of direct neurological involvement are secondary to either metastatic spread via meningeal vessels or by direct tumor extension [8]. CNS involvement can be seen at any time during the course of systemic HL. Occasionally, impaired neurological function can be the first and only presenting feature prior to the development of any other evidence of systemic lymphoma [8–12] Earlier series suggested that CNS HL was most often seen in the context of relapsed, disseminated systemic disease [5, 7, 13]. However, one of the largest reported series suggested that CNS disease could be seen at presentation or as an isolated site of relapse [14]. Very rarely, the CNS is the sole site of disease (primary CNS HL). Primary CNS HL is exceedingly rare and comprises a very small subset of primary CNS lymphomas. Very little is known about etiology, optimal management, and prognosis of this condition [15–17].

Indirect involvement usually occurs as a paraneoplastic syndrome. but can also be secondary to vascular, infectious, or iatrogenic causes. Since paraneoplastic syndromes are discussed elsewhere in this book, this chapter will focus on direct and other indirect complications of CNS HL, while only briefly mentioning paraneoplastic syndromes associated with HL. Iatrogenic neurological complications can be occasionally associated with therapy for HL. For example, 5-year survivors of systemic HL, treated with radiotherapy to the neck and mediastinum, have a substantially higher risk of transient ischemic attacks and stroke [18].

Direct Involvement of the CNS by Hodgkin Lymphoma

Pathogenesis

Tumor cells obtain access to the CNS via direct extension from dural or osseous sites of disease, or by hematogenous spread. There are no known risk factors for CNS spread in patients with HL, but a role for immunosuppression and EBV infection has been suggested [15, 17, 19, 20]. In the largest series of CNS HL reported, five of six patients with immune system dysregulation had disease limited to the brain when CNS HL was diagnosed, perhaps suggesting the CNS is a sanctuary site in these patients [14]. Mixed cellularity histology has also been associated with CNS spread, but this has not been confirmed in all series [5, 13, 14, 21, 22].

Intracranial Involvement

HL produces intraparenchymal brain lesions less frequently than other lymphomas known to invade the CNS. These lesions can present as solitary masses (Fig. 17.1) or, uncommonly, as multiple small lesions in the course of disseminated disease [15, 23, 24]. The cerebral hemispheres are the most commonly affected parts of the brain, followed by the brainstem, pituitary, and cerebellum [5, 25, 26]. Intracranial masses can also develop from the expansion of meningeal deposits and via hematogenous spread to involve optic nerve and chiasm [8, 27], orbit [28, 29], and cavernous sinus [30]. Intraparenchymal mass lesions may be more common than leptomeningeal disease [14].

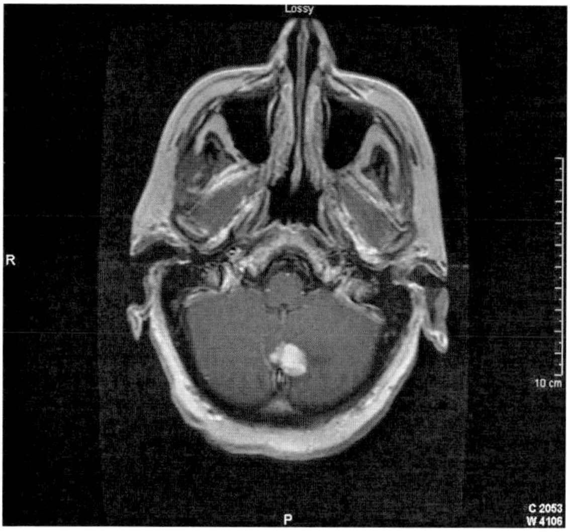

Fig. 17.1 Gadolinium-enhanced MRI scan from a patient with a cerebellar metastasis from Hodgkin lymphoma (Courtesy of Dr. Tracy Batchelor, Department of Neurology, Massachusetts General Hospital, Boston, MA)

Signs and Symptoms

Similar to other lymphomas, CNS signs and symptoms from HL depends upon the site of involvement: the leptomeninges, parenchyma, epidural space, or infiltration of blood vessels or peripheral nerves. Cranial nerve palsies, pain/sensory symptoms, motor deficits, altered mental status, and headache are often reported. Autonomic deficits and Horner's syndrome have also been described [8, 11, 31]. B symptoms (fevers, night sweats, weight loss) usually occur if there is concomitant systemic disease.

Spinal Cord Involvement

Both intramedullary spinal cord involvement and epidural spinal cord compression have been described [32, 33]. Epidural lymphoma involves the CNS by compression of the spinal cord in up to 5% of cases [34]. Mixed cellularity histology may have the greatest predilection for epidural compression [13, 35–37].

Most epidural lesions are diagnosed when extranodal disease already exists [34]. Similar to other cancers, the thoracic spinal cord is the most frequently involved part of the spine. HL often spreads from the paraspinal region into the epidural space via intervertebral foramina, which can result in spinal cord compression, without destruction of the vertebral body resulting in normal plain films or bone scans [34]. Epidural spinal cord compression due to HL presents with similar signs and symptoms to other causes of spinal cord compression, such as back pain, and leg weakness and numbness.

Leptomeningeal Disease

Although it can occur at any time during the course of disease, lymphomatous involvement of the leptomeninges is rare in HL [36, 38–40]. Tumor implants are distributed along the leptomeninges in an inhomogeneous fashion that usually results in gross thickening of these membranes. Infiltration is most commonly present at the base of the skull and around the adjacent spinal cord [41, 42]. Occasionally, cells can infiltrate into the adjacent brain or spinal cord parenchyma, resulting in intraparenchymal masses. Areas around the blood vessels and points of exit of the cranial nerves from the skull are particularly prone to lymphomatous spread. Most patients present with symptoms reflecting global cerebral dysfunction and cranial nerve palsies such as headache, altered mental status, and facial nerve palsy [41].

Diagnosis

Diagnostic evaluation includes neuro-imaging, lumbar puncture, and biopsy if the diagnosis is uncertain. Contrast enhanced CT or MRI (preferred) may show single or multiple contrast-enhancing brain masses, leptomeningeal enhancement, subependymal enhancement, or nerve root enlargement. Hydrocephalus may be present if cerebrospinal fluid (CSF) pathways are obstructed; however, elevated intracranial pressure can occur even in the absence of hydrocephalus. The entire neuraxis should be imaged to determine the extent of CNS involvement. Lumbar puncture for CSF analysis may show Reed-Sternberg cells or other atypical/malignant cells, elevated white blood cell count, and elevated protein. Specifically, eosinophilic meningitis in a patient with HL should alert the clinician to possible CNS HL [40]. A biopsy may be required if the diagnosis is unclear, or if there is concern for another process such as an infection (Fig. 17.2).

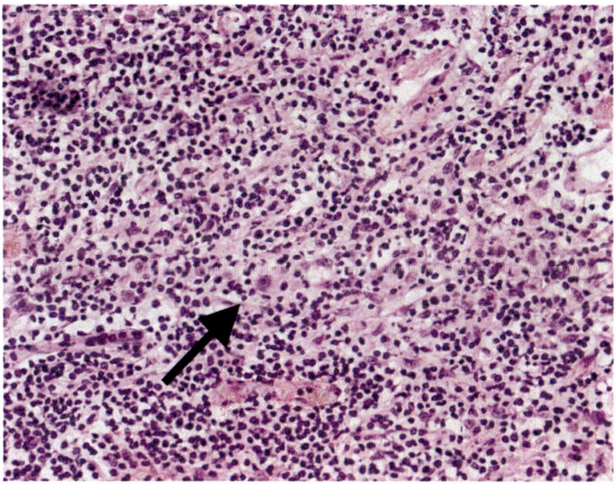

Fig. 17.2 Biopsy specimen from a patient with nodular sclerosis Hodgkin lymphoma involving the cerebellum. A Reed-Sternberg cell (*black arrow*) is seen in the *center* of the panel (40X, hematoxylin-eosin stain). This was originally published in [14]. © the American Society of Hematology

Treatment and Prognosis

Due to its rarity, there is no consensus on how to treat CNS HL and no clinical trials have been conducted. Surgery, radiation, and several different chemotherapy regimens have been used. Corticosteroids cause tumor lysis, so may help control acute symptoms, but should be deferred until CSF or, if necessary, a biopsy has been obtained because these drugs can disrupt cellular morphology and obscure the pathological diagnosis. Both whole brain radiation and stereotactic focal radiation have been utilized. The standard regimen for intracranial metastasis is 30 Gy delivered to the whole brain in ten fractions [38]. Chemotherapy regimens have included MVPP (mustine, vinblastine, procarbazine, prednisone); Stanford V (mechlorethamine, doxorubicin, vinblastine, vincristine, bleomycin, etoposide, prednisone); ABVD (doxorubicin, bleomycin, vinblastine, dacarbazine); ifosfamide; rituximab, high dose methotrexate; IVAC (ifosfamide, etoposide, and high-dose cytarabine); and lomustine, procarbazine, prednisone, and cyclophosphamide [14]. High dose chemotherapy followed by autologous stem cell transplantation has also been tried [14]. There are no compelling data to favor one modality versus another or a particular combination of chemotherapy agents, but fortunately, durable responses are usually achieved with treatment. It appears that improved response rates and survival can be seen when early diagnosis and aggressive chemotherapy and radiation are used in combination [5]. As reported by Biagi et al [15], the short term prognosis following treatment of CNS HL is excellent. In their series, seven of eight patients were alive and progression free after follow-up ranging from 6 to 36 months. Recently, Gerstner et al. reported a series of 16 patients with CNS HL where 12 achieved a complete or partial response to CNS directed therapy [14]. Median overall survival was 43.8 months from diagnosis of CNS disease, and patients with relapsed disease limited to the brain or with CNS involvement at initial diagnosis of HL had better prognoses.

Epidural HL deposits respond promptly to radiation. Surgery is reserved for diagnosis when epidural disease is the first presentation of HL, or when spinal instability is present [38]. Severity of weakness at diagnosis remains the single most important prognostic factor for outcome and recovery of function after treatment may be achieved in some patients who are paraplegic at presentation. Durable remissions may be obtained if systemic disease is controlled with chemotherapy or radiation.

Although not studied systematically, intrathecal chemotherapy may have a role in patients with leptomeningeal dissemination from HL. If untreated, the median survival after diagnosis of leptomeningeal HL is usually measured in weeks to months. Therefore, an aggressive diagnostic and therapeutic approach is usually warranted in appropriate patients. Despite focal symptomatology, meningeal HL is a diffuse disease. The entire neuraxis must be treated to insure complete tumor eradication. The combination of steroids, radiation, local, or systemic chemotherapy can control disease in many patients [5, 35].

Indirect Involvement of the CNS by Hodgkin Lymphoma

HL can produce neurological symptoms indirectly via a number of mechanisms (Table 17.1). Many of the indirect complications of HL are similar for both non-Hodgkin and Hodgkin lymphomas and will be described in detail in other chapters. Complications preferentially developing in HL will be described in the paragraphs that follow.

Primary Angiitis of the CNS

Primary angiitis of the CNS is a rare and potentially fatal vasculitis, exclusively confined to the brain and spinal cord. It was first described in association with HL by Cravioto and Feigin in 1959 [43]. The pathogenesis of primary CNS angiitis is not well known, but an association with viral infections and HL has been described [44–47].

Clinical presentation depends on the site of CNS involvement. Headaches, seizures, confusion, and focal neurological deficits have all been described. Rare cases of spinal cord involvement have been reported, including transverse myelitis [44]. Diagnosis is difficult due to diverse clinical manifestations and lack of specific confirmatory laboratory tests. Cerebral angiography usually reveals multifocal and segmental narrowing or microaneurysm formation [44, 48].

Biopsy of the leptomeninges and underlying brain parenchyma is often the only definite way to make a diagnosis [49]. When affected vessels are sampled, the specificity of the biopsy approaches 100%; pathology reveals segmental granulomatous and nongranulomatous inflammation of leptomeningeal vessels [50]. Treatment consists of steroids and immunosupression, but results are usually disappointing. Roggerone et al. reported a case of CNS angiitis in the setting of HL that presented as recurrent cerebral venous thrombosis and the patient responded dramatically to rituximab and steroids [48].

Infectious Complications

Patients with HL are frequently immunosuppressed and susceptible to opportunistic CNS infections. Immunity is altered not only by the disease, but also by its treatment. Functional and quantitative defects, mainly involving CD4+ T-helper cells, represent the basic intrinsic immunologic alterations in HL [4]. Staging splenectomies further predispose patients to infections with encapsulated bacteria; fortunately, this is rarely done in the modern era. Cell-mediated immunity is also deficient, which increases susceptibility to opportunistic infections. One of the most severe CNS infections associated with HL is progressive multifocal leukoencephalopathy (PML), which is caused by a polyomavirus (JC virus). The syndrome can have a variable presentation with progressive motor weakness, sensory abnormalities, visual defects, headaches, dysarthria, ataxia, and alteration of consciousness. MRI scans reveal multiple confluent T2/FLAIR hyperintense areas, predominantly in the periventricular white matter with variable contrast enhancement. Brain biopsy is often diagnostic, but can be avoided if viral DNA is detected by PCR in CSF. Other than reversing immunosuppression if possible, there are no effective treatments, although responses have been reported with cytarabine and alfa-interferon [51, 52].

HL also predisposes patients to a number of other CNS infections. The most common entities are meningitis or meningoencephalitis caused by *Listeria monocytogenes* and *Cryptococcus neoformans*; encephalitis due to herpes viruses (*Varicella zoster, cytomegalovirus, Herpes simplex 1 and 2)*, measles virus, or *Toxoplasma gondii*; and brain abscess associated with *Nocardia asteroides*. Tuberculosis has also been reported [53].

Herpes zoster infection may occur at any time in the course of HL and accounts for 25% of infections in these patients. Disease can be disseminated in 20% of cases, resulting in more complications [54]. Most patients suffer from ophthalmic, visceral, or CNS involvement. The most severe neurological complications include encephalitis and meningitis, followed by shingles and post herpetic neuralgia syndromes. In patients with post-herpetic neuralgia, the most commonly affected dermatomes are lower thoracic, followed by lumbar and cranial [55]. Motor radiculopathies are also common, with weakness corresponding to the distribution of the rash. Postviral meningoencephalitis leading to progressive encephalopathy has been described [38]. Infectious vasculopathy causing stroke has also been described as a sequel of zoster, usually affecting the ophthalmic division of the trigeminal nerve [38, 56]. In patients who are not severely immunocompromised, prognosis for recovery is generally good. Treatment with acyclovir should be initiated promptly, especially in cases of disseminated disease.

Paraneoplastic Syndromes

Paraneoplastic syndromes occur in approximately 1–5% of patients with HL [57]. Virtually any paraneoplastic syndrome can be encountered, although the neurologic syndromes most frequently associated with HL include paraneoplastic cerebellar degeneration (PCD), subacute sensorineuropathy, and Lambert-Eaton syndrome (Table 17.2). All syndromes can develop before the diagnosis of HL is evident. For a more detailed description of the paraneoplastic syndromes associated with HL, see Chapter 19.

Table 17.2 Paraneoplastic neurological syndromes associated with Hodgkin lymphoma

Syndrome	Associated antibodies	References
Limbic encephalitis	Anti-Hu	[59–61]
Subacute cerebellar degeneration	Anti-Yo Anti-Tr	[61–68]
Chorea	Unknown	[69]
Inflammatory myopathy	Unknown	[70]
Acquired neuromyotonia (Isaacs' syndrome)	Anti-VGKC (voltage-gated potassium channels)	[71, 72]
Lambert-Eaton myasthenic syndrome	Anti-VGCC (voltage-gated calcium channels)	[73, 74]
Stiff person syndrome	Anti-amphiphysin	[73, 75]
Opsoclonus-myoclonus	Anti-Hu Anti-Ri	[76]
Memory loss (Ophelia syndrome)	Unknown	[77, 78]
Subclinical autonomic dysfunction	Unknown	[31]

Acknowledgment MMM would like to thank Dr. Lawrence Recht for guidance during writing of the original version of this chapter for the first edition of *Lymphoma of the Nervous System.*

References

1. Jaffe ES, Lee Harris N, Stein H, Vardiman J (eds) (2001) Tumours of Haematopoietic and Lymphoid Tissues: pathology and genetics. WHO Classification of Tumours. IARC Press, Lyon
2. Tierney L, McPhee S, Papadakis M (eds) (1997) Current Medical Diagnosis and Treatment, 36th edn. Appleton & Lange, New York, NY

3. Murchison C (1870) Case of "lymphadenoma" of the lymphatic system, spleen, liver, lungs, heart, diaphragm, dura mater. Trans Pathol Soc Lond 21:372–389
4. Abate G, Corazzelli G, Ciarmiello A, Monfardini S (1997) Neurologic complications of Hodgkin's disease: a case history. Ann Oncol 8:593–600
5. Sapozink MD, Kaplan HS (1983) Intracranial Hodgkin's disease. A report of 12 cases and review of the literature. Cancer 52:1301–1307
6. Re D, Fuchs M, Schober T et al (2007) CNS Involvement in Hodgkin's Lymphoma. J Clin Oncol 25:3181
7. Hirmiz K, Foyle A, Wilke D et al (2004) Intracranial presentation of systemic Hodgkin's disease. Leuk Lymphoma 45:1667–1671
8. McFadzean RM, McIlwaine GG, McLellan D (1990) Hodgkin's disease at the optic chiasm. J Clin Neuroophthalmol 10:248–254
9. Sparling H, Adams R (1946) Primary Hodgkin's sarcoma of the brain. Arch Pathol 42: 338–344
10. Schircker J, Smith D (1955) Primary intracerebral Hodgkin's disease. Cancer 8:629–633
11. Burstein SD, Kernohan JW, Uihlein A (1963) Neoplasms of the reticuloendothelial system of the brain. Cancer 16:289–305
12. Cambier J, Boivin P, Girauld A et al (1973) Cerebral lesions in Hodgkin's disease. Ann Med Interne (Paris) 124:65–74
13. Cuttner J, Meyer R, Huang Y (1979) Intracerebral involvement in Hodgkin's disease: a report of 6 cases and review of the literature. Cancer 43:1497–1506
14. Gerstner ER, Abrey LE, Schiff D et al (2008) CNS Hodgkin lymphoma. Blood 112: 1658–1661
15. Biagi J, MacKenzie RG, Lim MS et al (2000) Primary Hodgkin's disease of the CNS in an immunocompetent patient: a case study and review of the literature. Neurooncol 2:239–243
16. Bender BL, Mayernik DG (1986) Hodgkin's disease presenting with isolated craniospinal involvement. Cancer 58(8):1745–1748
17. Herrlinger U, Klingel K, Meyermann R et al (2000) Central nervous system Hodgkin's lymphoma without systemic manifestation: case report and review of the literature. Acta Neuropathol 99:709–714
18. De Bruin ML, Dorresteijn LD, van't Veer MB et al (2009) Increased risk of stroke and transient ischemic attack in 5-year survivors of Hodgkin lymphoma. J Natl Cancer Inst 101:928–937
19. Klein R, Mullges W, Bendszus M et al (1999) Primary intracerebral Hodgkin's disease: report of a case with Epstein-Barr virus association and review of the literature. Am J Surg Pathol 23:477–481
20. Alexander FE, Jarrett RF, Lawrence D et al (2000) Risk factors for Hodgkin's disease by Epstein-Barr virus (EBV) status: prior infection by EBV and other agents. Br J Cancer 82:1117–1121
21. Akyuz C, Yalcin B, Atahan IL et al (2005) Intracranial involvement in Hodgkin's disease. Pediatr Hematol Oncol 22:589–596
22. Antonio G, Dahlstrom J, Chandran KN, O'Neil R (2000) Cerebellopontine angle Hodgkin's disease. Australas Radiol 44:115–117
23. Nakayama H, Tokuuye K, Kagami Y et al (2000) Brain involvement in Hodgkin's disease: case reports and review of the literature. Radiat Med 18:205–208
24. Kalinka E, Robak T, Wrzesien-Kus A et al (2002) Diagnostic and therapeutic quandaries in primary manifestation of Hodgkin's disease in the central nervous system. Ann Hematol 81:289–291
25. King DP, Richardson JS (1950) Hodgkin's disease of the cerebellum. St Thomas Hosp Rep 6:273–275
26. Lascelles RG, Burston J (1962) Hodgkin's disease presenting with symptoms of cranial nerve involvement. Arch Neurol 7:359–364
27. Litvak J, Leder MM, Kauvar AJ (1964) Hodgkin's disease involving optic nerve and brain. J Neurosurg 21:798–801

28. Fratkin JD, Shammas HF, Miller SD (1978) Disseminated Hodgkin's disease with bilateral orbital involvement. Arch Ophthalmol 96:102–104
29. Sahjupaul R, Elisevich K, Allen L (1996) Hodgkin's disease of the orbit with intracranial extension. Ophthalmic Surg Lasers 27:239–242
30. Kasner SE, Galetta SL, Vaughn DJ (1996) Cavernous sinus syndrome in Hodgkin's disease. J Neuroophthalmol 16:204–207
31. Turner ML, Boland OM, Parker AC, Ewing DJ (1993) Subclinical autonomic dysfunction in patients with Hodgkin's disease and non-Hodgkin's lymphoma. Br J Haematol 84:623–626
32. Citow JS, Rini B, Wollmann R, Macdonald RL (2001) Isolated, primary extranodal Hodgkin's disease of the spine: case report. Neurosurgery 49:453–456; discussion 6–7
33. Higgins SA, Peschel RE (1995) Hodgkin's disease with spinal cord compression. A case report and a review of the literature. Cancer 75:94–98
34. Friedman N, Kim T, Panahon A (1976) Spinal cord compression in malignant lymphoma: treatment and results. Cancer 37:1485–1491
35. Orlowski EP, Hansen RM, Anderson T et al (1984) Hodgkin's disease with leptomeningeal involvement. Report of a case with long survival. Cancer 53:1833–1835
36. Dillman R, Mueh J, Greco C, Green M (1980) Leptomeningeal Hodgkin's disease. Ann Intern Med 92:714–715
37. Rabhi M, Ennibi K, Chaari J, Toloune F (2007) Hodgkin's disease presenting with spinal cord compression. Rev Neurol (Paris) 163:1109–1112
38. Recht L (1995) Neurological complications of lymphoma. In: Wiley R (ed) Neurological Complications of Cancer. Marcel Dekker, New York, NY, pp 465–87
39. Cervantes F, Montserrat E, Rozman C (1979) Eosinophilic meningitis in Hodgkin's disease. Ann Intern Med 91:930
40. Patchell R, Perry MC (1981) Eosinophilic meningitis in Hodgkin disease. Neurology 31: 887–8
41. Lokich J, Galbo C (1981) Leptomeningeal lymphoma: perspectives on management. Cancer Treat Rev 8:103–110
42. Bunn PA Jr, Schein PS, Banks PM, DeVita VT Jr (1976) Central nervous system complications in patients with diffuse histiocytic and undifferentiated lymphoma: leukemia revisited. Blood 47:3–10
43. Cravioto H, Feigin I (1959) Noninfectious granulomatous angiitis with a predilection for the nervous system. Neurology 9:599–609
44. Yuen RW, Johnson PC (1996) Primary angiitis of the central nervous system associated with Hodgkin's disease. Arch Pathol Lab Med 120:573–576
45. Rosen CL, DePalma L, Morita A (2000) Primary angiitis of the central nervous system as a first presentation in Hodgkin's disease: a case report and review of the literature. Neurosurgery 46:1504–1508; discussion 8–10
46. Inwards DJ, Piepgras DG, Lie JT et al (1991) Granulomatous angiitis of the spinal cord associated with Hodgkin's disease. Cancer 68:1318–1322
47. Yoong MF, Blumbergs PC, North JB (1993) Primary (granulomatous) angiitis of the central nervous system with multiple aneurysms of spinal arteries. Case report. J Neurosurg 79: 603–607
48. Roggerone S, Traverse-Glehen A, Derex L et al (2008) Recurrent cerebral venous thrombosis revealing paraneoplastic angiitis in Hodgkin's lymphoma. J Neurooncol 89:195–198
49. Volmer T, Guarnaccia J, Harrington W et al (1993) Idiopathic granulomatous angiitis of the central nervous system: diagnositic challenges. Arch Neurol 50:925–930
50. Calabrese LH, Furlan AJ, Gragg LA, Ropos TJ (1992) Primary angiitis of the central nervous system: diagnostic criteria and clinical approach. Cleve Clin J Med 59:293–306
51. Portegies P, Algra PR, Hollak CE et al (1991) Response to cytarabine in progressive multifocal leucoencephalopathy in AIDS. Lancet 337:680–1
52. Steiger MJ, Tarnesby G, Gabe S et al (1993) Successful outcome of progressive multifocal leukoencephalopathy with cytarabine and interferon. Ann Neurol 33:407–411

53. Shet AS, Saba N, Rausch D, Belzer M (2004) Intra-cranial lesions in a patient with Hodgkin lymphoma. Leuk Lymphoma 45:419–422
54. Mazur MH, Dolin R (1978) Herpes zoster at the NIH: a 20 year experience. Am J Med 65:738–744
55. Correale J, Monteverde DA, Bueri JA, Reich EG (1991) Peripheral nervous system and spinal cord involvement in lymphoma. Acta Neurol Scand 83:45–51
56. Guerreiro CA, Guerreiro MM (1984) Ocular herpes zoster and delayed cerebrovascular accident: report of a case. Arq Neuropsiquiatr 42:402–407
57. Vickers SM, Niederhuber JE (1997) Hodgkin's disease associated with neurologic paraneoplastic syndrome. South Med J 90:839–844
58. Cipriani D, Landonio G, Canepari C (1989) A case of Vogt-Koyanagi-Harada syndrome in a patient affected by Hodgkin's disease. J Neurol 236:303–4
59. Arasaki K, Kwee IL, Nakada T (1987) Limbic lymphoma. Neuroradiology 29:389–392
60. Deodhare S, O'Connor P, Ghazarian D, Bilbao JM (1996) Paraneoplastic limbic encephalitis in Hodgkin's disease. Can J Neurol Sci 23:138–140
61. Grisold W, Drlicek M, Liszka-Setinek U, Wondrusch E (1995) Anti-tumour therapy in paraneoplastic neurological disease. Clin Neurol Neurosurg 97:106–111
62. Cehreli C, Payzin B, Undar B et al (1995) Paraneoplastic cerebellar degeneration in association with Hodgkin's disease: a report of two cases. Acta Haematol 94:210–213
63. Hammack J, Kotanides H, Rosenblum MK, Posner JB (1992) Paraneoplastic cerebellar degeneration. II. Clinical and immunologic findings in 21 patients with Hodgkin's disease. Neurology 42:1938–1943
64. Cavo M, Zaccaria A, d'Alessandro R et al (1984) Hodgkin's disease and subacute cerebellar degeneration. A case report and review of the literature. Nouv Rev Fr Hematol 26:197–199
65. Graus F, Dalmau J, Valldeoriola F et al (1997) Immunological characterization of a neuronal antibody (anti-Tr) associated with paraneoplastic cerebellar degeneration and Hodgkin's disease. J Neuroimmunol 74:55–61
66. Graus F, Gultekin SH, Ferrer I et al (1998) Localization of the neuronal antigen recognized by anti-Tr antibodies from patients with paraneoplastic cerebellar degeneration and Hodgkin's disease in the rat nervous system. Acta Neuropathol 96:1–7
67. Arkenau HT, Gordon C, Murphy F, Cunningham D (2007) Paraneoplastic syndrome: subacute cerebellar degeneration in Hodgkin's disease. Leuk Lymphoma 48:819–822
68. Ypma PF, Wijermans PW, Koppen H, Sillevis Smitt PA (2006) Paraneoplastic cerebellar degeneration preceding the diagnosis of Hodgkin's lymphoma. Neth J Med 64:243–247
69. Batchelor TT, Platten M, Palmer-Toy DE et al (1998) Chorea as a paraneoplastic complication of Hodgkin's disease. J Neurooncol 36:185–190
70. Dansey RD, Hammond-Tooke GD, Lai K, Bezwoda WR (1988) Subacute myelopathy: an unusual paraneoplastic complication of Hodgkin's disease. Med Pediatr Oncol 16: 284–286
71. Lahrmann H, Albrecht G, Drlicek M et al (2001) Acquired neuromyotonia and peripheral neuropathy in a patient with Hodgkin's disease. Muscle Nerve 24:834–838
72. Caress JB, Abend WK, Preston DC, Logigian EL (1997) A case of Hodgkin's lymphoma producing neuromyotonia. Neurology 49:258–9
73. Dropcho EJ (1998) Neurologic paraneoplastic syndromes. J Neurol Sci 153:264–278
74. O'Neill JH, Murray NM, Newsom-Davis J (1988) The Lambert-Eaton myasthenic syndrome. A review of 50 cases. Brain 111(Pt 3):577–596
75. Grimaldi LM, Martino G, Braghi S et al (1993) Heterogeneity of autoantibodies in stiff-man syndrome. Ann Neurol 34:57–64
76. Kay CL, Davies-Jones GA, Singal R, Winfield DA (1993) Paraneoplastic opsoclonus-myoclonus in Hodgkin's disease. J Neurol Neurosurg Psychiatry 56:831–2
77. Carr I (1982) The Ophelia syndrome: memory loss in Hodgkin's disease. Lancet 1:844–5
78. Pfliegler G, Posan E, Glaub D et al (1990) Hodgkin's disease and memory loss: another case of the Ophelia syndrome. Br J Haematol 74:232

Chapter 18
Neurological Complications of Plasma Cell Disorders

Jan Drappatz and Kurt A. Jaeckle

Introduction

Neurological complications of plasma cell disorders primarily involve the peripheral nervous system (PNS) and presentations range from mild sensory neuropathies to severe and disabling motor neuropathies. The central nervous system (CNS) is directly affected due to disease infiltration, or indirectly due to complications from hyperviscosity or hypercalcemia. The major neurological complications that occur in patients with plasma cell disorders are summarized in Table 18.1.

Central Nervous System Complications

The most common cause of CNS dysfunction in patients with plasma cell disorders is related to tumor mass effect, especially compression of the spinal cord, but also cranial nerves [1, 2]. Leptomeningeal metastases have been reported in patients with multiple myeloma (MM), usually in the late phase of the disease [3–6]. Neurological symptoms may also occur as a consequence of hypercalcemia [7] or hyperviscosity [8].

Hyperviscosity Syndrome

M protein in high concentration can lead to the hyperviscosity syndrome. Most cases are observed in Waldenstrom macroglobulinemia (WM) with IgM [9], followed by IgA myeloma and IgG myeloma [10, 11]. The syndrome is typically observed when serum viscosity exceeds 4.0 centipoule (cp) units, about three times the normal viscosity of 1.4–1.8 cp. It usually manifests with diffuse, reduced

J. Drappatz (✉)
Department of Neurology, Harvard Medical School, Center for Neuro-Oncology, Dana Farber Cancer Institute, Brigham and Women's Hospital, Boston, MA 02115, USA
e-mail: jan_drappatz@dfci.harvard.edu

T. Batchelor, L.M. DeAngelis (eds.), *Lymphoma and Leukemia of the Nervous System*, DOI 10.1007/978-1-4419-7668-0_18,

Table 18.1 Summary of neurologic complications associated with plasma cell disorders (modified with permission from [59]

PNS complications	CNS complications
1. *Peripheral neuropathies* o Sensory > motor demyelinating neuropathy: • *Anti-MAG present* – often IgM-MGUS related • *Anti-MAG absent* – often IgG & IgA-MGUS related • Waldenstrom macroglobulinemia o Sensory > motor axonal neuropathy: • Cryoglobulinemia (with demyelinating + axonal features) • Chemotherapeutic agents o Motor > sensory demyelinating neuropathy: • In Myeloma, POEMS syndrome o Sensory > motor neuropathy ± autonomic dysfunction • Amyloidosis 2. *Polyradiculopathies* due to epidural or leptomeningeal disease	1. *Epidural spinal cord compression* back pain, paralysis, sensory loss, loss of bowel and bladder function 2. *Leptomeningeal infiltration* multiple cranial neuropathies, headaches, confusion, hydrocephalus 3. *Paraneoplastic disorders* cerebellar degeneration, motor neuron disease (see chapter paraneoplastic diseases) 4. *Hyperviscosity syndrome* headache, vertigo, ataxia, confusion, hearing loss, strokes 5. *Bing-Neel-Syndrome* encephalopathy with seizures, altered mental status and focal neurologic symptoms 6. *Hypercalcemia* headaches, weakness, seizures, lethargy, confusion and coma

flow in the cerebral and retinal circulation, and symptoms are secondary to transient ischemia. Neurological symptoms include blurry vision, dizziness, headache, vertigo, ataxia, episodic confusion, hearing loss and, sometimes, stroke [12–14]. Funduscopic examination may reveal dilated and segmented, "sausage-shaped" retinal veins, flame-shaped hemorrhages, or papilledema [15]. Hyperviscosity syndrome may also be associated with bleeding complications, such as easy bruising, retinal, and mucosal hemorrhages, but it is only rarely associated with intracranial hemorrhage [16]. Plasmapheresis can rapidly reduce the plasma levels of M protein and lead to prompt relief of symptoms. In addition, chemotherapy should be considered as early as possible to decrease paraprotein production. Treatment options include alkylating agents, particularly chlorambucil, cyclophosphamide and bendamustine, purine nucleoside analogs, such as fludarabine or cladribine, the proteasome inhibitor bortezomib [17], and the monoclonal antibodies alemtuzumab or rituximab [18, 19].

Bing-Neel Syndrome

The association of WM with nervous system infiltration by malignant lymphoplasmacytoid cells is called the Bing-Neel syndrome [20, 21], and usually represents

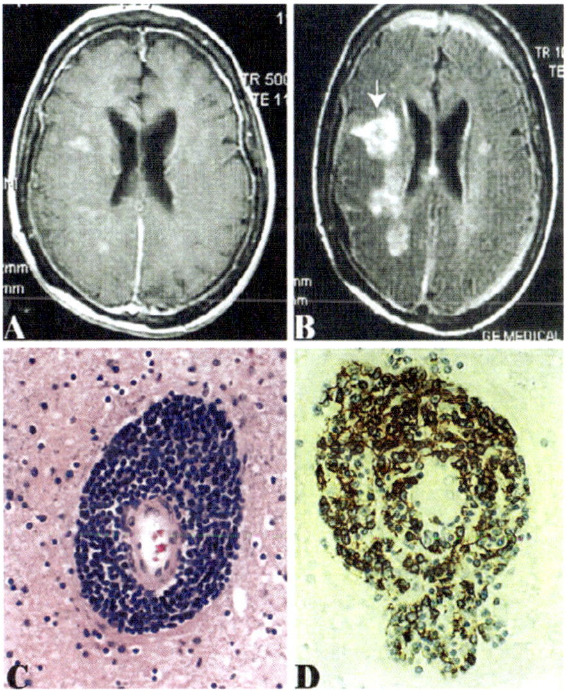

Fig. 18.1 82 year old man with Waldenstrom macroglobulinemia and progressive cognitive decline over a 2-month period. MRI demonstrates multiple lesions in the white matter that were minimally enhancing with gadolinium (**a**) and associated with white matter edema on the FLAIR images (**b**). Microscopic examination at autopsy showed prominent perivascular infiltrates (**c**) that were immunohistochemically positive for CD20 (**d**) (reproduced from Welch et al. [25] with kind permission of the College of American Pathologists)

a late complication of advanced disease. Pathology shows areas of demyelination and perivascular plasma cell and lymphocytic infiltrates [22–25], or positive CSF cytology. Imaging usually demonstrates enhancing abnormalities involving the meninges or brain parenchyma (Fig. 18.1) [26]. Patients often present with confusion, somnolence, focal neurological deficits, and seizures. Treatment is based on anecdotal evidence and may include radiation, intrathecal chemotherapy, alkylating agents, rituximab, and high dose methotrexate [21, 23, 24].

CNS Involvement by Multiple Myeloma

Direct involvement of the CNS by MM is extremely rare. Only 109 cases have been described in the literature, and the overall frequency of this neurological complication is estimated at approximately 1% [27, 28]. CNS myelomatosis is usually associated with unfavorable cytogenetic abnormalities, such as deletions of chromosome 17p13.1 (p53), high tumor burden, plasmablastic morphology, additional extramedullary myeloma manifestations, and circulating plasma cells [28]. It more commonly presents as diffuse leptomeningeal involvement than a localized cerebral mass. Hydrocephalus due to leptomeningeal infiltration has also been reported [29, 30]. The diagnosis, if not evident from the imaging studies, is made by examination of the CSF, as all patients with meningeal involvement show plasma cells within the CSF, and the CSF protein is usually increased; the paraprotein can also be detected in the CSF.

The most common presenting symptoms are altered mental status, headaches, cranial nerve palsies, and limb weakness [28]. The prognosis is poor, despite the use of aggressive local and systemic treatments, including autologous stem cell transplants [27, 31, 32].

Cranial nerve signs in MM patients are more commonly due to involvement of cranial nerve foramina in myelomatous skull base lesions, or from compression or distortion of nerves by tumor masses arising from the sphenoid or petrous bones [33–35]. The most commonly affected cranial nerves are II, V, VI, VII, and VIII [33]. Unilateral chin hypoesthesia ("numb chin syndrome") is attributed to involvement of the mandible, which has an incidence of 10–15% in MM [36].

Epidural Disease in Multiple Myeloma

Epidural spinal cord compression (ESCC) occurs in approximately 20% of MM patients [37, 38], accounting for about 5–10% of all cases of neoplastic ESCC [39]. Although ESCC is usually caused by vertebral body collapse, a small percentage of patients may develop spinal cord compression from MM, extending into the epidural space. A substantial number of patients present with ESCC as the initial disease manifestation of myeloma. In proportion to the volume of bone in the spinal regions, thoracic spine and lumbosacral spine are more commonly involved than the cervical spine. The most common presenting symptom is bone pain, which initially is localized, and typically increases in intensity with time, and often will eventually take on a radicular quality. Many patients have considerable weakness and are non-ambulatory at diagnosis [39]. Additional signs and symptoms include a sensory level, Lhermitte's sign, and bowel and bladder disturbances. Since neurological function prior to treatment is the best predictor of outcome, recognition of early neurological signs and symptoms of ESCC is very important.

Management of ESCC requires immediate diagnosis, so that appropriate treatment may begin before irreversible motor or sensory deficits occur. To detect early evidence of ESCC and to define the area of involvement, patients should undergo an MRI of the entire spine without delay (Fig. 18.2).

The mainstay of treatment is radiotherapy (RT) in combination with corticosteroids. Surgical decompression is controversial. Early studies comparing the efficacy of laminectomy to that of RT found no difference in outcome or survival [40]. However, a subsequent randomized, prospective trial demonstrated that ESCC patients with solid tumors, treated with the combination of surgery, followed by RT can remain ambulatory longer, and those who are not ambulatory at presentation have a better chance of regaining ambulatory function than those treated with RT alone, although no significant survival benefit could be demonstrated [41]. The role of surgery in hematopoietic tumors, such as MM, is less clearly defined and is often reserved for those with spinal instability, or when the diagnosis is unknown.

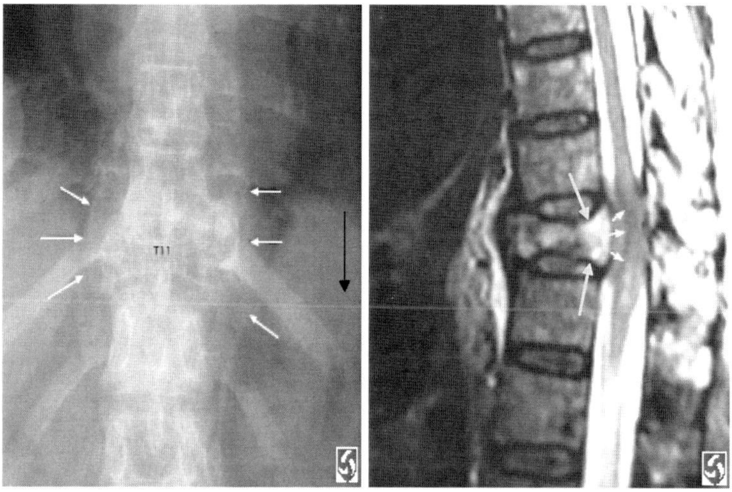

Fig. 18.2 The anteroposterior radiograph of the thoracolumbar spine of a 64-year-old woman with multiple myeloma shows a lytic, destructive lesion of T11 with vertebral collapse (*left*). Widening of the paraspinal lines (*white arrows*) indicates extension of a soft tissue mass from the marrow. In the sagittal T2 weighted MRI of T11 (*right*), the pathologic fracture and paraspinal hematoma appear bright (*long arrows*). Areas of high signal in vertebrae other than T11 suggest diffuse marrow abnormality. The spinal cord is encroached by the mass (*short arrows*) and bright CSF surrounding the cord has been replaced (printed with permission of Department of Radiology, Brigham and Women's Hospital, Boston, MA, http://brighamrad.harvard.edu)

Percutaneous vertebroplasty and kyphoplasty are methods used in the treatment of osteolytic lesions of vertebral bodies. Viscous cement is injected into the cavity, which restores most of the original height of the vertebral body, and can improve the quality of life, reduce pain, and increase overall functioning in patients with vertebral compression fractures [42]. These treatment options are only considered if the ESCC patient is free of neurological signs and symptoms caused by vertebral body collapse or tumor extension, which are relative contraindications. Therefore, their main role may be the prompt treatment of vertebral disease before the onset of compression fractures [43].

Pain control can be achieved with nonsteroidal anti-inflammatory drugs, opiates, and corticosteroids. In addition, bisphosphonates reduce pain associated with osteolytic changes in MM, and may also significantly reduce recurrent pathologic fractures [44].

Hypercalcemia

Hypercalcemia is common in MM and results from increased bone resorption by osteoclasts. A review of 1,027 newly diagnosed MM patients identified hypercalcemia in 13% [45], and it occurs in approximately one third of MM patients at some point during the course of the disease [46].

CNS symptoms include progressive lethargy and confusion, particularly with serum calcium levels greater than 14 mg/dl. Headache, elevated CSF protein, and seizures may also occur [47]. Patients with hypercalcemia complain of nausea, vomiting, weakness, constipation and abdominal discomfort. Polydipsia and polyuria result from hypercalcemia-induced nephrogenic diabetes insipidus. Hypercalcemia should be treated urgently. Hydration is important to improve renal function and to increase renal calcium excretion. The addition of loop diuretics can boost urinary calcium excretion. Inhibition of bone resorption through bisphosphonates is the second mainstay of treatment.

Peripheral Nervous System Complications

Peripheral neuropathies (PN) are one of the most common neurological manifestations of plasma cell disorders. 8–36% of patients with monoclonal gammopathy of unknown significance (MGUS) have symptomatic neuropathy [48, 49]. Earlier studies suggested that 3–13% of MM patients have subclinical PN, detected by abnormalities in electrophysiologic studies or histopathologic findings of nerve [50, 51]. A phase II study of bortezomib in previously untreated MM patients showed pretreatment neuropathy in 20% of patients [52]. Conversely, approximately 10% of patients with an idiopathic neuropathy have an associated plasma cell disorder, a prevalence six to ten times higher than that observed in the general population [53].

PN in plasma cell disorders constitute a heterogeneous group of diseases. In addition to the nerve damaging effects of monoclonal proteins, peripheral nerve dysfunction may also occur as a consequence of direct infiltration of the peripheral nerves by malignant cells, and may result in mononeuropathies. In addition, thalidomide and bortezomib, drugs used in the treatment of MM, can cause neuropathy.

Neuropathies Associated with Monoclonal Gammopathies of Undetermined Significance (MGUS)

IgM monoclonal gammopathy of undetermined significance (MGUS) is the most commonly found monoclonal gammopathy associated with neuropathy and PN is often the only clinical manifestation of the underlying hematological disorder. Although IgG is the most common paraprotein in MGUS, IgM is more frequently found in the subset of patients with neuropathy. Up to 50% of patients with IgM MGUS have a symptomatic neuropathy [54]. Immunohistochemistry has shown direct binding of the IgM protein to nerve myelin, causing separation of the outer layers of compacted myelin [55–57]. The antibody is directed against myelin-associated glycoprotein (MAG), which comprises approximately 1% of peripheral nerve myelin and can be detected in the serum [49]. MAG acts as an adhesion molecule for interactions between Schwann cells and axons [58]. Patients with anti-MAG are typically older men who present with slowly progressive distal sensory loss, paresthesias, and mild distal weakness as result of a symmetric sensorimotor demyelinating PN. Features of large-fiber sensory dysfunction, such as ataxia, loss of joint position, Romberg's sign and imbalance are often also present. Distal deep tendon reflexes are absent [54]. The CSF protein level is elevated and electrodiagnostic studies show demyelinating features. Of the remaining cases of IgM MGUS-related neuropathies, some will have antibodies against additional myelin or other nerve components, such as sulfate-3-glucuronyl-paragloboside (SGPG) and sulfoglucuronyl-lactosaminyl-paragloboside, neurofilaments, sulfatides, gangliosides, P0 (a myelin associated protein) or chondroitin sulfate [59]. Many patients will not have any detectable antibodies. Whether the measurement of these antibodies has any practical implications in the management of patients, is unclear. In one study, antibody tests did not have an independent prognostic value, in addition to electrophysiologic data and clinical presentation in terms of future neurological deficit, or outcome in polyneuropathy associated with IgM monoclonal gammopathy [60]. Others, however, argue that the detection of anti-MAG antibodies may help to confirm a favorable prognosis [61], and therefore aid in treatment decisions.

In general, treatment should be reserved for patients who have progressive and disabling symptoms. Treatments that may be considered include plasma exchange, steroids, cytotoxic drugs, such as nucleoside analogues and alkylating agents, intravenous immunoglobulin (IVIG), and monoclonal antibodies, specifically rituximab, which targets the B cell surface antigen CD20 [54, 62]. A Cochrane database review on the treatment of anti-MAG associated neuropathy concluded that IVIG may produce some short-term benefits, but longer trials were needed [63]. Rituximab may have a more significant impact [64]. The most recent clinical trial for anti-MAG demyelinating polyneuropathy evaluated rituximab in a double-blind, placebo-controlled design [65]. Thirteen patients were randomized to 4 weekly infusions of 375 mg/m^2 rituximab and 13 to placebo. Although the results were not significant, there was a trend favoring the rituximab group due to lower disability scores and improved timed walking, especially in those patients with the highest anti-MAG titers and worse sensory dysfunction at baseline. However, the small number of patients enrolled in this study do not allow one to draw definitive conclusions regarding the role of rituximab in the treatment of this disorder.

Neuropathies associated with IgG and IgA MGUS, but without anti-MAG antibodies, are far less common. They have a more heterogeneous clinical phenotype, yet are more responsive to treatment [66]. Most patients develop a distal, symmetric, sensorimotor polyneuropathy with predominantly sensory symptoms. The neuropathy in IgG and IgA MGUS is responsive to plasma exchange or IVIG [67, 68]. If this does not lead to objective benefit, the agents listed above for the anti-MAG syndrome may be considered.

MGUS related neuropathies can be indistinguishable from chronic inflammatory demyelinating polyradiculoneuropathy, clinically, electrophysiologically, and in response to treatment [69].

Neuropathy in Multiple Myeloma (MM)

Polyneuropathy is a fairly common complication of MM, affecting approximately 20% of newly diagnosed patients [52]. In most cases, it manifests as a mild distal sensorimotor polyneuropathy. Perineural immunoglobulin deposition, specifically IgM or IgG kappa, with or without amyloidosis, may be responsible for polyneuropathy in approximately 30% of MM-associated neuropathy cases [70]. In neuropathies without evidence of amyloid infiltration, the etiology is likely multifactorial, possibly related to nutritional and metabolic factors, i.e., uremia secondary to renal failure [71]. The neuropathy associated with MM is not usually responsive to treatment of the underlying illness and in fact, may be worsened by neurotoxic drugs [54].

In the less common variant of myeloma, the solitary plasmacytoma of bone (also known as Crow-Fukase syndrome), PN occurs in the majority of cases. The typical features of the POEMS syndrome (*p*olyneuropathy – primarily motor, *o*rganomegaly, *e*ndocrinopathy, *M* protein, and *s*kin changes) usually lead to the diagnosis. The disease affects a younger patient population, and is typically more debilitating due to weakness and sensory loss of the distal limbs that can appear over a period of weeks. There is a disproportionate loss of vibration and proprioception compared to pain and temperature sensation. The M protein is found in the majority of cases and CSF protein levels are often more than 100 mg per deciliter, although the cell count is normal [72]. The cause of the frequent association of this neuropathy with osteosclerotic myeloma remains poorly understood. Electrophysiologic studies and pathological specimens present a mixed picture of axonal degeneration and demyelination.

Treatment involves targeting the underlying plasma cell disorder with local radiation therapy or surgical resection. This approach has been successful for patients with isolated lesions. In the majority of cases, local radiotherapy leads to considerable improvement of symptoms after 3–6 months [73]. The prognosis for patients with widespread disease is less favorable. There are isolated reports of responses with melphalan, thalidomide, prednisolone, tamoxifen, and retinoic acid [59, 74, 75]. For refractory neuropathy, more aggressive combination regimens, including high-dose chemotherapy and stem cell rescue, from either autologous or allogeneic sources, are being explored [76–78].

Treatment of the underlying MM can also cause PN. Thalidomide and bortezomib cause a length-dependent, predominantly sensory, and often partially reversible axonal neuropathy that affects large and small fibers in a dose dependent fashion [52, 79, 80].

Neuropathy of Waldenstrom's Macroglobulinemia

Sensorimotor PN occurs with a frequency of 5–10% in patients with Waldenstrom's macroglobulinemia, and the presentation is similar to the neuropathy seen in IgM MGUS described above [81–83]. Antibodies to myelin-associated glycoprotein

(MAG) are found in some of these patients. Electrophysiologic studies demonstrate demyelination, comparable to the neuropathy seen in IgM MGUS, and the treatment options are also similar and include plasma exchange, rituximab, purine analogues (fludarabine, cladribine), thalidomide, bortezomib, and R-CHOP (rituximab, cyclophosphamide, doxorubicin, vincristine and prednisone) based chemotherapy.

Amyloid Polyneuropathy

Painful PN symptoms are characteristic of amyloidosis, a multisystem disorder characterized by IgG or IgA lambda paraproteinemia and deposition of immunoglobulin light chains in kidney, heart, and liver. The presumptive cause of the neuropathy is either a direct neurotoxic effect or vascular insufficiency [84]. About 30% of PNs in MM are associated with amyloid, and a small number of cases of Waldenstrom's macroglobulinemia have been associated with amyloid. Amyloid PN frequently presents as a progressive sensory or sensorimotor polyneuropathy often accompanied by autonomic dysfunction, such as orthostatic hypotension, impotence, and bladder dysfunction. Patients typically complain of burning or painful electrical sensations [84]. On examination, pain and temperature loss are characteristic. Consistent with a predominant effect on small-diameter sensory fibers, vibration, and position sense are usually spared [1].

Nerve biopsy will establish the diagnosis by identifying amyloid deposits in the endoneurium associated with an axonal neuropathy [84]. The prognosis for patients with amyloid polyneuropathy is poor [85]. Chemotherapy aims to destroy the amyloid-producing plasma cells. Symptomatic treatment can be helpful and includes use of elastic stockings, fluorinated steroids for orthostatic hypotension, and medications such as carbamazepine, gabapentin or amitriptyline to control pain.

Cryoglobulinemic Neuropathy

Cryoglobulins are immunoglobulins that reversibly precipitate at temperatures below 37°C and are associated with Waldenstrom macroglobulinemia, MM, or MGUS. For example, 5–7% of patients with MM have an associated cryoglobulinemia [86]. Neurological presentations range from a subacute mononeuritis multiplex to a chronic distal symmetric sensorimotor polyneuropathy [87]. Nerve biopsy demonstrates epineurial vasculitis, which is probably responsible for ischemic nerve damage [88]. Therapy should be directed at the underlying plasma cell disorder.

Diagnostic Approach to Neuropathies in Patients with Plasma Cell Disorders

The work-up of adult onset neuropathy should always include serum and urine electrophoresis. If an M-Protein is found, a careful evaluation for the presence of myeloma or macroglobulinemia should be the next step and usually includes a peripheral blood count with smear, renal function tests, a skeletal survey to rule out lytic or blastic lesions, testing for cryoglobulins, LDH, β2-microglobulin, and a 24 hour urine collection for protein. If the skeletal survey is abnormal or an elevated M-protein level is detected, then a bone marrow biopsy should be performed.

The measurement of antibodies can help to identify any of the distinct clinical syndromes listed above and to differentiate these from CIDP. Testing for antibodies against MAG, SGPG, GD1b ganglioside, GalNAc-GD1a, GM2 gangliosides, neurofilament, sulfatides, and others can be achieved through commercial or academic specialty laboratories [89].

If the neuropathy is asymmetric, a nerve biopsy is indicated to rule out plasma cell infiltration of the nerve. A body PET scan may help localize the site of nerve infiltration prior to biopsy. A nerve biopsy can also help to identify vasculitis associated with cryoglobulin deposits or amyloid deposition.

References

1. Dispenzieri A, Kyle RA (2005) Neurological aspects of multiple myeloma and related disorders. Best Pract Res Clin Haematol 18:673–688
2. Spinazze S, Caraceni A, Schrijvers D (2005) Epidural spinal cord compression. Crit Rev Oncol Hematol 56:397–406
3. Maghfoor I, Perry MC (2000) Malignancy: meningeal myeloma: a case report and review of literature. Hematology 5:47–52
4. Roddie P, Collie D, Johnson P (2000) Myelomatous involvement of the dura mater: a rare complication of multiple myeloma. J Clin Pathol 53:398–399
5. Savage DG, Mears JG, Balmaceda C et al (2002) Leptomeningeal relapse of multiple myeloma following allogeneic stem cell transplantation. Leuk Res 26:689–692
6. Slager UT, Taylor WF, Opfell RW, Myers A (1979) Leptomeningeal myeloma. Arch Pathol Lab Med 103:680–682
7. Oyajobi BO (2007) Multiple myeloma/hypercalcemia. Arthritis Res Ther 9(Suppl 1):S4
8. Mehta J, Singhal S (2003) Hyperviscosity syndrome in plasma cell dyscrasias. Semin Thromb Hemost 29:467–471
9. Johnson SA, Oscier DG, Leblond V (2002) Waldenstrom's macroglobulinaemia. Blood Rev 16:175–184
10. Preston FE, Cooke KB, Foster ME et al (1978) Myelomatosis and the hyperviscosity syndrome. Br J Haematol 38:517–530
11. Pruzanski W, Watt JG (1972) Serum viscosity and hyperviscosity syndrome in IgG multiple myeloma. Report on 10 patients and a review of the literature. Ann Intern Med 77:853–860
12. Adams BD, Baker R, Lopez JA, Spencer S (2009) Myeloproliferative disorders and the hyperviscosity syndrome. Emerg Med Clin North Am 27:459–476
13. Pavy MD, Murphy PL, Virella G (1980) Paraprotein-induced hyperviscosity. A reversible cause of stroke. Postgrad Med 68:109–112
14. Stone MJ (2009) Waldenstrom's macroglobulinemia: hyperviscosity syndrome and cryoglobulinemia. Clin Lymphoma Myeloma 9:97–99
15. Bernard A, Rousselie F (1986) Macular manifestations of monoclonal dysgammaglobulinemias. Apropos of 3 cases. J Fr Ophthalmol 9:805–810
16. Alatoom A, Elsabrouty R, Willis J et al (2009) Fatal cerebral hemorrhage in a patient with CD19-positive IgM-producing aggressive plasma cell myeloma, hyperviscosity syndrome and cryoglobulinemia. Int J Clin Exp Pathol 2:498–507

17. Chen C, Kouroukis CT, White D et al (2009) Bortezomib in relapsed or refractory Waldenstrom's macroglobulinemia. Clin Lymphoma Myeloma 9:74–76
18. Dimopoulos MA, Gertz MA, Kastritis E et al (2009) Update on treatment recommendations from the Fourth International Workshop on Waldenstrom's Macroglobulinemia. J Clin Oncol 27:120–126
19. Treon SP (2009) How I treat Waldenstrom macroglobulinemia. Blood 114:2375–2385
20. Bing JN, Fog M, Neel AV (1937) Report of a third case of hyperglobulinemia with affection of the central nervous system on a toxi-infectious basis, and some remarks on the differential diagnosis. Acta Med. Scand 91:409–427
21. Fintelmann F, Forghani R, Schaefer PW et al (2009) Bing-Neel syndrome revisited. Clin Lymphoma Myeloma 9:104–106
22. Edgar R, Dutcher TF (1961) Histopathology of the Bing-Neel syndrome. Neurology 11:239–245
23. Grewal JS, Brar PK, Sahijdak WM et al (2009) Bing-Neel syndrome: a case report and systematic review of clinical manifestations, diagnosis, and treatment options. Clin Lymphoma Myeloma 9:462–466
24. Malkani RG, Tallman M, Gottardi-Littell N et al (2009) Bing-Neel syndrome: an illustrative case and a comprehensive review of the published literature. J Neurooncol 96(3):301–312
25. Welch D, Whetsell WO Jr., Weil RJ (2002) Pathologic quiz case. A man with long-standing monoclonal gammopathy and new onset of confusion. Central nervous system involvement by Waldenstrom macroglobulinemia-Bing-Neel syndrome. Arch Pathol Lab Med 126:1243–1244
26. Drappatz J, Akar S, Fisher DC et al (2008) Imaging of Bing-Neel syndrome. Neurology 70:1364
27. Fassas AB, Ward S, Muwalla F et al (2004) Myeloma of the central nervous system: strong association with unfavorable chromosomal abnormalities and other high-risk disease features. Leuk Lymphoma 45:291–300
28. Nieuwenhuizen L, Biesma DH (2008) Central nervous system myelomatosis: review of the literature. Eur J Haematol 80:1–9
29. Dennis M, Chu P (2000) A case of meningeal myeloma presenting as obstructive hydrocephalus – a therapeutic challenge. Leuk Lymphoma 40:219–220
30. Pontikoglou C, Fragos C, Kolyvaki E et al (2005) Multiple myeloma involving the central nervous system: a report of two cases with unusual manifestations. Leuk Lymphoma 46:737–741
31. Quach H, Ryan G, Ganju V, Prince HM (2005) Effective treatment of leptomeningeal multiple myeloma with total craniospinal irradiation supported by second allogeneic donor stem cell infusion. Bone Marrow Transplant 35:423–424
32. Veinstein A, Brizard A, Randriamalala E et al (1997) Central nervous system relapses after autologous stem cell transplantation for myeloma. Report of two cases. Hematol Cell Ther 39:327–330
33. Hogan MC, Lee A, Solberg LA, Thome SD (2002) Unusual presentation of multiple myeloma with unilateral visual loss and numb chin syndrome in a young adult. Am J Hematol 70:55–59
34. Knapp AJ, Gartner S, Henkind P (1987) Multiple myeloma and its ocular manifestations. Surv Ophthalmol 31:343–351
35. Shone GR (1985) Facial palsy due to myeloma of the temporal bone. J Laryngol Otol 99:907–908
36. Witt C, Borges AC, Klein K, Neumann HJ (1997) Radiographic manifestations of multiple myeloma in the mandible: a retrospective study of 77 patients. J Oral Maxillofac Surg 55: 450–453; discussion 454–455
37. Colak A, Cataltepe O, Ozgen T, Erbengi A (1989) Spinal cord compression caused by plasmacytomas. A retrospective review of 14 cases. Neurosurg Rev 12:305–308
38. Spiess JL, Adelstein DJ, Hines JD (1988) Multiple myeloma presenting with spinal cord compression. Oncology 45:88–92

39. Schiff D (2003) Spinal cord compression. Neurol Clin 21:67–86
40. Young RF, Post EM, King GA (1980) Treatment of spinal epidural metastases. Randomized prospective comparison of laminectomy and radiotherapy. J Neurosurg 53:741–748
41. Patchell RA, Tibbs PA, Regine WF et al (2005) Direct decompressive surgical resection in the treatment of spinal cord compression caused by metastatic cancer: a randomised trial. Lancet 366:643–648
42. Witham TF, Khavkin YA, Gallia GL et al (2006) Surgery insight: current management of epidural spinal cord compression from metastatic spine disease. Nat Clin Pract Neurol 2:87–94; quiz 116
43. Sun H, Nemecek AN (2009) Optimal management of malignant epidural spinal cord compression. Emerg Med Clin North Am 27:195–208
44. Costa L, Major PP (2009) Effect of bisphosphonates on pain and quality of life in patients with bone metastases. Nat Clin Pract Oncol 6:163–174
45. Kyle RA, Gertz MA, Witzig TE et al (2003) Review of 1027 patients with newly diagnosed multiple myeloma. Mayo Clin Proc 78:21–33
46. Mundy GR (1998) Myeloma bone disease. Eur J Cancer 34:246–251
47. Riggs JE (2002) Neurologic manifestations of electrolyte disturbances. Neurol Clin 20: 227–239
48. Nobile-Orazio E, Barbieri S, Baldini L et al (1992) Peripheral neuropathy in monoclonal gammopathy of undetermined significance: prevalence and immunopathogenetic studies. Acta Neurol Scand 85:383–390
49. Vrethem M, Cruz M, Wen-Xin H et al (1993) Clinical, neurophysiological and immunological evidence of polyneuropathy in patients with monoclonal gammopathies. J Neurol Sci 114:193–199
50. Silverstein A, Doniger DE (1963) Neurologic complications of myelomatosis. Arch Neurol 9:534–544
51. Walsh JC (1971) The neuropathy of multiple myeloma. An electrophysiological and histological study. Arch Neurol 25:404–414
52. Richardson PG, Xie W, Mitsiades C et al (2009) Single-agent bortezomib in previously untreated multiple myeloma: efficacy, characterization of peripheral neuropathy, and molecular correlations with response and neuropathy. J Clin Oncol 27: 3518–3525
53. Kelly JJ Jr., Kyle RA, O'Brien PC, Dyck PJ (1981) Prevalence of monoclonal protein in peripheral neuropathy. Neurology 31:1480–1483
54. Ramchandren S, Lewis RA (2009) Monoclonal gammopathy and neuropathy. Curr Opin Neurol 22:480–485
55. Latov N, Braun PE, Gross RB et al (1981) Plasma cell dyscrasia and peripheral neuropathy: identification of the myelin antigens that react with human paraproteins. Proc Natl Acad Sci USA 78:7139–7142
56. Latov N, Hays AP, Sherman WH (1988) Peripheral neuropathy and anti-MAG antibodies. Crit Rev Neurobiol 3:301–332
57. Ellie E, Vital A, Steck A et al (1996) Neuropathy associated with "benign" anti-myelin-associated glycoprotein IgM gammopathy: clinical, immunological, neurophysiological pathological findings and response to treatment in 33 cases. J Neurol 243:34–43
58. Yeung KB, Thomas PK, King RH et al (1991) The clinical spectrum of peripheral neuropathies associated with benign monoclonal IgM, IgG and IgA paraproteinaemia. Comparative clinical, immunological and nerve biopsy findings. J Neurol 238:383–391
59. Drappatz J, Batchelor T (2004) Neurologic complications of plasma cell disorders. Clin Lymphoma 5:163–171
60. Eurelings M, Moons KG, Notermans NC et al (2001) Neuropathy and IgM M-proteins: prognostic value of antibodies to MAG, SGPG, and sulfatide. Neurology 56:228–233
61. Nobile-Orazio E, Carpo M (2001) Neuropathy and monoclonal gammopathy. Curr Opin Neurol 14:615–620

62. Zivkovic SA, Lacomis D, Lentzsch S (2009) Paraproteinemic neuropathy. Leuk Lymphoma 50:1422–1433
63. Lunn MP, Nobile-Orazio E (2003) Immunotherapy for IgM anti-Myelin-associated glycoprotein paraprotein-associated peripheral neuropathies. Cochrane Database Syst Rev 1:CD002827
64. Pestronk A, Florence J, Miller T et al (2003) Treatment of IgM antibody associated polyneuropathies using rituximab. J Neurol Neurosurg Psychiatry 74:485–489
65. Dalakas MC, Rakocevic G, Salajegheh M et al (2009) Placebo-controlled trial of rituximab in IgM anti-myelin-associated glycoprotein antibody demyelinating neuropathy. Ann Neurol 65:286–293
66. Vrethem M, Reiser N, Lauermann C, Svanborg E (2009) Polyneuropathy associated with IgM vs IgG monoclonal gammopathy: comparison between clinical and electrophysiological findings. Acta Neurol Scand 122(1):52–57
67. Gorson KC, Ropper AH, Weinberg DH, Weinstein R (2002) Efficacy of intravenous immunoglobulin in patients with IgG monoclonal gammopathy and polyneuropathy. Arch Neurol 59:766–772
68. Wicklund MP, Kissel JT (2001) Paraproteinemic neuropathy. Curr Treat Options Neurol 3:147–156
69. Hadden RD, Nobile-Orazio E, Sommer C et al (2006) European Federation of Neurological Societies/Peripheral Nerve Society guideline on management of paraproteinaemic demyelinating neuropathies: report of a joint task force of the European Federation of Neurological Societies and the Peripheral Nerve Society. Eur J Neurol 13:809–818
70. Victor M, Banker BQ, Adams RD (1958) The neuropathy of multiple myeloma. J Neurol Neurosurg Psychiatry 21:73–88
71. Briemberg HR, Amato AA (2003) Neuromuscular complications of cancer. Neurol Clin 21:141–165
72. Nakanishi T, Sobue I, Toyokura Y et al (1984) The Crow-Fukase syndrome: a study of 102 cases in Japan. Neurology 34:712–720
73. Kelly JJ Jr., Kyle RA, Miles JM, Dyck PJ (1983) Osteosclerotic myeloma and peripheral neuropathy. Neurology 33:202–210
74. Kuwabara S, Misawa S, Kanai K et al (2008) Thalidomide reduces serum VEGF levels and improves peripheral neuropathy in POEMS syndrome. J Neurol Neurosurg Psychiatry 79:1255–1257
75. Steck AJ, Czaplinski A, Renaud S (2008) Inflammatory demyelinating neuropathies and neuropathies associated with monoclonal gammopathies: treatment update. Neurotherapeutics 5:528–534
76. Creange A, Chater A, Brouet JC et al (2008) A case of POEMS syndrome treated by autologous hematopoietic stem-cell transplantation. Nat Clin Pract Neurol 4: 686–691
77. Gupta S, Rana V, Chandra D et al (2006) Autologous peripheral stem cell transplant for POEMS syndrome: a case report. Hematology 11:361–363
78. Mahdi-Rogers M, Kazmi M, Ferner R et al (2009) Autologous peripheral blood stem cell transplantation for chronic acquired demyelinating neuropathy. J Peripher Nerv Syst 14:118–124
79. Plasmati R, Pastorelli F, Cavo M et al (2007) Neuropathy in multiple myeloma treated with thalidomide: a prospective study. Neurology 69:573–581
80. Richardson PG, Briemberg H, Jagannath S et al (2006) Frequency, characteristics, and reversibility of peripheral neuropathy during treatment of advanced multiple myeloma with bortezomib. J Clin Oncol 24:3113–3120
81. Julien J, Vital C, Vallat JM et al (1978) Polyneuropathy in Waldenstrom's macroglobulinemia. Deposition of M component on myelin sheaths. Arch Neurol 35:423–425
82. Rudnicki SA, Harik SI, Dhodapkar M et al (1998) Nervous system dysfunction in Waldenstrom's macroglobulinemia: response to treatment. Neurology 51:1210–1213

83. Vital C, Deminiere C, Bourgouin B et al (1985) Waldenstrom's macroglobulinemia and peripheral neuropathy: deposition of M-component and kappa light chain in the endoneurium. Neurology 35:603–606
84. Adams D (2001) Hereditary and acquired amyloid neuropathies. J Neurol 248:647–657
85. Kyle RA, Greipp PR (1983) Amyloidosis (AL). Clinical and laboratory features in 229 cases. Mayo Clin Proc 58:665–683
86. Bloch KJ, Franklin E (1982) Plasma cell dyscrasias and cryoglobulins. JAMA 248:2670–2676
87. Garcia-Bragado F, Fernandez JM, Navarro C et al (1988) Peripheral neuropathy in essential mixed cryoglobulinemia. Arch Neurol 45:1210–1214
88. Nemni R, Corbo M, Fazio R et al (1988) Cryoglobulinaemic neuropathy. A clinical, morphological and immunocytochemical study of 8 cases. Brain 111(Pt 3):541–552
89. Vernino S, Wolfe GI (2007) Antibody testing in peripheral neuropathies. Neurol Clin 25:29–46

Chapter 19
Neurological Complications of Acute and Chronic Leukemia

Marc C. Chamberlain

Introduction

Leukemia is classified into acute and chronic types, and is further separated into lymphoid and myeloid forms, and whether tumors are comprised of cells that appear mature (chronic leukemia) or immature (acute leukemia) (see Chapter 2) [1–3]. Within each category, leukemia is defined according to a combination of morphology, immunophenotype, and cytogenetic features, in addition to clinical syndrome. An estimated, 30,800–33,400 new case of leukemia will be diagnosed in the United States each year. Acute leukemia, a clonal disease of hematopoietic stem cells, accounts for slightly more than half of all new leukemia diagnoses in the United States, annually. Hematopoietic stem cells may differentiate along lymphoid or myeloid lines. In adults, acute myelogenous leukemia (AML), also called acute non-lymphocytic leukemia, is three times more common than acute lymphocytic leukemia (ALL) and represents 60–70% all acute leukemia with 11,000–12,000 new cases diagnosed annually in the United States. AML is most common in individuals older than 50 years of age, whereas ALL is more common in children and young adults. Approximately one third of patients with either ALL or AML achieve long-term survival; however, outcome is highly dependent upon cytogenetic profile. Chronic lymphocytic leukemia (CLL) is the second most common adult leukemia and affects 8,000–9,000 persons in the United States, annually. Like AML, CLL is more common in the elderly. CLL represents a monoclonal disorder with expansion of small lymphocytes of B-cell (95%) or T-cell (5%) lineage. Median survival is 6 years, but is dependent upon staging (as per the Rai staging system) at disease presentation. CLL only rarely progresses to a more malignant phenotype. Chronic myelogenous leukemia (CML) is characterized by excessive clonal proliferation of myeloid cells and affects 4,000–5,000 adults annually in the United States. The

---

M.C. Chamberlain (✉)
Department of Neurology and Neurological Surgery, University of Washington, Seattle, WA, USA;
Division of Neuro-Oncology, Department of Neurology, Fred Hutchinson Research Cancer Center,
Seattle Cancer Care Alliance, Seattle, WA 98109-1023, USA
e-mail: chambemc@uw.edu

T. Batchelor, L.M. DeAngelis (eds.), *Lymphoma and Leukemia of the Nervous System*, DOI 10.1007/978-1-4419-7668-0_19,

Table 19.1 Neurological complications of leukemia outlined by nervous system compartment

- Direct
  - Meningeal
    - Leukemic
  - Parenchymal
    - Tumor
    - Hemorrhage
      - Vascular slugging/stasis due to hyperleukocytosis
      - Thrombocytopenia due to leukemia or treatment
  - Epidural
    - Leukemic
- Indirect
  - Meningeal
    - Infectious
      - Bacterial meningitis
      - Fungal meningitis
      - Chemical meningitis
    - Headache
      - Low-pressure headache (post-lumbar puncture)
      - Subdural hematoma
  - Parenchymal
    - Hemorrhage
      - Treatment-induced sinus thrombosis (l-asparaginase)
      - Treatment-induced thrombocytopenia
      - Post cranial irradiation-Moyamoya disease
      - Disseminated intravascular coagulopathy (DIC)
      - Fungal-related
        - Mycotic aneurysm
        - Vasculitis
    - Encephalopathy
      - Radiation-related
      - Methotrexate-related
      - Toxic-metabolic
      - Organ failure
      - Posterior reversible encephalopathy syndrome (PRES)
      - Multifocal necrotizing leukoencephalopathy
      - Thrombotic thrombocytopenic purpura (TTP)
      - Infectious (Human Herpes Virus-6)
  - Spinal
    - Treatment-related (intra-thecal drugs) myelopathy
  - Epidural
    - Hemorrhage
      - Treatment-induced thrombocytopenia
      - Post-LP hematoma
    - Steroid-related epidural lipomatosis
  - Peripheral neuropathy
    - Treatment-related (vinca alkaloids)
  - Myopathy
    - Treatment-related (corticosteroids)

disease can be divided into two phases; an initial chronic phase, in which cell maturation is normal, followed by an acute phase (blast crisis), characterized by maturation arrest. Median survival of CML is 4 years. For a more detailed overview of the leukemias, the reader is referred to Chapter 2.

The neurological manifestations of leukemia are diverse and reflect either direct tumor involvement, or indirect complications of immunosuppression or therapy. The following discussion of the neurological complications of leukemia highlights the most frequently observed syndromes (Table 19.1).

Chloromas

AML may give rise to solid tumors consisting of myeloid leukemic blasts called granulocytic sarcomas or chloromas [4–6] (Fig. 19.1). The term chloroma results from the greenish color of these tumors caused by the presence of myeloperoxidase. Chloromas usually have a dural attachment, and although rare, parenchymal brain tumors have been reported. These tumors are hypercellular and avidly enhance after contrast administration on either cranial MR or CT imaging. Neurological findings are dependent upon tumor location. Chloromas most often occur in bone, which may lead to epidural spinal cord compression, or proptosis and a restrictive ophthalmopathy with involvement of the orbit; intracranial dural infiltration may simulate a meningioma. Although chloromas are very radiosensitive, their presence

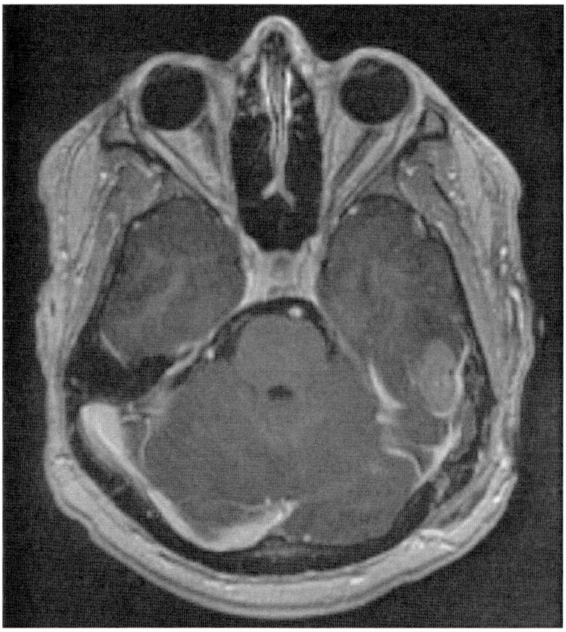

Fig. 19.1 Left temporal lobe chloroma in a patient with AML. Axial T1-weighted, post-contrast cranial MRI

typically heralds aggressive systemic disease, such that disease control is a function of extracranial therapy and response.

Intracranial Hemorrhage

Hemorrhagic complications are common in patients with acute leukemia (approximately 20% of all patients) and constitute the second most common cause of death in such patients. Approximately 20% of all leukemic deaths occur as a result of intracranial hemorrhage (ICH) [4, 7–15]. ICH is the most common hemorrhagic complication in acute promyelocytic leukemia (APL) and is common in AML and ALL (ranging in incidence from 2 to 18% of all patients with acute leukemia). ICH may occur at diagnosis of leukemia (early hemorrhage), or subsequent to diagnosis, and following initial treatment (late hemorrhage). Disseminated intravascular coagulation (DIC), disseminated aspergillosis or mucormycosis, leukemic cell infiltration, thrombocytopenia or l-asparaginase-related thrombosis, in that order, are the most common etiologies for ICH. Both DIC (especially common in the M3 subtype of AML) and thrombocytopenia typically result in a solitary, often-massive ICH, whereas ICH associated with disseminated fungal infection occurs during neutropenia, and is the result of hemorrhagic infarction. Leukemic cell infiltration occurs with marked leukocytosis (defined as >300,000 leukemic cells/μL), and results in multiple intracranial hemorrhages. L-asparaginase may induce hyperfibrinogenemia and result in cortical vein or sinus thrombosis, with resulting venous infarction. Fungal-related mycotic aneurysms and ICH may occur in patients with fungemia (blood culture positive for fungus) and are often fatal. Topographically, the majority of ICH is intraparenchymal with cerebral hemorrhage more common than cerebellar. Subdural hematoma is relatively infrequent except as a complication following stem cell transplantation. Aside from symptomatic treatment of ICH, treatment is directed at the underlying cause of the hemorrhage (for example correction of an underlying coagulopathy, whole brain irradiation or systemic chemotherapy for hyperleukocytosis and brain leukemic infiltration). In general, ICH in the patient with leukemia portends short survival.

Encephalopathy

A variety of etiologies may account for encephalopathy (defined as an alteration in consciousness, neurobehavioral abnormalities, seizures or focal neurological deficits) in the leukemic patient. Most commonly, toxic/metabolic (narcotic overmedication, hyponatremia, uremia, organ failure) causes are identified; however, consideration of other possible causes including DIC, sinus thrombosis, ICH, chemotherapy (either high dose methotrexate or cytarabine), or radiation toxicity and infections (disseminated *Candida* or *Aspergillus, Human Herpes Virus-6*) is necessary [4, 7–15]. Evaluation for DIC is warranted in any patient with leukemia and encephalopathy, and should include a coagulopathy evaluation. Rarely, thrombotic thrombocytopenic purpura (TTP) may complicate the treatment of leukemia, causing neurological symptoms [16, 17]. TTP is characterized clinically by the pentad of a microangiopathic hemolytic anemia, thrombocytopenia, fever, renal dysfunction, and encephalopathy. Serum fibrinogen is low in TTP as a consequence of a prothrombotic state induced by abnormal aggregation of von Willebrand factor (prothrombotic). It is a consequence of congenital or acquired deficiency in the von Willebrand factor cleaving protease (ADAMTS-13). Treatment is with plasma exchange, though mortality remains high (10–20%).

Sinus thrombosis is occasionally due to leukemic infiltration of the superior sagittal sinus (SSS), but more often occurs with dehydration, sepsis-related coagulopathy, or l-asparaginase chemotherapy. Clinical presentation may be an isolated headache, raised intracranial pressure syndrome (headache, nausea, vomiting, transient visual obscurations, and diplopia), hemiparesis, or encephalopathy. Cranial imaging most often demonstrates a venous hemorrhagic stroke and occlusion of the SSS.

Chemotherapy-related encephalopathy is seen following high-dose methotrexate as either a transient diffuse encephalopathy or a more chronic diffuse leukoencephalopathy. High-dose cytarabine (ara-C), used in the treatment of AML, causes either a pure cerebellar syndrome or diffuse encephalopathy, and is more common in the elderly patient (age > 60 years) and in patients with renal impairment.

Radiation-related encephalopathy occurs in two contexts: as an early-delayed side effect or more commonly, as a late-delayed radiation complication [4, 12, 18]. In both instances, radiation therapy is given as prophylactic whole brain radiotherapy in high-risk (for leukemic meningitis) patients. Early-delayed radiation syndrome, occurring weeks after completion of radiation therapy, is a generalized demyelinating syndrome that presents with hypersomnolence, is benign, and resolves with steroid treatment. Late-delayed radiation toxicity (occurring months to years after radiotherapy) has two major forms: mineralizing arteriopathy (usually seen in children) and a necrotizing leukoencephalopathy (seen in adults). The former is reflected as dystrophic calcification in small blood vessels and is commonly seen in the basal ganglia, dentate nuclei, thalami, and subcortical white matter. Necrotizing leukoencephalopathy is an admixture of demyelination, astrogliosis, and necrosis presenting with either a static or progressive encephalopathy. Neither condition is treatable; however, they are related to both chemotherapy (in particular methotrexate, both systemic and intra-CSF) and radiation dose, and therefore potentially modifiable as acute leukemia induction regimens are tailored to the risk of CNS relapse.

Leukemic patients treated with high dose systemic chemotherapy regimens may develop the posterior reversible leukoencephalopathy syndrome (PRES) [19–22]. The cardinal features of PRES are both clinical (i.e. hypertension, headaches, seizures, altered mental status and visual disturbances) and radiological. The radiological findings are characterized by cortical abnormalities best visualized by FLAIR and T2-weighted MRI, and topography of involvement. PRES is usually limited to the white matter of the parietal and occipital lobes, however, anterior and infratentorial involvement have also been described. Most often, PRES is associated with malignant hypertension or eclampsia; however, PRES is a well-described complication of high-dose chemotherapy and tacrolimus and related immunophilins (i.e. cyclosporine) administered in conjunction with stem cell transplantation [20, 21]. The precipitating event in the development of PRES is acute endothelial cell damage, resulting in a microangiopathy, cerebrovascular dysregulation, and vasogenic edema. The clinical and radiographic findings are reversible with treatment of the underlying hypertension or withdrawal of the offending agent.

Another rare cause of encephalopathy in leukemic patients is multifocal necrotizing leukoencephalopathy (MNL) [23]. MNL is a rare neurological treatment-related complication infrequently observed in patients treated for acute leukemia, acquired immunodeficiency syndromes such as AIDS, and chronic steroid-requiring diseases such as collagen vascular diseases. Most commonly, the lesions of MNL are located in the pons, but may occasionally be extrapontine. Due to the predominantly pontine location of MNL, most reported series are postmortem analyses. Histology reveals scattered infiltration by lipid-laden macrophages, accompanied by focal vacuolation, occasional axonal spheroids, and dystrophic calcification. Reactive astrocytosis is noted in the periphery, and the lesions display myelin loss. MRI reveals contrast-enhancement on T1-weighted images and often scattered calcification best identified by cranial CT.

Meningitis

Meningitis in leukemia patients may result from leptomeningeal infiltration of tumor (LM), subarachnoid hemorrhage, chemical (treatment-related following intra-CSF instillation of chemotherapy), or infectious (bacterial or fungal) causes [4–6, 10, 11, 13–15, 24–30]. Subarachnoid hemorrhage often occurs in the context of ICH, either in isolation or more frequently as more diffuse hemorrhage secondary to DIC. Spinal subarachnoid hemorrhage may occur in the context of DIC and APL (M3) and presents primarily with back pain that migrates rostrocaudally.

Chemical meningitis (typically due to intra-CSF cytarabine, especially the liposomal preparation, or methotrexate and most often given intraventricularly) is temporally related to intra-CSF chemotherapy. Chemical meningitis begins 1–2 days after intra-CSF chemotherapy administration, is transient, typically lasting less than 5 days, and demonstrates no evidence of infection with CSF culture. Like other meningitis syndromes, patients complain of headache, fever, nausea, vomiting, photophobia, and meningismus. Notwithstanding an inflammatory CSF, chemical meningitis rapidly abates and is both treated and prevented by steroids.

Infectious meningitis occurs in leukemia due to immunosuppression, both as a result of the underlying disease and its treatment. *Listeria*, *Candida* and *Aspergillus* are common infectious etiologies, however, clinical presentation differs. *Listeria* typically presents as a meningitic syndrome, whereas *Candida* presents with a diffuse encephalopathy and multiple small brain abscesses, and *Aspergillus* presents with progressive hemorrhagic stroke confined to a single or multiple vascular territories.

LM is the most common cause of a meningeal process in patients with leukemia. Acute leukemia, in particular ALL, has the highest propensity to invade the meninges and result in leukemic meningitis (LM) (Figs. 19.2 and 19.3) [12, 14, 24]. This is also true for Burkitt's lymphoma and lymphoblastic lymphoma (2–3% all adult NHL), two subtypes of what is now considered ALL [6]. Although AML infrequently results in LM, an unusual subtype, acute myelomonocytic leukemia (AMML) has a high risk (estimated at 20%) for the development of LM [5, 26]. Prior to CNS prophylaxis, 70% of ALL patients undergoing autopsy had postmortem evidence of LM. However, using contemporary induction protocols with CNS prophylaxis, only 5–10% of adult patients with acute leukemia develop CNS disease [14, 15]. Nonetheless, patients who develop CNS recurrence with leukemia, have a poor prognosis. Chronic leukemias (CLL and CML), the most common adult leukemias encountered, rarely cause LM [10, 11, 25].

Leukemic meningitis may be observed at diagnosis (3–5% all adult patients with ALL), or at relapse (5–7% of adult patients with ALL and prior CNS prophylaxis) [13, 24]. Three groups of patients with LM at relapse are recognized: CNS only (53%), bone marrow followed by CNS relapse (24%), and simultaneous CNS and

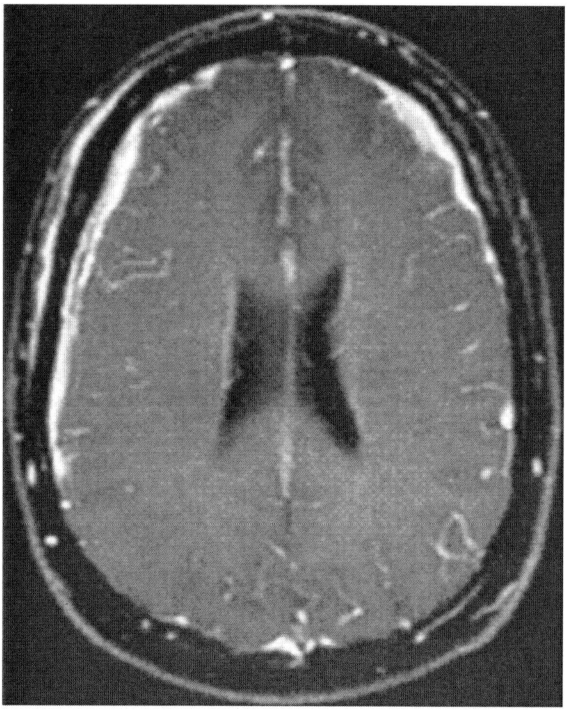

Fig. 19.2 Leptomeningeal enhancement over the cerebral convexities in a patient with recurrent ALL. Axial T1-weighted, post-contrast cranial MRI

Fig. 19.3 Spinal subarachnoid nodules in a patient with ALL. Sagittal post-contrast T1-weighted, cervical spine MRI

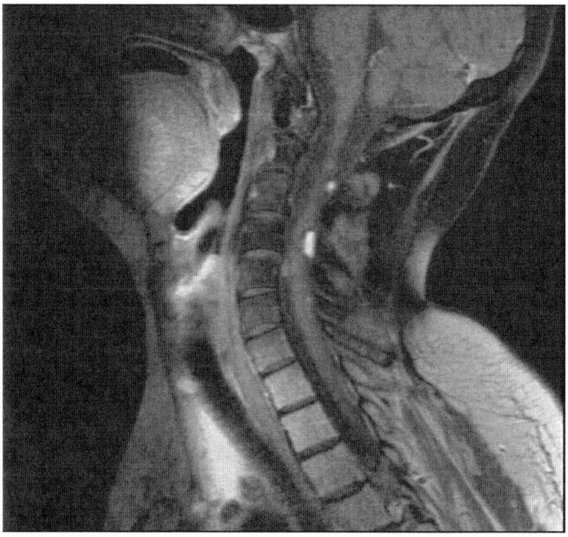

bone marrow relapse (27%). In the series of Surapaneni et al., of 527 consecutive adult patients with ALL, amongst those with isolated LM, 88% subsequently relapsed in the bone marrow [24]. As a consequence, the development of LM, regardless of time after induction therapy, predicts for systemic recurrence and poor outcome. Therefore, the treatment of adult acute leukemia is increasingly defined by CNS risk stratification, and CNS prophylaxis is accordingly tailored to prevent CNS relapse [31].

Risk of LM relapse is associated with several prognostic factors in adults including young age, leukocytosis, presence of extramedullary disease, a high leukemia cell proliferation rate (S+GM fraction >14%), an elevated serum LDH level (>600 U/L), mature B-cell immunophenotype (L3), Philadelphia chromosome positivity [t(9;22)], + CD56 expression by leukemia cells, and an elevated serum β2-microglobulin level (>4 mg/dl) [31–36]. Kantarjian et al. assessed 3 risk factors (elevated serum LDH, elevated serum β2-microglobulin, and a high leukemia cell proliferation rate) in adult ALL and determined the risk of CNS relapse [31, 32]. Four groups were identified and in patients with one risk factor, the incidence of LM at 1 year exceeded 13% and increased to >20% if two or more risk factors were present. This approach has resulted in CNS disease risk stratification and intensification of CNS prophylaxis in adult ALL, in an attempt to reduce the incidence of LM [31]. Similar to data with lymphomatous meningitis, once LM has occurred, prognosis is poor with a median survival of 6 months, although there are occasional long-term survivors [24].

In ALL, the presence of CSF leukemic blasts at diagnosis (3–5% of all patients with ALL), determines survival, according to CSF category. The CSF categories are as follows: normal CSF without blast cells (CNS1), normal CSF i.e. no evidence of pleocytosis (<5 WBC/microliter of CSF) and blasts (CNS2), CSF pleocytosis and blasts (CNS3), traumatic LP with blasts (TLP+), and traumatic lumbar puncture without blasts (TLP-) [37]. Patients with CNS1, CNS2 and TLP- have similar overall survival, whereas patients with CNS3 have a markedly worse prognosis and reduced survival. Patients with TLP+ have intermediate survival relative to CNS1/2 and CNS3. These data suggest two groups of patients (CNS3 and TLP+) who may benefit from more aggressive CNS prophylaxis than the typical regimen administered to CNS1 (and CNS2 and TLP-) patients.

The clinical presentation of LM in patients with leukemia is similar to that observed in patients with LM from solid tumors [26, 29, 30, 38]. However, patients with hematologic malignancies present with a higher frequency of cranial nerve signs (for example trigeminal, oculomotor or optic neuropathies) as initial manifestations of neoplastic meningitis [26]. LM is pleomorphic in its clinical presentation as it affects all levels of the CNS [26, 27, 29, 30, 38]. In general, 3 domains of neurological disturbance are recognized in patients with LM, including: (1) the cerebral hemispheres (2) the cranial nerves, and (3) the spinal cord and nerve roots. The common symptoms and signs of cerebral hemispheric dysfunction are headache, mental status change, including confusion, and seizures.

The single most useful laboratory test in diagnosing LM is an examination of the CSF, usually obtained by lumbar puncture [26, 27, 29, 30, 38, 39]. In nearly all patients with LM, the CSF is abnormal regardless of the results of CSF cytology. A CSF cytological examination positive for malignant cells is the standard method in most clinical series by which LM is diagnosed. Numerous biochemical markers have been evaluated, but in general, their use has been limited by poor sensitivity and specificity [40–46]. In leukemia, monoclonal antibodies against cell surface markers can be used to distinguish between reactive versus neoplastic lymphocytes in the CSF [47, 48]. Furthermore, the demonstration by immunohistochemistry of monoclonality of CSF cells is as compelling as a positive cytology. Lastly, the finding of CSF lymphocytes of B-cell lineage is highly suggestive of LM as reactive lymphocytes in CSF are of T-cell lineage. Cytogenetic studies have also been evaluated in an attempt to improve the diagnostic accuracy of LM. Flow cytometry and DNA single cell cytometry, techniques that measure the chromosomal contents of cells, and fluorescent *in* situ hybridization (FISH) that detects numerical and structural genetic aberrations as a sign of malignancy can give additional diagnostic information, but still have a low sensitivity [49–51]. Polymerase chain reaction (PCR) can establish a correct diagnosis when cytology is inconclusive, but the genetic alteration of the specific leukemia must be known for it to be amplified with this technique; this is particularly pertinent in hematological malignancies [48–51].

A variety of radiographic methods are available to evaluate patients with suspected LM including cranial computed tomography, brain and spine magnetic resonance imaging (S-MR), computerized tomographic myelography (CT-M), and radionuclide CSF flow studies [52–57]. Despite the superiority of cranial contrast-enhanced MR (MR-Gd) or CT in the evaluation of LM, both studies have a high incidence of false negatives (30% by MR-Gd and 58% by CE-CT). Thus, normal studies by either methodology do not exclude a diagnosis of LM, even in patients with negative CSF cytologies; however positive MR-Gd or CE-CT may both be suggestive and diagnostic of LM [26, 27, 29, 30]. MR-Gd and CE-CT are most useful in demonstrating bulky disease, a pattern of disease most responsive to radiotherapy and least responsive to intra-CSF chemotherapy, though less commonly seen with LM from hematologic malignancies than LM in patients with solid tumors. Radionuclide CSF flow studies (FS), or so-called radionuclide ventriculography, provide a safe physiological assessment of the functional anatomy of the CSF spaces [30, 57]. FS have in prior reports demonstrated superiority in detecting interruption of CSF flow in patients with LM when compared with CT-myelography and contrast-enhanced spine MR. However, FS are informative only with respect to compartmentalization of CSF and provide no information regarding bulky leptomeningeal disease, an aspect of LM best addressed by CT-M or S-MR. In addition, CT-M and S-MR are clearly superior to FS in detecting epidural spinal cord compression or intraparenchymal spinal cord metastases, two rare CNS complications of leukemia requiring emergency radiotherapy.

Therefore, patients suspected of LM should undergo: (1) 1 or 2 lumbar punctures for CSF cytology and flow cytometry and if negative, proceed to either a ventricular or lateral cervical CSF analysis in patients strongly suspected to have the disease on clinical grounds; (2) contrast enhanced cranial imaging (MR preferred to CT); (3) contrast enhanced spine MR; and (4) CSF flow study either by lumbar or ventricular radioisotope administration; the ventricular route is preferred if plans include intra-CSF chemotherapy administration via an Ommaya reservoir.

Increasingly, clinicians have adopted a risk-oriented approach to prophylaxis against LM, with therapeutic regimens tailored to the risk of the individual leukemia patient. This approach is a reflection of the poor patient survival following the development of LM (2–6 month median survival) [31].

A compilation of studies from adult patients with ALL using a risk-oriented approach to CNS prophylaxis treatment regimens suggest the following: regimens without cranial irradiation are effective; high-dose systemic therapy for low-risk disease is sufficient without intrathecal therapy; intrathecal methotrexate or alternating with cytarabine is effective without need for triple intrathecal therapy; intrathecal therapy and high-dose systemic chemotherapy are effective for high-risk disease, but the optimal CNS regimen for the high-risk leukemic patient remains undefined and under investigation.

The goal of treatment of LM is palliative and is meant to improve or delay progression of neurological symptoms and signs. The treatment of LM includes craniospinal irradiation, systemic chemotherapy, intrathecal chemotherapy, and high-dose chemotherapy with hematopoietic stem cell rescue (Table 19.2). Since most CNS disease in ALL occurs in the setting of advanced or relapsed systemic disease, control of both CNS and systemic disease is critical.

Table 19.2 Intra-CSF chemotherapy (drugs and drug schedules) for leukemic meningitis

Drugs	Induction regimens		Consolidation regimen		Maintenance regimen	
	Bolus regimen	*CxT regimen	Bolus regimen	*CxT regimen	Bolus regimen	*CxT regimen
Methotrexate	10–15 mg twice weekly (Total 4 weeks)	2 mg/day for 5 days every other week (Total 8 weeks)	10–15 mg once weekly (total 4 weeks)	2 mg/day for 5 days every other week (Total 4 weeks)	10–15 mg once a month	2 mg/day for 5 days once a month
Cytarabine	25–100 mg 2 times weekly (Total 4 weeks)	25 mg/day for 3 days weekly (Total 4 weeks)	25–100 mg once weekly (Total 4 weeks)	25 mg/day for 3 days every other week (Total 4 weeks)	25–100 mg once a month	25 mg/day for 3 days once a month
DepoCyt®	50 mg every 2 weeks (Total 8 weeks)		50 mg every 4 weeks (Total 24 weeks)			
Thiotepa	10 mg 2 times weekly (Total 4 weeks)	10 mg/day for 3 days weekly (Total 4 weeks)	10 mg once weekly (Total 4 weeks)	10 mg/day for 3 days every other week (Total 4 weeks)	10 mg once a month	10 mg/day for 3 days once a month
α-Interferon#	1×10^6 U 2 times weekly (Total 4 weeks)		1×10^6 U 3 times weekly every other week (Total 4 weeks)		1×10^6 U 3 times weekly 1 week per month)	
Etoposide#		0.5 mg/day for 5 days every other week (Total 8 weeks)		0.5 mg/day for 5 days every other week (Total 4 weeks)		0.5 mg/day for 5 days once a month
Topotecan#	0.4 mg 2 times weekly (Total 4 weeks)		0.4 mg 2 times weekly every other week (Total 4 weeks)		0.4 mg 2 times weekly once a month	
Rituximab#	25 mg 2 times weekly (Total 4 weeks)		25 mg 2 times weekly every other week (Total 4 weeks)		25 mg 2 times weekly once a month	

*CxT, Concentration times time method of administration, rarely used; #Considered experimental; U, Units.

Epidural Spinal Cord Compression

Leukemic epidural spinal cord compression (ESCC) is relatively rare (1% occurrence) with two exceptions: Burkitt's lymphoma and lymphoblastic lymphoma (incidence 10–18%), both of which are presently considered as part of the ALL spectrum and similarly treated [4, 6, 15]. Unlike solid cancers that initially metastasize to the vertebral body, leukemic ESCC originates in the paravertebral space and extends through the intervertebral foramina with resultant spinal cord or cauda equina compression. As a consequence, bone involvement by neuroimaging is absent. Additionally and unlike solid cancer, there are no issues of spinal instability due to the lack of vertebral body involvement. Otherwise, the presentation of leukemic ESCC is similar to that commonly seen with lymphoma and solid cancer beginning with pain (local, referred or radicular), and evolving to myelopathy. Surgery is rarely contemplated (unless the primary is unknown) as leukemic ESCC is radiosensitive and responds to systemic chemotherapy. However, chemotherapy alone is reserved for patients with pain-only ESCC syndromes. Most importantly, the presence of ESCC in patients with leukemia does not negatively affect survival as treatment most often results in complete tumor eradication. Two other diagnostic considerations in leukemic patients with ESCC include an epidural hematoma seen most often in the thrombocytopenic patient, following a lumbar puncture and the patient on chronic steroids with steroid-induced epidural lipomatosis.

Radiculopathy

Herpes zoster is a common cause of dermatomal vesicular rash in leukemic patients and is most common in CLL where 7% of patients have at least one *Herpes zoster* infection during the course of their disease [4, 5, 10, 11]. The pain associated with an acute *Herpes zoster* infection may evolve into post-herpetic neuralgia, a chronic and disabling pain syndrome. Disseminated infection may occur in up to 20% of cases during which neurological involvement is observed in 50%. Neurological manifestations occurring in the context of disseminated *Herpes zoster* may include encephalitis, meningitis and motor neuropathies.

Peripheral Neuropathy

Peripheral neuropathies occur in two contexts in leukemia, either by direct tumor infiltration of a nerve or as a consequence of chemotherapy [4, 12]. Optic neuropathy, either unilateral or bilateral, is a common presentation of LM (incidence 20–30%) and warrants emergency radiotherapy to preserve vision. Another common cranial neuropathy is the numb chin syndrome, wherein leukemic cells infiltrate the mental nerve, a subdivision of the mandibular branch of the trigeminal nerve, as it exits the mental foramen in the mandible; leukemic infiltration of the bone results in compromise of the nerve and focal numbness of the chin and lip. It may also be an early indication of LM and warrants CSF evaluation. The most common peripheral neuropathy in leukemic patients is a length-dependent axonal sensorimotor neuropathy caused by vinca alkaloids. Initial symptoms are paresthesias of the hands and feet followed by progressive motor dysfunction, culminating in foot and wrist drop. Occasionally, symptoms may be transiently worsened by administration of granulocyte- or granulocyte macrophage colony stimulating factor. Though the neuropathy may resolve after drug discontinuation, early dose modification based on clinical symptoms and signs may mitigate the development of a disabling chronic neuropathy. Cranial neuropathies from vincristine are uncommon, but may affect the oculomotor, trigeminal, facial, or recurrent laryngeal nerves manifested as ptosis, diplopia, jaw pain, facial paresis, and vocal cord paralysis. These vincristine-related nerve injuries should not be confused with LM. Lastly, transient autonomic neuropathy is common (20–30%) in patients receiving vinca alkaloids; the most common symptoms are abdominal pain and constipation. Rarely, patients treated with high-dose cytarabine develop an acute demyelinating neuropathy, which resembles the Guillain-Barre syndrome and may require transient respiratory support.

Myopathy

Myopathy is observed in the majority of leukemic patients after several weeks (>2 weeks) of therapy, though in susceptible individuals (elderly, deconditioned or malnourished), it may appear within days of steroid therapy [4, 12]. The myopathy is proximal and preferentially affects the lower extremities; over time, shoulder weakness is also observed. It is characterized histologically by bland atrophy of type 2 (fast twitch) fibers. Therapy entails steroid reduction and if possible, discontinuation. Recovery after steroid taper may require months before power returns to normal.

References

1. Xie Y, Davies SM, Xiang Y et al (2004) Trends in leukemia incidence and survival in the United States (1973–1998). Cancer 97(9):2229–2235
2. Hoelzer D, Gokbuget N, Ottmann O et al (2002) Acute lymphoblastic leukemia. Hematology 1:162–171
3. Pui CH, Carroll WL, Meshinchi S, Arceci RJ (2011) Biology, risk stratification, and therapy of pediatric acute leukemias: An update. J Clin Oncol 29(5):551–565
4. Recht L, Mrugala M (2003) Neurologic complications of hematologic neoplasms. Neurol Clin N Am 21:87–105
5. Meyer RJ, Ferreira PP, Cuttner J et al (1980) Central nervous system involvement at presentation in acute granulocytic leukemia. A prospective cytocentrifuge study. Am J Med 68:691–694
6. Teshima T, Akashi K, Shibuka T et al (1990) Central nervous system involvement in adult T-cell leukemia/lymphoma. Cancer 65:327–332

7. Kim H, Lee J-H, Choi S-J et al (2004) Analysis of fatal intracranial hemorrhage in 792 acute leukemia patients. Haematologica 89:622–624
8. Kawanami T, Kurita K, Yamakawa M et al (2002) Cerebrovascular disease in acute leukemia: a clinicopathological study of 14 patients. Intern Med 41(12):1130–1134
9. Sostak P, Padovan CS, Yousry TA et al (2003) Prospective evaluation of neurological complications after allogeneic bone marrow transplantation. Neurology 60:842–848
10. Bower JH, Hammack JE, McDonnell SK, Tefferi A (1997) The neurologic complications of B-cell chronic lymphocytic leukemia. Neurology 48:407–412
11. Cramer SC, Glaspy JA, Efird JT, Louis DN (1996) Chronic lymphocytic leukemia and the central nervous system: A clinical and pathological study. Neurology 46:19–25
12. Plotkin SR, Wen PY (2003) Neurologic complications of cancer therapy. Neurol Clin N Am 21:279–318
13. Cortes J (2001) Central nervous system involvement in adult acute lymphocytic leukemia. Hematol Oncol Clin North Am 15:145–162
14. Wolk RW, Masse SR, Conklin R, Freireich EJ (1974) The incidence of central nervous system leukemia in adults with acute leukemia. Cancer 33:863–871
15. Stewart DJ, Keating MJ, McCredie KB et al (1981) Natural history of central nervous system acute leukemia in adults. Cancer 47:184–196
16. Rachmani R, Avidor A, Youkla P et al (1998) Thrombotic thrombocytopenic purpura complicating chronic myelogenous leukemia treated with alpha-interferon-A report of two successfully treated patients. Acta Haematol 100:204–206
17. Byrnes JJ, Baquerizo H, Gonzalez GT et al (1986) Thrombotic thrombocytopenic purpura subsequent to acute myelogenous leukemia. Am J Hematol 21:299–304
18. Chen C-Y, Zimmerman RA, Faro S et al (1996) Childhood Leukemia: central nervous system abnormalities during and after treatment. AJNR 17:295–310
19. Hinchey J, Chaves C, Appignani B et al (1996) A reversible posterior leukoencephalopathy syndrome. N Engl J Med 334:494
20. Shin RK, Stern JW, Janss AJ et al (2001) Reversible posterior leukoencephalopathy during the treatment of acute lymphoblastic leukemia. Neurology 56:388–391
21. Lavigne CM, Shrier DA, Ketkar M, Powers JM (2004) Tacrolimus leukoencephalopathy: a neuropathological confirmation. Neurology 2:1132–1133
22. Lamy C, Oppenheim C, Meder JF, Mas JL (2004) Neuroimaging in posterior reversible encephalopathy syndrome. J Neuroimaging 14:89–96
23. Anders KH, Becker SP, Holden JK et al (1993) Multifocal necrotizing leukoencephalopathy with pontine predilection in immunosuppressed patients: a clinicopathologic review of 16 cases. Hum Pathol 24(8):897–904
24. Surapaneni UR, Cortes JE, Thomas D et al (2002) Central Nervous System Relapse in Adults with Acute Lymphoblastic Leukemia. Cancer 94(3):773–780
25. Cash J, Fehir KM, Pollack MS (1987) Meningeal involvement in early stage chronic lymphocytic leukemia. Cancer 59:798–800
26. Dekker AW, Elderson A, Punt K, Sixma JJ (1985) Meningeal involvement in patients with acute non-lymphocytic leukemia. Cancer 985(56):2078–2082
27. Kaplan JG, DeSouza TG, Farkash A et al (1990) Leptomeningeal metastases: comparison of clinical features and laboratory data of solid tumors, lymphomas and leukemias. J Neurooncol 9:225–229
28. Chamberlain M (1996) Leptomeningeal metastases. In: Levin V (ed) Cancer in the Nervous System. Churchill Livingstone, New York, NY, pp 282–290
29. Grossman SA, Krabak MJ (1999) Leptomeningeal carcinomatosis. Cancer Treat Rev 25(2):103–119
30. Chamberlain MC (1998) Leptomeningeal metastases: a review of evaluation and treatment. J Neurooncol 37:271–284
31. Kantarjian HM, Walters RS, Smith TL et al (1988) Identification of risk groups for development of central nervous system leukemia in adults with acute lymphocytic leukemia. Blood 72:1784–1789

32. Kantarjian HM, Smith T, Estey E et al (1992) Prognostic significance of elevated serum beta 2-microglobulin levels in acute lymphocytic leukemia. Am J Med 93:599–604
33. Ravandi F, Cortes J, Estrov Z et al (2002) CD56 expression predicts occurrence of CNS disease in acute lymphoblastic leukemia. Leuk Res 26:643–649
34. Kantarijian HM, O'Brien S, Smith TL et al (2000) Results of treatment with hyper-CVAD, a dose-intensive regimen, in adult a cute lymphocytic leukemia. J Clin Oncol 18:547–561
35. Mavlight GM, Stuckey SE, Cabanillas FF et al (1980) Diagnosis of leukemia or lymphoma in the central nervous system by beta 2-microglobulin determination. N Engl J Med. 303: 718–722
36. Kersten MJ, Evers LM, Dellemijn PL et al (1996) Elevation of cerebrospinal fluid soluble CD27 levels in patients with meningeal localization of lymphoid malignancies. Blood 87:1985–1999
37. Burger B, Zimmermann M, Mann G et al (2003) Diagnostic cerebrospinal fluid examination in children with acute lymphoblastic leukemia: significance of low leukocyte counts with blasts or traumatic lumbar puncture. J Clin Oncol 21(2):184–188
38. Wasserstrom W, Glass J, Posner J (1982) Diagnosis and treatment of leptomeningeal metastases from solid tumors experience with 90 patients. Cancer 49:759–772
39. Van Oostenbrugge RJ, Twijnstra A (1999) Presenting features and value of diagnostic procedures in leptomeningeal metastases. Neurology 53:382–385
40. Wasserstrom WR, Schwartz MK, Fleisher M et al (1981) Cerebrospinal fluid biochemical markers in central nervous system tumors: a review. Ann Clin Lab Sci 11(3):239–251
41. Van Zanten AP, Twijnstra A, Hart AA et al (1986) Cerebrospinal fluid lactate dehydrogenase activities in patients with central nervous system metastases. Clin Chim Acta 161(3): 259–268
42. Klee GG, Tallman RD, Goellner JR et al (1986) Elevation of carcinoembryonic antigen in cerebrospinal fluid among patients with meningeal carcinomatosis. Mayo Clin Proc 61(1): 9–13
43. Twijnstra A, van Zanten AP, Hart AA et al (1987) Serial lumbar and ventricle cerebrospinal fluid lactate dehydrogenase activities in patients with leptomeningeal metastases from solid and haematological tumours. J Neurol Neurosurg Psychiatry 50(3):313–320
44. Twijnstra A, Ongerboer de VBW, van Zanten AP et al (1989) Serial lumbar and ventricular cerebrospinal fluid biochemical marker measurements in patients with leptomeningeal metastases from solid and hematological tumors. J Neurooncol 7(1):57–63
45. Chamberlain MC (1998) Cytologically negative carcinomatous meningitis: usefulness of CSF biochemical markers. Neurology 50(4):1173–1175
46. Garson JA, Coakham HB, Kemshead JT et al (1985) The role of monoclonal antibodies in brain tumour diagnosis and cerebrospinal fluid (CSF) cytology. J Neurooncol 3(2):165–171
47. Boogerd W, Vroom TM, van Heerde P et al (1988) CSF cytology versus immunocytochemistry in meningeal carcinomatosis. J Neurol Neurosurg Psychiatry 51(1):142–145
48. Van Oostenbrugge RJ, Hopman AH, Ramaekers FC et al (1998) In situ hybridization: a possible diagnostic aid in leptomeningeal metastasis. J Neurooncol 38(2–3):127–133
49. Cibas ES, Malkin MG, Posner JB et al (1987) Detection of DNA abnormalities by flow cytometry in cells from cerebrospinal fluid. Am J Clin Pathol 88(5):570–577
50. Biesterfeld S, Bernhard B, Bamborschke S et al (1993) DNA single cell cytometry in lymphocytic pleocytosis of the cerebrospinal fluid. Acta Neuropathol (Berl) 86(5):428–432
51. Van Oostenbrugge RJ, Hopman AH, Arends JW et al (1998) The value of interphase cytogenetics in cytology for the diagnosis of leptomeningeal metastases. Neurology 51(3):906–908
52. Chamberlain M, Sandy A, Press G (1990) Leptomeningeal metastasis a comparison of gadolinium-enhanced MR and contrast-enhanced CT of the brain. Neurology 40:435–438
53. Gomori JM, Heching N, Siegal T (1998) Leptomeningeal metastases: evaluation by gadolinium enhanced spinal magnetic resonance imaging. J Neuro Oncol 36:55–60
54. Sze G, Soletsky S, Bronen R et al (1989) MR imaging of the cranial meninges with emphasis on contrast enhancements and meningeal carcinomatosis. AJNR 10:965–975

55. Chamberlain MC (1995) Comparative spine imaging in leptomeningeal metastases. Neurooncol 23:233–238
56. Kramer E, Rafto S, Packer R et al (1991) Comparison of myelography with CT follow-up versus gadolinium MRI for subarachnoid metastatic disease in children. Neurology 41:46–50
57. Chamberlain M, Corey-Bloom J (1991) Leptomeningeal metastases Indium-DTPA CSF flow studies. Neurology 41:1765–1769

Chapter 20
Paraneoplastic Neurological Disorders in Leukemia and Lymphoma

Myrna R. Rosenfeld and Josep Dalmau

Introduction

Paraneoplastic neurological disorders (PND) are an extensive group of neurological syndromes related to the presence of a tumor, but not caused by metastases or other complications such as coagulopathy, infections, nutritional or metabolic disorders, or side effects of cancer treatment [1]. Currently, most PND are considered to be immune-mediated by antibodies (onconeuronal antibodies), cytotoxic T-cells, or cytokines released by inflammatory cells or the tumor. When using this definition, the frequency of PND in patients with leukemia or lymphoma is much lower than the 0.1–1% estimated for patients with solid tumors. PND related to leukemia or lymphoma more frequently involves the peripheral nervous system than the central nervous system. Given that most PND of the peripheral nervous system are not associated with onconeuronal antibodies, most patients with leukemia and lymphoma who develop PND do not harbor these antibodies. Therefore, in these patients, the diagnosis of PND is strongly based on clinical findings.

Diagnostic Approach

Diagnostic criteria for PND have been proposed recently and include 2 categories: definite and possible (Table 20.1) [2]. These criteria take into consideration the syndrome itself (Table 20.2), the response to treatment of the underlying cancer, the temporal relationship of the neurological complaint to the discovery of a cancer, and whether onconeuronal antibodies are present. Some large series of patients, with a specific type of PND (e.g., cerebellar degeneration, limbic encephalitis), contain a few patients who had leukemia or lymphoma. Occasionally, some of these patients had onconeuronal antibodies e.g., Ma2 [3] and CRMP5 [4], but detection

J. Dalmau (✉)
Division of Neuro-Oncology, Department of Neurology, Hospital of the University of Pennsylvania, Philadelphia, PA 19104, USA
e-mail: josep.dalmau@uphs.upenn.edu

T. Batchelor, L.M. DeAngelis (eds.), *Lymphoma and Leukemia of the Nervous System*, DOI 10.1007/978-1-4419-7668-0_20,

of these and other classical ononeuronal antibodies is extremely rare except for anti-Tr antibodies in patients with Hodgkin lymphoma and cerebellar degeneration [5]. Therefore, the above indicated criteria are applicable to some of these patients, but because classical syndromes, as well as onconeuronal antibodies are uncommon, most leukemia and lymphoma patients will fall into the category of possible paraneoplastic syndrome, usually related to a neuropathy of uncertain etiology.

Table 20.1 Diagnostic criteria of PND of the CNS [2]

Definite PND
(1) Classical syndrome *with* cancer diagnosed within 5 years of neurologic symptom development
(2) Non-classical syndrome that resolves or significantly improves after cancer treatment without concomitant immunotherapy, provided that the syndrome is not susceptible to spontaneous remission
(3) Non-classical syndrome *with* cancer diagnosed within 5 years of neurologic symptom development *and* positive antineuronal antibodies
(4) Neurological syndrome (classical or not) *without* cancer and *with* well-characterized antineuronal antibodies (Hu, Yo, CV2/CRMP5, Ri, Ma2, or amphiphysin)
Possible PND
(1) Classical syndrome *with* high risk of cancer, *without* antineuronal antibodies
(2) Neurological syndrome (classical or not) *without* cancer and *with* partially-characterized antineuronal antibodies
(3) Non-classical syndrome *with* cancer diagnosed within 2 years of neurologic symptom development, *without* antineuronal antibodies

One of the criteria of PND is the development of neurological symptoms of unclear etiology that respond to successful treatment of the tumor [2]. A caveat in applying these criteria to patients with leukemia or lymphoma is that these malignancies can occasionally infiltrate and track along the peripheral nerves and nerve roots (neurolymphomatosis) [6–8], which can be difficult to demonstrate with neuroimaging, FDG-PET, or even biopsy, and this may falsely suggest a paraneoplastic syndrome. Moreover, since leukemia and lymphoma often respond to treatment [6], the neurological improvement of these patients may suggest a PND when, in fact, the cause is metastatic invasion of the nerves. A similar problem occurs in the interpretation of dramatic improvements of "limbic encephalitis" in some patients with leukemia or lymphoma [9, 10]. A careful review of the clinical, MRI, and cerebrospinal fluid (CSF) of these patients may show that the MRI abnormalities are different from those found in typical limbic encephalitis (e.g. involving areas of the brain other than the limbic system), and that the improvement of symptoms was likely related to a direct anti-tumor effect on neoplastic cells involving the brain.

Different from patients with solid tumors in whom PND often precede the diagnosis of the tumor, the timing of symptom development is not well established in patients with leukemia or lymphoma. Two exceptions include: anti-Tr associated

Table 20.2 Paraneoplastic syndromes of the nervous system

	Paraneoplastic neurological disorders	
Location of pathological findings	Classical	Non-classical
Brain, cranial nerves and retina	Cerebellar degeneration Limbic encephalitis Encephalomyelitis Opsoclonus-myoclonus	Brainstem encephalitis Optic neuritis Cancer-associated retinopathy Melanoma-associated retinopathy
Spinal cord		Stiff-person syndrome Myelitis Necrotizing myelopathy Motor neuron syndromes
Neuromuscular junction	Lambert-Eaton myasthenic syndrome	Myasthenia gravis
Peripheral nerves or muscle	Sensory neuronopathy Intestinal pseudoobstruction Dermatomyositis	Sensorimotor neuropathy Neuropathy and paraproteinemia Neuropathy with vasculitis Acquired neuromyotonia Autonomic neuropathies Polymyositis Acute necrotizing myopathy

cerebellar degeneration that often precedes the diagnosis of Hodgkin lymphoma, and peripheral neuropathies related to monoclonal gammopathies of uncertain significance (MGUS), which may precede the transformation into a malignant B- or plasma cell disorder.

Patients with leukemia or lymphoma often undergo autologous or heterologous hematopoietic stem cell transplant that may cause a large variety of neurological complications, that could be incorrectly attributed to a PND (see Chapter 23) [11]. Some complications related to drugs to increase blood cell counts (colony stimulating factors) and complications of graft versus host disease may result in inflammatory or immune mediated disorders (myasthenia gravis, dermatomyositis, acute polyradiculoneuritis) that may be mistakenly attributed to an underlying paraneoplastic disorder (Fig. 20.1). Infections that predominantly occur in the post-transplant period or in immunocompromised patients, such as human herpesvirus 6 (HHV6) encephalitis, may cause a limbic encephalitis that is clinically and radiologically indistinguishable from a paraneoplastic syndrome (Fig. 20.2) [12, 13].

Overall, the above considerations should bring a note of caution when applying the standard clinical criteria of PND (mainly developed for solid tumors) to patients with leukemia or lymphoma. In most instances, the diagnosis will depend on the exclusion of other disorders, rather than on supportive tests (e.g., presence of onconeuronal antibodies).

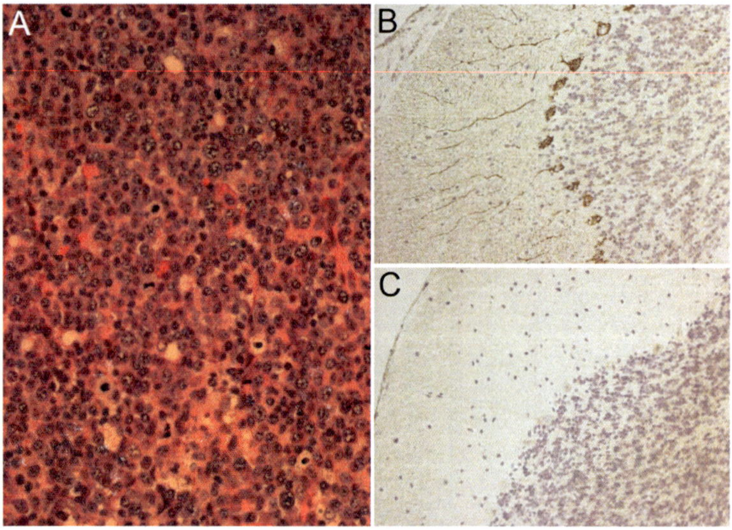

Fig. 20.1 Post-transplant lymphoproliferative disorder and Tr antibodies. This patient had a history of liver transplant and chronic treatment with tacrolimus, when she developed a neuropathy in the lower extremities. She was diagnosed with a post-transplant lymphoproliferative disorder (PTLD, **panel a**) and had rapid worsening of the neuropathy. Serum studies revealed Epstein–Barr virus and antibodies to Tr (**panel b**, an antibody that usually associates with paraneoplastic cerebellar degeneration and Hodgkin lymphoma). Decreased immunosuppression and treatment with rituximab led to complete remission of the PTLD and substantial improvement of the neuropathy, along with reduction of levels of Epstein–Barr virus and Tr antibodies (**panel c**). **Panel a** shows the lymph node biopsy, with extensive infiltration of plasma cells, a few atypical lymphoid cells, and a few scattered macrophages. **Panels b** and **c**, show the reactivity of the patient's serum Tr antibodies with Purkinje cells in sections of rat brain, before (**b**) and after (**c**) treatment

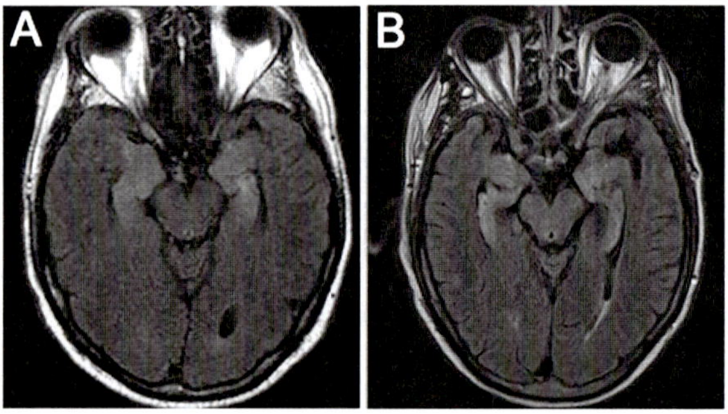

Fig. 20.2 Paraneoplastic limbic encephalitis and human herpesvirus 6 limbic encephalitis. **Panel a** shows typical increased fluid-attenuated inversion recovery (FLAIR) signal involving the hippocampi of a patient with paraneoplastic limbic encephalitis. For comparison **panel b** shows medial temporal lobe FLAIR abnormalities along with atrophy in a patient who developed human herpesvirus 6 limbic encephalitis

Specific Paraneoplastic Neurological Disorders

Cerebellar Degeneration

This disorder may occur in patients with Hodgkin or non-Hodgkin lymphoma and is characterized by the subacute onset of dizziness, vertigo, oscillopsia, gait unsteadiness that in a few days or weeks, evolve to gait and limb ataxia. Other clinical features may include dysarthria, dysphagia, diplopia (often without obvious oculoparesis), and downbeating nystagmus. The CSF usually demonstrates lymphocytic pleocytosis, moderate increase of protein concentration, and in approximately 60% of patients, oligoclonal bands or elevated IgG index. MRI of the brain is often normal at symptom onset, but shows progressive cerebellar atrophy as the disease evolves. However, in some patients, early MRI studies show cerebellar cortical fluid-attenuated inversion recovery (FLAIR) and T2 hyperintensities with contrast enhancement that may suggest leptomeningeal lymphoma.

Patients with Hodgkin lymphoma and, rarely, non Hodgkin lymphoma, develop antibodies (anti-Tr) that predominantly react with the cytoplasm and dendrites of Purkinje cells [14, 15]. The target autoantigen is unknown. Any patient who develops cerebellar degeneration in association with these antibodies should be carefully evaluated for an underlying Hodgkin lymphoma [5, 16]. However, the same antibody-related cerebellar syndrome may occur without a tumor association, and rarely the antibody has been found in patients with other symptoms, such as peripheral neuropathy. Some patients with anti-Tr antibodies develop transient encephalitis in association with mild cerebellar symptoms, tremor, and myoclonus, preceding the diagnosis of Hodgkin lymphoma. The diagnosis of anti-Tr associated cerebellar degeneration is important because these patients often respond to treatment of the tumor and immunotherapy with corticosteroids, intravenous immunoglobuin (IVIg), or plasma exchange [5, 16].

Another autoimmune response described in two patients with acute cerebellar degeneration is directed against the metabotropic glutamate receptor (mGluR1) [17]. The two patients developed symptoms while in remission of a Hodgkin lymphoma and neither improved with immunotherapy. Passive transfer of antibodies to rodents reproduced the cerebellar dysfunction.

There are no convincing patients reported with leukemia and immune-mediated paraneoplastic cerebellar degeneration.

Limbic Encephalitis

This disorder has been reported in multiple single case reports of patients with Hodgkin lymphoma (the "Ophelia syndrome) [18–24] and rarely with non-Hodgkin lymphoma [25–27]. There are no convincing cases in association with leukemia. Patients usually develop progressive alteration of mood, irritability, depression, sleep disturbances, seizures, hallucinations, and short-term memory loss [28, 29]. Patients may be agitated or quietly confused, repeating the same questions, sometimes with episodes of staring, and psychomotor or temporal lobe seizures. Less frequently, patients are agitated with delirium, delusional thoughts and paranoid ideation [21]. Regardless of the type of presentation, the EEG is almost always abnormal, revealing foci of epileptic activity in one or both temporal lobes or focal or generalized slow activity. In general, the neurological symptoms precede the diagnosis of Hodgkin lymphoma, although it has been reported during remission in some patients.

In 80% of the patients, the CSF shows mild to moderate lymphocytic pleocytosis, usually less than 100 white blood cells/μl, increased protein concentration (usually <150 mg/dl), normal glucose concentration, and frequently elevated IgG index and oligoclonal bands. In 70–80% of patients with a typical syndrome of limbic encephalitis, the MRI FLAIR or T2 sequences demonstrate hyperintense signal in the medial aspect of the temporal lobes. Some patients may have additional MRI abnormalities in other brain regions, including the thalamus ("pulvinar sign"), which along with symptoms of rapidly progressive cognitive decline and memory deficits may suggest Creutzfeldt-Jakob disease [26].

Overall, the information provided by the combination of clinical, EEG, MRI, and CSF studies suggests the diagnosis of limbic encephalitis in most patients with a classic presentation of the syndrome [30]. Some patients have antibodies to neuronal cell surface antigens with a pattern of immunoreactivity that suggest that the target antigen is a synaptic protein (Fig. 20.3).

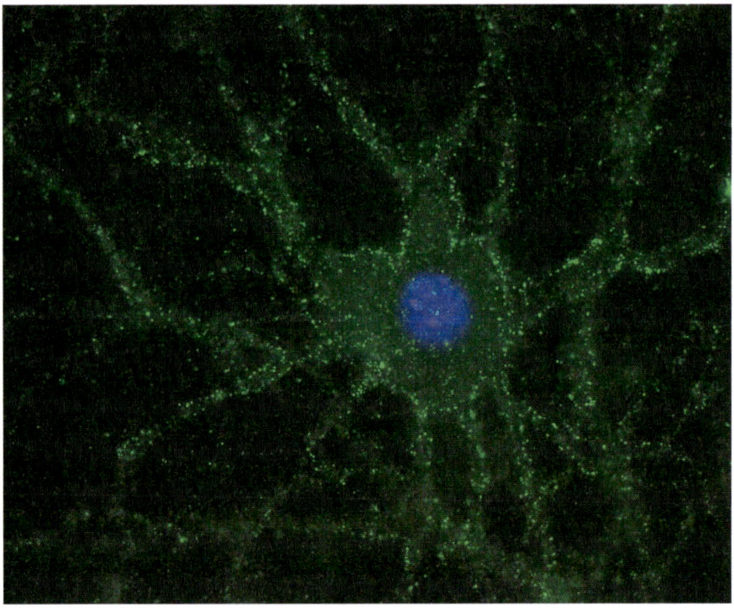

Fig. 20.3 Antibodies to neuronal cell surface antigens in a patient with Hodgkin lymphoma and limbic encephalitis (Ophelia syndrome). Immunolabeling of live, non-permeabilized cultured hippocampal rat neurons with CSF of a patient with Hodgkin disease and limbic encephalitis indicating that the target epitopes are on the cell surface. The antigen is unknown

There are a few patients with Hodgkin lymphoma who have presented with diffuse paraneoplastic encephalitis [31], or a combination of several paraneoplastic syndromes, including, limbic encephalitis, stiff-person syndrome and demyelinating neuropathy [24].

Limbic encephalitis associated with Hodgkin lymphoma frequently responds to treatment of the tumor and immunotherapy [20, 21, 31, 32]. If the disorder is not recognized and treated, it may evolve to hippocampal sclerosis and dementia [23].

Miscellaneous Paraneoplastic Syndromes of the Central Nervous System

Other paraneoplastic syndromes of the central nervous system related to lymphoma include stiff-person syndrome [33], myelopathy [34], motor neuron disease, and retinopathy. A patient with primary hypothalamic lymphoma developed stiff-person syndrome in association with panhypopituitarism [35]. Patients with Hodgkin lymphoma may develop a subacute myelopathy associated with intense vasculitis of the spinal cord [36]. It is unclear whether these old case reports represent a viral process, such as varizella-zoster infection, common in immunosuppressed patients. Other reports of patients with Hodgkin lymphoma and subacute myelopathy were characterized by neurological improvement after intrathecal administration of dexamethasone [37, 38].

In a report of 10 patients with motor neuron disease associated with Hodgkin or non-Hodgkin lymphoma, 7 had neurological improvement independent of the status of their malignancy. All but 1 patient had a pure lower motor neuron syndrome. In these patients, weakness tended to be asymmetric and greater in the legs than the arms [39]. However, in another report, only 1 of 9 patients had some neurological improvement. The patient who improved had only lower motor neuron features, as well as proximal conduction block on nerve conduction studies; the other 8 patients had either probable or definite upper and lower motor neuron dysfunction [40]. These reports suggest that patients with lymphoma who develop a pure lower motor neuron syndrome may have a relatively benign neurological course, but if they have upper and lower motor neuron dysfunction, the syndrome is severe and progresses in a fashion typical of amyotrophic lateral sclerosis.

Paraneoplastic retinopathy has been reported in a few patients with chronic lymphocytic leukemia, some of whom have enolase antibodies [41], and in patients with Hodgkin [42] and non-Hodgkin lymphoma [43]. Some of these patients had recoverin antibodies, while in others, the target retinal antigen was unknown.

Polyradiculoneuritis (Guillain-Barré) and Brachial Neuritis

Patients with Hodgkin lymphoma are at increased risk of developing an acute polyradiculoneuritis identical to Guillain-Barré syndrome (GBS) [44]. In some patients, the GBS may be the first manifestation of tumor relapse. Treatment is the same as for the non-cancer related forms of GBS and consists of plasma exchange and IVIg neither of which is contraindicated in patients with cancer [44]. There is some evidence suggesting that patients with cancer-associated GBS have a worse neurological outcome compared to patients with GBS and no underlying cancer [44].

One patient with acute lymphoblastic leukemia and chronic graft versus host disease (cGVHD) developed an inflammatory demyelinating polyradiculoneuropathy that responded to high-dose immunoglobulin therapy [45]. Another patient with a Burkitt-like lymphoma developed a neuropathy suggestive of an axonal GBS [46]. In both cases, the authors suggested that immunological mechanisms triggered by the cGVHD or the lymphoma were involved in the development of the neuropathy. There may be an increased risk of GBS following hematopoietic stem cell transplantation (HSCT), although the mechanisms are unclear [47]. When GBS occurs early in the post-transplant period, it has been attributed to cytosine arabinoside in the conditioning regimen [48]. The development of an axonal GBS, during the period of rapid immune reconstitution, following an allogenic HSCT was attributed to immune dysregulation [49].

One patient with Hodgkin lymphoma developed bilateral brachial plexopathies 2 months after radiation therapy, and surgical exploration showed perineural edema and mononuclear cell infiltrates; treatment with prednisone led to complete resolution of neurological symptoms [50]. Another patient with Hodgkin lymphoma developed brachial neuritis shortly after chemotherapy, and a Lhermitte's sign after radiation therapy; despite successful treatment of the tumor, the patient did not recover from the neuropathy [51].

Paraneoplastic Vasculitis of Nerve and Muscle

In a review of the literature, 3 of 13 patients with this disorder had lymphoma [52]. One study reported a patient who presented with multiple cranial neuropathies and later, mononeuritis multiplex of the extremities [53]. A nerve biopsy revealed microvasculitis and the patient was treated with prednisone, IVIg, azathioprine, and cyclosporine without benefit. Three years following the initial presentation, the patient developed a gammopathy and a bone marrow biopsy revealed a B-cell lymphoma. Repeat nerve biopsy demonstrated near total destruction of axons, with replacement within the axon of IgM-related material, without evidence for vasculitis; similar IgM material was found around the blood vessels.

Patients with chronic lymphoid leukemia may develop peripheral neuropathy as a result of paraneoplastic leukocytoclastic vasculitis (Fig. 20.4) [54]. Paraneoplastic vasculitis resulting in neuropathy is important to recognize because it usually responds to treatment of the tumor, corticosteroids, or cyclophosphamide.

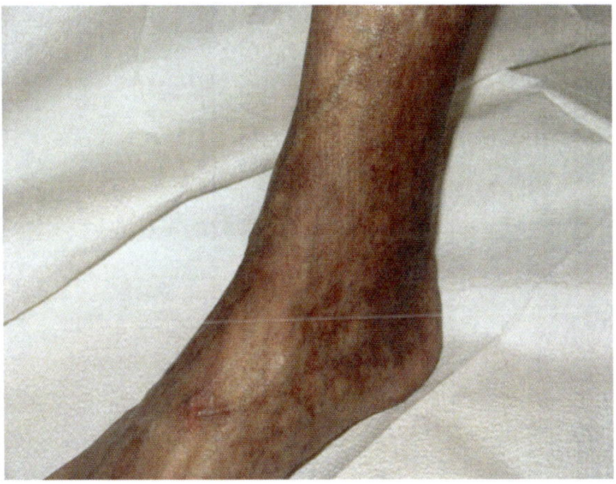

Fig. 20.4 Paraneoplastic leukocytoclastic vasculitis and neuropathy. Skin purpura caused by leukocytoclastic vasculitis involving the lower extremities of a patient with marginal-zone lymphoma. The patient developed a sensorimotor neuropathy with predominantly axonal features selectively involving the lower extremities. The skin lesions and neuropathy resolved completely after treatment of the lymphoma with cyclophosphamide, adriamycin, rituximab and prednisone

Miscellaneous Paraneoplastic Syndromes of the Peripheral Nervous System

Neuromyotonia or Isaacs syndrome, a disorder characterized by spontaneous and continuous muscle fiber activity of peripheral nerve origin, has been reported in patients with Hodgkin lymphoma. In one case, symptoms involving bulbar muscles developed while the tumor was in remission; the patient responded to treatment with carbamazepine [55]. In another patient, the neurological symptoms were the first manifestation of the Hodgkin lymphoma [56].

Lymphoproliferative disorders including Hodgkin and non-Hodgkin lymphoma, and Castleman's disease may occur in association with the Lambert-Eaton myasthenic syndrome (LEMS) [57]. In a review of the literature, Tyagi et al identified 9 patients with LEMS and lymphoproliferative disorders [58]. The neurological symptoms usually respond to treatment of the neoplastic disease along with medication to increase the release of acetylcholine, and immunomodulation.

The association of myasthenia gravis with tumors other than thymoma is controversial. However, in some instances, the association appears more than coincidental. A patient with acetylcholine receptor antibody positive myasthenia gravis had limited response to pyridostigmine; 2 years later, a lymphoma was diagnosed and treated with resolution of the myasthenia [59].

Multiple case reports of lymphoma and leukemia associated with dermatomyositis and polymyositis suggest that these are true paraneoplastic syndromes [60–64]. Although paraneoplastic dermatomyositis is extremely rare in children, a 14 year old girl developed a B-cell lymphoma arising from a calcinoid lesion [65]. In another child, polymyositis was the presenting symptom of an immunoblastic sarcoma [66].

Neuropathies Associated with Malignant Monoclonal Gammopathies

The neuropathies associated with monoclonal gammopathies or paraproteinemia are a varied group of disorders that are potentially treatable [67]. Approximately 10% of patients with multiple myeloma develop neuropathy that may be in the form of a mild sensorimotor axonal neuropathy, a pure sensory neuropathy or a subacute monophasic, or relapsing and remitting neuropathy. If the myeloma is associated with amyloidosis, neuropathic symptoms often include autonomic dysfunction and lancinating, and burning dysesthesias [68]. The onset of the neuropathy often precedes the myeloma diagnosis, and treatment of the myeloma does not usually alter the course of the neuropathy; the impact of immunotherapies is unknown.

In contrast, more than 50% of patients with osteosclerotic myeloma develop a symmetrical, predominantly motor peripheral neuropathy similar to a chronic inflammatory demyelinating polyradiculoneuropathy (CIDP). Some patients will develop additional symptoms indicative of the POEMS syndrome (polyneuropathy, organomegaly, endocrinopathy and skin changes). Radiological evaluation often reveals one or a few osteosclerotic lesions most commonly found in the truncal and proximal long bones, and radiation often results in improvement of the neuropathy. Systemic chemotherapy, with or without corticosteroids, should be considered for patients with diffuse sclerotic lesions, or those with no obvious bone lesions [69, 70]. In one report, patients with POEMS syndrome and a rapidly progressive neuropathy improved after peripheral blood stem cell transplant [71]. Plasma exchange or IVIg have not been shown to be effective in isolated cases [72], although there is a single patient in whom IVIg with corticosteroids produced a dramatic improvement [73].

Castleman's disease (angiofollicular lymph node hyperplasia) is a rare disorder that overlaps with the POEMS syndrome. Patients develop several types of neuropathies, including a painful sensorimotor neuropathy, a chronic relapsing sensorimotor neuropathy, and a predominantly motor neuropathy [74]. Variable benefit has been reported with resection of the involved lymph nodes, chemotherapy, interferon-alpha, rituximab, anti-IL-6 receptor antibodies, thalidomide, or plasma exchange [75]. There is an increased incidence of Castleman's disease in patients with HIV, usually in association with the human herpes virus-8. Specific serum antibodies are absent and serum levels of interleukin-6 are often elevated [76].

Approximately 10% of patients with Waldenström's macroglobulinemia develop a progressive distal sensorimotor polyneuropathy with initial involvement, predominantly of large sensory fibers, especially those for vibration. The neuropathy may result from an IgM protein against myelin-associated glycoprotein (MAG) or various gangliosides, including GD1b and GM1 [77]. The neuropathy in some patients may also be due to amyloid deposition or cryoglobulinemia. In addition to treatment aimed at the Waldenström's macroglobulinemia, there are reports of patients with anti-MAG IgM who improved with fludarabine, rituximab, or after autologous peripheral stem cell transplant [78–80]. In general, most patients require aggressive chemotherapy, which may result in improvement or stabilization of the neuropathy [79, 81].

Patients with monoclonal gammopathy of undetermined significance (MGUS) develop one of several neuropathic syndromes, and require close observation as they are at risk for transformation of the gammopathy to a malignant hematologic disorder (most commonly lymphoma, multiple myeloma or Waldenström's macroglobulinemia). While the risk for transformation varies, depending on the study and length of follow-up, in general, the risk of progression is estimated at 1% per year and patients remain at risk even after 25 years or more of follow-up [82, 83].

Plasma exchange may be efficacious for the peripheral neuropathy associated with MGUS due to elevated IgG or IgA, but not IgM, proteins [84] There is a report of one patient who responded to peripheral blood stem cell transplantation [85]. Some patients with MGUS develop a chronic inflammatory demyelinating polyneuropathy (CIDP-MGUS), and these patients appear to respond to the same treatment utilized for idiopathic CIDP, including IVIg, plasma exchange, and corticosteroids [86, 87].

Patients with IgM-MGUS comprise a separate clinical category and in general, have worse responses to therapy than IgA or IgG-MGUS. About 50% of patient's with IgM-MGUS have anti-MAG antibodies and of those without these antibodies, many will have monoclonal antibodies that react with gangliosides [88]. Antibodies to GM1 ganglioside are primarily associated with motor neuropathies or a lower motor neuron syndrome [89, 90], while antibodies to GD1b have been associated with a sensory ataxic neuropathy [91].

The neuropathies associated with IgM-MGUS are usually chronic, slowly progressive, and in general, refractory to therapies. However, there are reports of responses to fludarabine or rituximab [80, 92]. A recent prospective trial of 17 patients with disabling IgM-MGUS polyneuropathy compared outcomes after treatment with rituximab, intermittent cyclophosphamide with prednisone or fludarabine. For all three treatments, approximately 10% of subjects responded by the primary outcome measurement of improvement of 1 point or more on the Overall Disability Sum Score [93]. In contrast, a study of two patients with a chronic motor neuropathy associated with anti-ganglioside IgM antibodies demonstrated no response to 1 year of treatment with rituximab [94], and one patient with anti-MAG antibodies had significant worsening of their neuropathy, temporally related to treatment with rituximab [95]. The utility of IVIg in MGUS neuropathy remains controversial with conflicting reports in the literature, although there is one class I study suggesting short-term benefit in some patients [96]. One study of patients with MAG associated IgM-MGUS compared IVIg to interferon-alpha and reported significant improvement with interferon-alpha, but not with IVIg [97].

References

1. Dalmau JO, Posner JB (1997) Paraneoplastic syndromes affecting the nervous system. Semin Oncol 24:318–328
2. Graus F, Delattre JY, Antoine JC et al (2004) Recommended diagnostic criteria for paraneoplastic neurological syndromes. J Neurol Neurosurg Psychiatry 75:1135–1140
3. Dalmau J, Graus F, Villarejo A et al (2004) Clinical analysis of anti-Ma2-associated encephalitis. Brain 127:1831–1844
4. Samii A, Dahlen DD, Spence AM et al (2003) Paraneoplastic movement disorder in a patient with non-Hodgkin's lymphoma and CRMP-5 autoantibody. Mov Disord 18:1556–1558
5. Bernal F, Shams'ili S, Rojas I et al (2003) Anti-Tr antibodies as markers of paraneoplastic cerebellar degeneration and Hodgkin's disease. Neurology 60:230–234
6. Baehring JM, Damek D, Martin EC et al (2003) Neurolymphomatosis. Neurooncol 5: 104–115
7. Gherardi R, Gaulard P, Prost C et al (1986) T-cell lymphoma revealed by a peripheral neuropathy. A report of two cases with an immunohistologic study on lymph node and nerve biopsies. Cancer 58:2710–2716
8. Odabasi Z, Parrott JH, Reddy VV et al (2001) Neurolymphomatosis associated with muscle and cerebral involvement caused by natural killer cell lymphoma: a case report and review of literature. J Peripher Nerv Syst 6:197–203
9. Markert A, May A, Weber J et al (2009) Bilateral renal lymphoma after paraneoplastic limbic encephalitis. J Clin Oncol 27:1142–1144
10. Rajappa S, Digumarti R, Immaneni SR et al (2007) Primary renal lymphoma presenting with paraneoplastic limbic encephalitis. J Clin Oncol 25:3783–3785
11. Rosenfeld MR, Pruitt A (2006) Neurologic complications of bone marrow, stem cell, and organ transplantation in patients with cancer. Semin Oncol 33:352–361
12. Seeley WW, Marty FM, Holmes TM et al (2007) Post-transplant acute limbic encephalitis: clinical features and relationship to HHV6. Neurology 69:156–165
13. Wainwright MS, Martin PL, Morse RP et al (2001) Human herpesvirus 6 limbic encephalitis after stem cell transplantation. Ann Neurol 50:612–619
14. Graus F, Dalmau J, Valldeoriola F et al (1997) Immunological characterization of a neuronal antibody (anti-Tr) associated with paraneoplastic cerebellar degeneration and Hodgkin's disease. J Neuroimmunol 74:55–61
15. Graus F, Gultekin SH, Ferrer I et al (1998) Localization of the neuronal antigen recognized by anti-Tr antibodies from patients with paraneoplastic cerebellar degeneration and Hodgkin's disease in the rat nervous system. Acta Neuropathol (Berl) 96:1–7
16. Hammack J, Kotanides H, Rosenblum MK et al (1992) Paraneoplastic cerebellar degeneration. II. Clinical and immunologic findings in 21 patients with Hodgkin's disease. Neurology 42:1938–1943
17. Sillevis SP, Kinoshita A, De Leeuw B et al (2000) Paraneoplastic cerebellar ataxia due to autoantibodies against a glutamate receptor. N Engl J Med 342:21–27
18. Carr I (1982) The Ophelia syndrome: memory loss in Hodgkin's disease. Lancet 1:844–845
19. de Bot ST, Dorresteijn LD, Haaxma CA et al (2008) From psychiatric symptoms to paraneoplastic syndrome. Tijdschr Psychiatry 50:603–609
20. Deodhare S, O'Connor P, Ghazarian D et al (1996) Paraneoplastic limbic encephalitis in Hodgkin's disease. Can J Neurol Sci 23:138–140
21. Kung S, Mueller PS, Geda YE et al (2002) Delirium resulting from paraneoplastic limbic encephalitis caused by Hodgkin's disease. Psychosomatics 43:498–501
22. Rosenbaum T, Gartner J, Korholz D et al (1998) Paraneoplastic limbic encephalitis in two teenage girls. Neuropediatrics 29:159–162
23. Shinohara T, Kojima H, Nakamura N et al (2005) Pathology of pure hippocampal sclerosis in a patient with dementia and Hodgkin's disease: the Ophelia syndrome. Neuropathology 25:353–360

24. Werbrouck B, Meire V, De Bleecker JL (2005) Multiple neurological syndromes during Hodgkin lymphoma remission. Acta Neurol Belg 105:48–50
25. Dogel D, Beuing O, Koenigsmann M et al (2008) Paraneoplastic limbic encephalitis resulting from non-Hodgkin lymphoma: two case reports. Fortschr Neurol Psychiatry 76:41–46
26. Mihara M, Sugase S, Konaka K et al (2005) The "pulvinar sign" in a case of paraneoplastic limbic encephalitis associated with non-Hodgkin's lymphoma. J Neurol Neurosurg Psychiatry 76:882–884
27. Thuerl C, Muller K, Laubenberger J et al (2003) MR imaging of autopsy-proved paraneoplastic limbic encephalitis in non-Hodgkin lymphoma. Am J Neuroradiol 24:507–511
28. Gultekin SH, Rosenfeld MR, Voltz R et al (2000) Paraneoplastic limbic encephalitis: neurological symptoms, immunological findings and tumour association in 50 patients. Brain 123:1481–1494
29. Tüzun E, Dalmau J (2007) Limbic encephalitis and variants: classification, diagnosis and treatment. Neurologist 13:261–271
30. Dalmau J, Bataller L (2006) Clinical and immunological diversity of limbic encephalitis: a model for paraneoplastic neurologic disorders. Hematol Oncol Clin North Am 20:1319–1335
31. Epaulard O, Courby S, Pavese P et al (2004) Paraneoplastic acute diffuse encephalitis revealing Hodgkin's disease. Leuk Lymphoma 45:2509–2512
32. Bernard P, Vinzio S, Talarmin F et al (2003) Hodgkin's disease manifesting as paraneoplastic limbic encephalitis. Rev Med Interne 24:257–260
33. Gutmann B, Crivellaro C, Mitterer M et al (2006) Paraneoplastic stiff-person syndrome, heterotopic soft tissue ossification and gonarthritis in a HLA B27-positive woman preceding the diagnosis of Hodgkin's lymphoma. Haematologica 91:ECR59
34. Anderson DW, Borsaru A (2008) Case report: lymphoma-related resolving paraneoplastic myelopathy with MRI correlation. Br J Radiol 81:e103–e105
35. Lee MT, Lee TI, Won JG et al (2004) Primary hypothalamic lymphoma with panhypopituitarism presenting as stiff-man syndrome. Am J Med Sci 328:124–128
36. Lester EP, Feld E, Kinzie JJ et al (1979) Necrotizing myelopathy complicating Hodgkin's disease. Arch Neurol 36:583–585
37. Dansey RD, Hammond-Tooke GD, Lai K et al (1988) Subacute myelopathy: an unusual paraneoplastic complication of Hodgkin's disease. Med Pediatr Oncol 16:284–286
38. Hughes M, Ahern V, Kefford R et al (1992) Paraneoplastic myelopathy at diagnosis in a patient with pathologic stage 1A Hodgkin disease. Cancer 70:1598–1600
39. Schold SC, Cho ES, Somasundaram M et al (1979) Subacute motor neuronopathy: a remote effect of lymphoma. Ann Neurol 5:271–287
40. Younger DS, Rowland LP, Latov N et al (1990) Motor neuron disease and amyotrophic lateral sclerosis: relation of high CSF protein content to paraproteinemia and clinical syndromes. Neurology 40:595–599
41. Adamus G, Aptsiauri N, Guy J et al (1996) The occurrence of serum autoantibodies against enolase in cancer-associated retinopathy. Clin Immunol Immunopathol 78:120–129
42. To KW, Thirkill CE, Jakobiec FA et al (2002) Lymphoma-associated retinopathy. Ophthalmology 109:2149–2153
43. Matus G, Dicato M, Focan C (2007) Cancer associated retinopathy (CAR). Two clinical cases and review of the literature. Rev Med Liege 62:166–169
44. Vigliani MC, Magistrello M, Polo P et al (2004) Risk of cancer in patients with Guillain-Barre syndrome (GBS). A population-based study. J Neurol 251:321–326
45. Wada S, Kimura T, Ikegame K et al (2008) Chronic inflammatory demyelinating polyradiculoneuropathy and hyponatremia in a patient with chronic graft versus host disease. Rinsho Shinkeigaku 48:426–429
46. Wanschitz J, Dichtl W, Budka H et al (2006) Acute motor and sensory axonal neuropathy in Burkitt-like lymphoma. Muscle Nerve 34:494–498
47. Wen PY, Alyea EP, Simon D et al (1997) Guillain-Barré syndrome following allogeneic bone marrow transplantation. Neurology 49:1711–1714

48. Rodriguez V, Kuehnle I, Heslop HE et al (2002) Guillain-Barré syndrome after allogeneic hematopoietic stem cell transplantation. Bone Marrow Transplant 29:515–517
49. Fujisaki G, Kami M, Murashige N et al (2006) Guillain-Barré syndrome associated with rapid immune reconstitution following allogeneic hematopoietic stem cell transplantation. Bone Marrow Transplant 37:617–619
50. Lachance DH, O'Neill BP, Harper CM Jr et al (1991) Paraneoplastic brachial plexopathy in a patient with Hodgkin's disease. Mayo Clin Proc 66:97–101
51. Symonds RP, Hogg RB, Bone I (1994) Paraneoplastic neurological syndromes associated with lymphomas. Leuk Lymphoma 15:487–490
52. Oh SJ (1997) Paraneoplastic vasculitis of the peripheral nervous system. Neurol Clin 15: 849–863
53. Turner MR, Warren JD, Jacobs JM et al (2003) Microvasculitic paraproteinaemic polyneuropathy and B-cell lymphoma. J Peripher Nerv Syst 8:100–107
54. Yadav BS, Sharma SC, Kapoor RK (2006) Paraneoplastic leukocytoclastic vasculitis in chronic lymphoid leukemia. J Cancer Res Ther 2:206–208
55. Lahrmann H, Albrecht G, Drlicek M et al (2001) Acquired neuromyotonia and peripheral neuropathy in a patient with Hodgkin's disease. Muscle Nerve 24:834–838
56. Caress JB, Abend WK, Preston DC et al (1997) A case of Hodgkin's lymphoma producing neuromyotonia. Neurology 49:258–259
57. Argov Z, Shapira Y, Averbuch-Heller L et al (1995) Lambert-Eaton myasthenic syndrome (LEMS) in association with lymphoproliferative disorders. Muscle Nerve 18:715–719
58. Tyagi A, Connolly S, Hutchinson M (2001) Lambert-Eaton myaesthenic syndrome: a possible association with Hodgkin's lymphoma. Ir Med J 94:18–19
59. Abrey LE (1995) Association of myasthenia gravis with extrathymic Hodgkin's lymphoma: complete resolution of myasthenic symptoms following antineoplastic therapy. Neurology 45:1019
60. Ambrosone L, Migliaresi S, Rambaldi A et al (1995) Adult polymyositis/dermatomyositis associated with acute myeloid leukemia. A case report. Clin Rheumatol 14:217–219
61. Langan SM, O'Briain S, Barnes L (2003) Dermatomyositis associated with angiotropic lymphoma. Clin Exp Dermatol 28:597–599
62. Lima M, Coutinho J, Bernardo L et al (2002) Philadelphia-positive T-cell acute lymphoblastic leukemia with polymyositis, migratory polyarthritis and hypercalcemia following a chronic myeloid leukemia. Ann Hematol 81:174–177
63. Salvatore JR, Sarid R, Harrington J et al (2003) Primary non-Hodgkin's lymphoma of the transverse colon presenting as dermatomyositis: case presentation and literature review. Med Oncol 20:413–424
64. Shen JK, Ding YM, Zhou WJ et al (2008) Polymyositis/dermatomyositis associated with acute myelocytic leukemia. Rheumatol Int 28:1265–1267
65. Morris P, Herrera-Guerra A, Parham D (2009) Lymphoma arising from a calcinotic lesion in a patient with juvenile dermatomyositis. Pediatr Dermatol 26:159–161
66. Sherry DD, Haas JE, Milstein JM (1993) Childhood polymyositis as a paraneoplastic phenomenon. Pediatr Neurol 9:155–156
67. Steck AJ, Erne B, Gabriel JM et al (1999) Paraproteinaemic neuropathies. Brain Pathol 9: 361–368
68. Ropper AH, Gorson KC (1998) Neuropathies associated with paraproteinemia. N Engl J Med 338:1601–1607
69. Dispenzieri A, Kyle RA, Lacy MQ et al (2003) POEMS syndrome: definitions and long-term outcome. Blood 101:2496–2506
70. Rotta FT, Bradley WG (1997) Marked improvement of severe polyneuropathy associated with multifocal osteosclerotic myeloma following surgery, radiation, and chemotherapy. Muscle Nerve 20:1035–1037

71. Dispenzieri A, Moreno-Aspitia A, Suarez GA et al (2004) Peripheral blood stem cell transplantation in 16 patients with POEMS syndrome, and a review of the literature. Blood 104:3400–3407
72. Silberstein LE, Duggan D, Berkman EM (1985) Therapeutic trial of plasma exchange in osteosclerotic myeloma associated with the POEMS syndrome. J Clin Apher 2:253–257
73. Henze T, Krieger G (1995) Combined high-dose 7S-IgG and dexamethasone is effective in severe polyneuropathy of the POEMS syndrome. J Neurol 242:482–483
74. Vingerhoets F, Kuntzer T, Delacretaz F et al (1995) Chronic relapsing neuropathy associated with Castleman's disease (angiofollicular lymph node hyperplasia). Eur Neurol 35:336–340
75. Ku A, Lachmann E, Tunkel R et al (1995) Severe polyneuropathy: initial manifestation of Castleman's disease associated with POEMS syndrome. Arch Phys Med Rehabil 76:692–694
76. Dispenzieri A, Gertz MA (2005) Treatment of Castleman's disease. Curr Treat Options Oncol 6:255–266
77. Dimopoulos MA, Panayiotidis P, Moulopoulos LA et al (2000) Waldenstrom's macroglobulinemia: clinical features, complications, and management. J Clin Oncol 18: 214–226
78. Rudnicki SA, Harik SI, Dhodapkar M et al (1998) Nervous system dysfunction in Waldenstrom's macroglobulinemia: response to treatment. Neurology 51:1210–1213
79. Weide R, Heymanns J, Koppler H (2000) The polyneuropathy associated with Waldenstrom's macroglobulinaemia can be treated effectively with chemotherapy and the anti-CD20 monoclonal antibody rituximab. Br J Haematol 109:838–841
80. Wilson HC, Lunn MP, Schey S et al (1999) Successful treatment of IgM paraproteinaemic neuropathy with fludarabine. J Neurol Neurosurg Psychiatry 66:575–580
81. Latov N (2000) Prognosis of neuropathy with monoclonal gammopathy. Muscle Nerve 23:150–152
82. Kyle RA, Rajkumar SV, Therneau TM et al (2005) Prognostic factors and predictors of outcome of immunoglobulin M monoclonal gammopathy of undetermined significance. Clin Lymphoma 5:257–260
83. Montoto S, Rozman M, Rosinol L et al (2003) Malignant transformation in IgM monoclonal gammopathy of undetermined significance. Semin Oncol 30:178–181
84. Dyck PJ, Low PA, Windebank AJ et al (1991) Plasma exchange in polyneuropathy associated with monoclonal gammopathy of undetermined significance. N Engl J Med 325:1482–1486
85. Lee YC, Came N, Schwarer A et al (2002) Autologous peripheral blood stem cell transplantation for peripheral neuropathy secondary to monoclonal gammopathy of unknown significance. Bone Marrow Transplant 30:53–56
86. Katz JS, Saperstein DS, Gronseth G et al (2000) Distal acquired demyelinating symmetric neuropathy. Neurology 54:615–620
87. Vital A, Lagueny A, Julien J et al (2000) Chronic inflammatory demyelinating polyneuropathy associated with dysglobulinemia: a peripheral nerve biopsy study in 18 cases. Acta Neuropathol 100:63–68
88. Ilyas AA, Quarles RH, Dalakas MC et al (1985) Monoclonal IgM in a patient with paraproteinemic polyneuropathy binds to gangliosides containing disialosyl groups. Ann Neurol 18:655–659
89. Latov N, Hays AP, Donofrio PD et al (1988) Monoclonal IgM with unique specificity to gangliosides GM1 and GD1b and to lacto-N-tetraose associated with human motor neuron disease. Neurology 38:763–768
90. Nardelli E, Steck AJ, Barkas T et al (1988) Motor neuron syndrome and monoclonal IgM with antibody activity against gangliosides GM1 and GD1b. Ann Neurol 23:524–528
91. Dalakas MC, Quarles RH (1996) Autoimmune ataxic neuropathies (sensory ganglionopathies): are glycolipids the responsible autoantigens? Ann Neurol 39:419–422
92. Goldfarb AR, Weimer LH, Brannagan TH III (2005) Rituximab treatment of an IgM monoclonal autonomic and sensory neuropathy. Muscle Nerve 31:510–515
93. Niermeijer JM, Eurelings M, Lokhorst HL et al (2009) Rituximab for polyneuropathy with IgM monoclonal gammopathy. J Neurol Neurosurg Psychiatry 80:1036–1039

94. Rojas-Garcia R, Gallardo E, de Andrés I et al (2003) Chronic neuropathy with IgM anti-ganglioside antibodies: lack of long term response to rituximab. Neurology 61:1814–1816
95. Broglio L, Lauria G (2005) Worsening after rituximab treatment in anti-MAG neuropathy. Muscle Nerve 32:378–379
96. Comi G, Roveri L, Swan A et al (2002) A randomised controlled trial of intravenous immunoglobulin in IgM paraprotein associated demyelinating neuropathy. J Neurol 249:1370–1377
97. Mariette X, Chastang C, Clavelou P et al (1997) A randomised clinical trial comparing interferon-alpha and intravenous immunoglobulin in polyneuropathy associated with monoclonal IgM. The IgM-associated Polyneuropathy Study Group. J Neurol Neurosurg Psychiatry 63:28–34

Part VI
Neurological Complications of Therapy for Lymphomas and Leukemias

Chapter 21
Neurological Complications of Radiation in Lymphoma and Leukemia Patients

Denise D. Correa and Lisa M. DeAngelis

Introduction

The side effects associated with radiation are of particular concern in patients with primary central nervous system lymphoma (PCNSL) given their relatively long survival. Whole-brain radiotherapy (WBRT) in combination with high-dose methotrexate-based chemotherapy (HD-MTX) is considered the standard treatment for PCNSL [1]. Favorable results have been demonstrated with this regimen, with a median survival of 40 months and a 30% 5-year survival, but several clinical trials reported delayed therapy-related neurotoxicity, particularly in long-term survivors over 60 years of age [2, 3]. When a combination of WBRT and chemotherapy is used, the incidence ranges from 8 to 50% of patients in different trials [2, 4, 5].

In adult patients with leukemia, CNS prophylaxis with intrathecal or high-dose chemotherapy, with or without cranial irradiation, is effective in reducing CNS relapse [6, 7]; these therapies have also been used in patients with CNS leukemia at diagnosis or at relapse. Although most studies have involved children, routine use of cranial irradiation in adults has been more limited to patients with high-risk disease due to increased neurotoxicity, and the efficacy of chemotherapy alone regimens [8–10]. Recently, chemotherapy alone has been shown to reduce subsequent CNS relapse in children, without the neurotoxicity associated with cranial irradiation [11].

Mechanisms of Radiation-Induced Neurotoxicity

In the process of treating a malignancy, radiation therapy (RT) often damages healthy tissue. RT-related factors that increase the risk of neurotoxicity have been identified, including volume of tissue irradiated, total dose, dose per fraction,

D.D. Correa (✉)
Department of Neurology, Memorial Sloan-Kettering Cancer Center, New York, NY 10021, USA
e-mail: corread@mskcc.org

T. Batchelor, L.M. DeAngelis (eds.), *Lymphoma and Leukemia of the Nervous System*, DOI 10.1007/978-1-4419-7668-0_21,

duration of therapy, and energy of radiation. Other contributing clinical factors include age, pre-existing neurological or systemic diseases (e.g., hypertension), genetic predisposition, and concomitant chemotherapy treatment [12, 13].

Suggested mechanisms include depletion of glial progenitor cells and perpetuation of oxidative stress induced by radiation [14]. Radiation may diminish the reproductive capacity of the O-2A progenitors of oligodendrocytes, disrupting the normal turnover of myelin [15]. Blood-vessel dilatation and wall thickening with hyalinization, increased blood-brain barrier (BBB) permeability due to endothelial cell loss and apoptosis, and a decrease in vessel density have also been hypothesized to lead to white matter necrosis [16]. The extent to which radiation damage is due to direct toxicity on cells or secondary to deleterious effects on the vasculature remains to be elucidated [17]. Progressive demyelination may take months to cause symptoms because of the slow turn-over of oligodendrocytes, contributing to the latency in onset of neurotoxicity. RT achieves therapeutic effect, in part, through DNA damage by introducing inter-strand DNA and DNA-protein crosslinks, single- and double-stranded DNA breaks, methylation, oxidation, and by increasing formation of reactive oxygen species (ROS). Increased numbers of reactive astrocytes and microglia have been shown to produce ROS, cytokines, and growth factors that may cause progressive inflammatory injury. The accumulation of DNA damage in neuronal cells, when unrepaired, can lead to the transcription of defective proteins, apoptosis, and neurodegeneration [18]. In addition, recent animal and human studies have documented that RT, as well as chemotherapy, can disrupt hippocampal neurogenesis [19, 20].

Clinical and Neuroimaging Findings

Radiation encephalopathy has been classified into three phases, according to the time between the administration of RT and the onset of the injury [13]. These are described as acute, early-delayed, and late-delayed (Table 21.1). *Acute* encephalopathy typically appears within days of initiation of RT, and the most common symptoms are nausea and vomiting, headache, drowsiness, and worsening of pre-existing neurological deficits. The pathogenesis most likely involves disruption of the BBB by endothelial apoptosis, and ensuing increased cerebral edema and intracranial pressure. Most neuroimaging studies show no evidence of cerebral edema, possibly due to decreased sensitivity to acute changes. Corticosteroids diminish the disruption of the BBB and often prevent clinical symptoms. *Early-delayed effects* occur 2 weeks to 6 months following RT, and are reversible in most cases. The symptoms include headache, lethargy, and resurgence of prior neurological signs; a transitory decline in cognitive functioning may also occur, but this is not predictive of cognitive problems that may develop later. Some patients may develop radiation somnolence syndrome or focal encephalopathy. Transient white matter hyperintensity, suggesting demyelination may be evident on magnetic resonance imaging (MRI), and is thought to be related to BBB disruption or injury to oligodendrocytes.

Table 21.1 Radiation injury[a]

Stage	Time after RT	Clinical findings	Pathogenesis	Outcome
Acute	Hours to days	Headache, vomiting Neurologic signs	Increased intracranial pressure (edema) BBB disruption	Recovery
Early-delayed	Two weeks to 6 months	Somnolence; headaches Increased focal signs Worsening MR scan	Demyelination Possibly cerebral edema	Recovery
Late-delayed	Months to years	Focal signs MR enhancement Memory loss Dementia Incontinence Gait ataxia MR atrophy, ventriculomegaly, leukoen-cephalopathy	Brain necrosis Possibly vascular Cellular loss Demyelination Possibly hydrocephalus	Responds to steroids Surgical removal Modest response to shunting in some cases

[a]Modified from DeAngelis and Posner [13].

The late-delayed effects of RT become apparent several months to many years after treatment, and often produce irreversible and progressive damage to the CNS through vascular injury causing chronic ischemia, cerebral atrophy, progressive demyelination of the white matter, and necrosis [13, 21]. The risk for developing radiation necrosis increases with irradiated volume, total dose and fraction size. There is variability in the reported incidence of necrosis, in part, due to diagnostic limitations as some patients are asymptomatic and imaging findings can be equivocal. MRI usually shows contrast enhancement at the original tumor site, and fluorodeoxyglucose (FDG) positron emission tomography (PET) scans may demonstrate hypometabolism in areas of necrosis and hypermetabolism in areas with tumor involvement [22]. Autopsy studies have demonstrated myelin and axonal loss, gliosis, spongiosis, and atherosclerosis of both large and small vessels, corresponding to the radiographic changes [23].

Most patients treated with WBRT or prophylactic irradiation for leukemia or small cell lung cancer eventually develop cerebral atrophy, ventricular dilatation, and leukoencephalopathy [21]. In some patients, communicating hydrocephalus may occur, but loss of cerebral mass from direct radiation damage to neurons and neuron precursors may occur. MRI typically shows hyperintensity in the periventricular white matter, and these changes are often more severe in the elderly (Fig. 21.1). Diffusion tensor MRI shows early dose-dependent progressive demyelination and axonal degeneration, and subsequent diffuse dose-independent demyelination [24]. Cognitive impairment is present in most patients treated with WBRT, and can be progressive in nature.

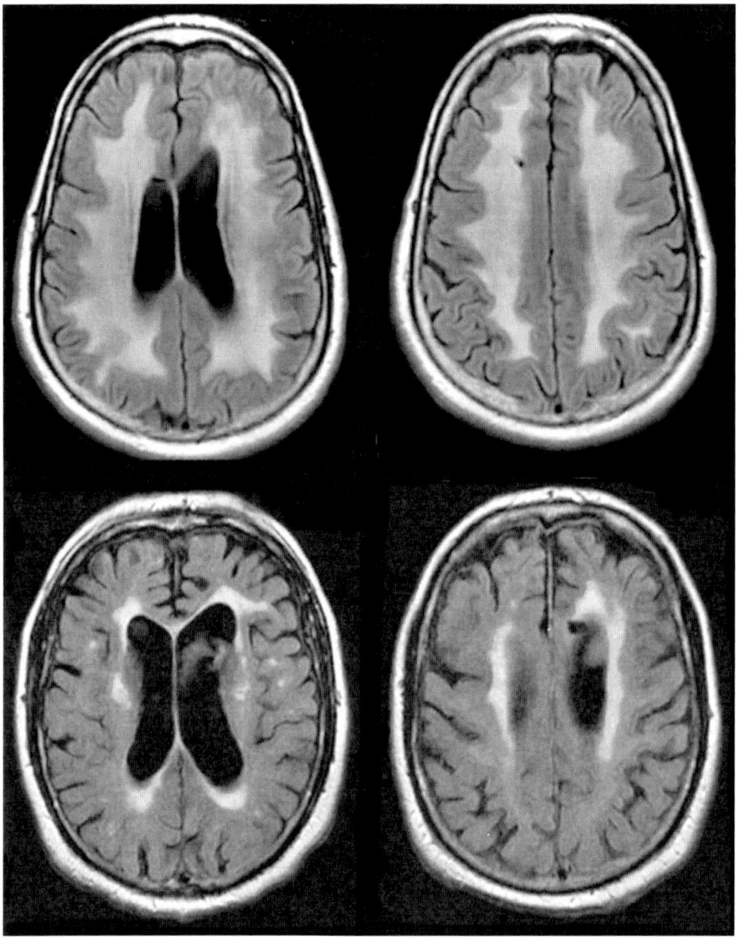

Fig. 21.1 FLAIR axial MRI scans showing periventricular white matter abnormalities in two PCNSL patients (first row and second row) treated with WBRT and HD-MTX-based chemotherapy

Neurological and Neurocognitive Adverse Effects

In patients with PCNSL, the specific contribution of the disease itself and the side effects of WBRT and chemotherapy to the development of neurological and cognitive sequelae are often difficult to ascertain. Neurological sequelae of treatment usually develop months to years after therapy [25], and can only be established in the absence of tumor. Therefore, its incidence is proportional to the percentage of patients with disease-free survival [1]. The neurologic sequelae of RT are predominantly cognitive, but several other post-treatment deficits may occur. Furthermore, the cognitive dysfunction seen with delayed treatment-induced neurotoxicity is often part of a syndrome, in which patients also develop gait disturbance and autonomic dysfunction [26]. A stereotypical gait disturbance is characterized by shuffling, wide base, impaired turning, and postural instability similar to that seen in Parkinsonism or normal pressure hydrocephalus. Urinary and fecal incontinence may be seen in approximately one-half of patients with delayed treatment-induced neurotoxicity. Other neurological symptoms that have been attributed at least in part to therapy include seizures, Parkinsonism, psychiatric disturbance, and cerebral and retinal ischemia. Although less well characterized, toxicity has been noted with CNS prophylaxis in adults, including decreased tolerance to systemic chemotherapy, infections due to immunosuppression, cerebral atrophy, and EEG abnormalities [6].

Neurocognitive Functions

A substantial number of brain tumor patients treated with RT alone or in combination with chemotherapy develop cognitive dysfunction that varies from mild to severe, and it is currently considered the most frequent complication among long-term survivors [12]. It often interferes with the patient's ability to function at premorbid levels professionally and socially, despite adequate disease control [27, 28]. The variability in the documented frequency of treatment-induced cognitive deficits may be partially associated with the insensitivity of the methods of assessment used, as most studies included only clinical observations, patient complaints, performance status ratings, and brief mental status examinations. These assessment methods have low sensitivity to detect cognitive dysfunction in this population [29]. Therefore, the incidence and severity of cognitive dysfunction associated with various treatment regimens in patients with disease-free survival remains unclear, and have most likely been significantly underestimated [25].

Overall, the literature suggests that the pattern of cognitive impairments associated with the delayed effects of WBRT and chemotherapy is diffuse and relatively independent of tumor location. The cognitive deficits are consistent with frontal-subcortical dysfunction, and domains particularly sensitive to treatment-induced dysfunction include attention, executive functions, learning and retrieval of new information, and graphomotor speed [27, 30, 31]. The side effects of medications, such as corticosteroids and antiepileptics often contribute to or exacerbate the cognitive difficulties. Most, but not all, studies suggest that in comparison to chemotherapy only regimens, RT alone or in combination with high-dose chemotherapy produces extensive white matter abnormalities that are associated with cognitive impairment [27, 32]. Although no information on adults with leukemia is available, children who underwent CNS prophylaxis with cranial irradiation and intrathecal or high-dose methotrexate have been shown to develop atrophy and leukoencephalopathy, and these abnormalities were associated with neuropsychological deficits [33].

Primary Central Nervous System Lymphoma

Cognitive dysfunction in PCNSL patients is related to multiple factors including the effects of the tumor itself, given its infiltrative and multifocal growth pattern, age, and the delayed effects of WBRT and HD-MTX, either combined or alone. Delayed treatment-related cognitive dysfunction is a significant problem, now that effective treatment for PCNSL has increased survival rates [2]. The specific contribution of the disease itself and various treatment modalities to cognitive dysfunction remains to be elucidated, as the neurotoxic potential of combined treatments is difficult to determine when each can produce CNS damage individually.

PCNSL patients treated with WBRT and HD-MTX-based chemotherapy, or with WBRT and chemotherapy with BBB disruption, had evidence of significant cognitive impairment [32]. The pattern of cognitive deficits was diffuse, and the domains most commonly disrupted included attention and executive functions, psychomotor speed, and learning and retrieval of new information. However, the retrospective nature of these studies limited the ability to examine the specific contributions of tumor versus the delayed effects of RT and chemotherapy to cognitive outcome.

Pels et al. [34] performed cognitive evaluations in twenty-seven patients (age range 27–74 years), subsequent to treatment with HD-MTX alone, WBRT alone, or combined modality therapy. Among the thirteen patients seen between 1 and 95 months after WBRT either alone or in combination with HD-MTX, eight had cognitive deficits (of these, five had progressive disease or partial treatment response, and two had complete treatment response); on subsequent follow-ups, nine patients declined (three had progressive disease or partial treatment response, and five had stable disease). Among the fourteen patients seen 10–38 months post-HD-MTX, ten had cognitive deficits (two had partial response and seven had complete response); on subsequent follow-ups, nine of the ten patients with complete response improved, and two patients with progressive disease declined. The authors concluded that treatment with WBRT either alone or in combination with chemotherapy, but not chemotherapy alone, was associated with cognitive deterioration. However, the inclusion of patients with progressive disease or partial response limited the ability to distinguish tumor from treatment effects on cognition.

Harder et al. [28] studied cognitive functions in nineteen PCNSL patients (median age=44 years, range 24–63) treated with HD-MTX followed by WBRT. Patients had a CR and were evaluated at a mean of 23 months after treatment completion. Eleven patients (58%) had impaired performance on 4 or more test indices of a total of 18 indices (defined as mild to moderate impairment), and four patients (21%) had impairment on more than 6 test indices (defined as severe impairment). In comparison to a non-CNS cancer control group, PCNSL patients had lower scores on verbal and non-verbal memory, attention, executive function, and motor speed. The authors concluded that combined modality therapy was associated with cognitive impairment, even in patients younger than 60 years.

Correa et al. [27] studied cognitive functions in twenty-eight PCNSL patients (mean age=60 years, range 36–85) treated with WBRT $\pm$ HD-MTX (n=18) or

HD-MTX alone (n=10). All patients were in disease remission and the mean time since treatment completion was 61 months for patients who had combined modality therapy and 18 months for patients treated with chemotherapy alone. Patients treated with WBRT ± chemotherapy had mild to moderate impairments (scores 1.5 sd below the normative mean) in attention/executive function, verbal memory, psychomotor speed, and language. Patients treated with chemotherapy only had moderate impairments in psychomotor speed as the only significant finding. The memory performance of patients treated with WBRT ± chemotherapy did not differ according to time since treatment completion ($\leq$ 60 months, n=9; $\geq$ 60 months, n=9), but was significantly ($p < 0.05$), more impaired than the performance of patients treated with chemotherapy only ($\leq$ 60 months). Quality of life assessment showed no differences according to treatment modality, but 50% of all patients were either unemployed or worked at a lower capacity. The authors concluded that WBRT ± chemotherapy was associated with more pronounced cognitive impairment than chemotherapy alone, regardless of time since treatment completion. In an ongoing prospective study involving 12 newly diagnosed PCNSL patients treated with induction chemotherapy (HD-MTX and rituximab) followed by dose-reduced WBRT [35], there has been no evidence of cognitive decline up to 2 years after completion of therapy.

In prospective studies of PCNSL patients treated with high-dose chemotherapy alone or with BBB disruption chemotherapy, there was evidence of diffuse cognitive impairment at baseline and prior to initiation of treatment. Post-treatment follow-ups were variable across studies, but several reported either stable or improved cognitive performance over the course of time [32]. However, methodological problems, such as small number of patients in each study, inclusion of patients with partial response to therapy or tumor recurrence, and incomplete reporting of cognitive test results limited the conclusions regarding the effects of chemotherapy on cognitive outcome.

Leukemia

The cognitive side effects of prophylactic cranial irradiation have been studied primarily in children with leukemia and adult survivors of childhood leukemia [36, 37]. However, there is a paucity of studies on neuropsychological outcome in adult leukemia patients treated with prophylactic irradiation. Tucker et al. [38] studied 23 patients with leukemia and non-Hodgkin lymphoma at a mean of 11 years after CNS prophylaxis with intrathecal chemotherapy and cranial irradiation. Mild concentration and memory difficulties, and lower performance IQ were reported; EEG abnormalities and cerebral atrophy were more common in older patients. However, in most studies with this clinical population, it is difficult to ascertain the specific contribution of each treatment modality to cognitive outcome, as most received prophylaxis with irradiation and chemotherapy. A recent study involving 498 children with acute lymphoblastic leukemia [11] reported that treatment with risk-adjusted systemic and intrathecal chemotherapy was associated with improved overall survival and reduced subsequent CNS relapse, without the neurotoxicity associated with cranial irradiation [11]; these findings were thought to support a treatment approach that excludes prophylactic cranial irradiation from the treatment of acute lymphoblastic leukemia without compromising overall survival.

Preventive or Treatment Interventions

There are no established preventive or therapeutic interventions for RT-induced injury. RT necrosis is usually treated with corticosteroids, and surgical resection for patients unresponsive to therapy [39]. There is preliminary evidence suggesting that bevacizumab may reduce abnormal enhancement associated with necrosis, possibly through the removal of vascular endothelial growth factor-induced reactive vascularization [40]. Treatments that target the vascular mechanism of RT damage, including hyperbaric oxygenation, anticoagulation, and aspirin have been attempted but without clear benefits [13].

Pharmacological treatments for RT-induced fatigue and cognitive dysfunction have been based primarily on therapies used for other neurological disorders that cause similar symptoms [41]. Although there are no studies targeting PCNSL or leukemia patients specifically, agents such as psychostimulants and acetylcholinesterase inhibitors have been used to treat cognitive dysfunction in patients with brain tumors. Improvement of fatigue and cognitive functions has been reported in high-grade glioma patients treated with methylphenidate [42, 43], and in patients with primary brain tumors treated with modafinil [44]. Donepezil has been shown to improve cognitive performance and mood in patients with brain tumors [45]. There are several ongoing trials using these medications, as well as cognitive rehabilitation and behavioral interventions. The prevention of cognitive deficits with agents that may protect neurons from treatment-induced damage is an area of growing interest, and trials to determine the potential neuroprotective effects of memantine and lithium in patients with brain metastases are being conducted [41].

References

1. DeAngelis LM, Yahalom J, Thaler HT, Kher U (1992) Combined modality therapy for primary CNS lymphoma. J Clin Oncol 10:635–643
2. Abrey LE, DeAngelis LM, Yahalom J (1998) Long-term survival in primary CNS lymphoma. J Clin Oncol 16:859–863
3. Poortmans PMP, Kluin-Nelemans HC, Haaxma-Reiche H et al (2003) High-dose methotrexate-based chemotherapy followed by consolidating radiotherapy in non-AIDS-related primary central nervous system lymphoma: European Organization for Research and Treatment of Cancer lymphoma group phase II Trial 20962. J Clin Oncol 21:4483–4488
4. O'Brien P, Roos D, Pratt G et al (2000) Phase II multicenter study of a brief single agent methotrexate followed by irradiation in primary CNS lymphoma. J Clin Oncol 18: 519–526

5. Sarazin M, Ameri A, Monjour A et al (1995) Primary central nervous system lymphoma: treatment with chemotherapy and radiotherapy. Eur J Cancer 31A:2003–2007
6. Cortes J (2001) Central nervous system involvement in adult acute lymphocytic leukemia. Hematol Oncol Clin N Am 15:145–162
7. Omura GA, Moffitt S, Vogler WR et al (1980) Combination chemotherapy of adult lymphoblastic leukemia with randomized central nervous system prophylaxis. Blood 2: 199–204
8. Sancho JM, Ribera JM, Oriol A et al (2006) Central nervous system recurrence in adult patients with acute lymphoblastic leukemia. Cancer 106:2540–2546
9. Sanders KE, Ha CS, Cortes-Franco JE et al (2004) The role of craniospinal irradiation in adults with a central nervous system recurrence of leukemia. Cancer 100:2176–2180
10. Surapanemi UR, Cortes JE, Thomas D et al (2002) Central nervous system relapse in adults with acute lymphoblastic leukemia. Cancer 94:773–779
11. Pui CH, Campana D, Pei D et al (2009) Treating childhood acute lymphoblastic leukemia without cranial irradiation. N Engl J Med 360:2730–2741
12. Behin A, Delattre J-Y (2003) Neurologic sequelae of radiotherapy on the nervous system. In: Schiff D, Wen PY (eds) Cancer Neurology in Clinical Practice. Humana Press, Inc., Totowa, NJ
13. DeAngelis LM, Posner JB (2009) Side effects of radiation therapy. In: DeAngelis LM, Posner JB (eds) Neurologic complications of cancer, 2nd edn. Oxford University Press, New York, NY
14. Tofilon PJ, Fike JR (2000) The radioresponse of the central nervous system: a dynamic process. Radiat Res 153:357–370
15. van der Maazen RW, Kleiboer BJ, Verhagen I, van der Kogel AJ (1993) Repair capacity of adult rat glial progenitor cells determined by an in vitro clonogenic assay after in vitro or in vivo fractionated irradiation. Int J Radiat Biol 63:661–666
16. Nordal RA, Wong CS (2005) Molecular targets in radiation-induced blood-brain barrier disruption. Int J Radiat Oncol Biol Phys 62:279–287
17. Noble M, Dietrich J (2002) Intersections between neurobiology and oncology: tumor origin, treatment and repair of treatment-associated damage. Trends Neurosci 25:103–107
18. Fishel ML, Vasko MR, Kelley MR (2007) DNA repair in neurons: so if they don't divide what's to repair. Mut Res 614:24–36
19. Dietrich J, Han R, Yang Y et al (2006) CNS progenitor cells and oligodendrocytes are targets of chemotherapeutic agents in vitro and vivo. J Biol 5:1–23
20. Monje ML, Palmer T (2003) Radiation injury and neurogenesis. Curr Opin Neurol 16: 129–134
21. Omuro AM, Ben-Porat LS, Panageas KS et al (2005) Delayed neurotoxicity in primary central nervous system lymphoma. Arch Neurol 62:1595–1600
22. Evans ES, Hahn CA, Kocak Z et al (2007) The role of functional imaging in the diagnosis and management of late normal tissue injury. Semin Radiat Oncol 17:72–80
23. Lai R, Abrey LE, Rosenblum MK, DeAngelis LD (2004) Treatment-induced leukoencephalopathy in primary CNS lymphoma. Neurology 62:451–456
24. Nagesh V, Tsien CI, Chenevert TL et al (2008) Radiation-induced changes in normal appearing white matter in patients with cerebral tumors: a diffusion tensor imaging study. Int J Radiat Oncol Biol Phys 70:1002–1010
25. Keime-Guibert F, Napolitano M, Delattre JY (1998) Neurological complications of radiotherapy and chemotherapy. J Neurol 245:695–708
26. Abrey LE, Correa DD (2005) Treatment-related neurotoxicity. Hematol Oncol Clin N Am 19:729–738
27. Correa DD, DeAngelis LM, Shi W et al (2004) Cognitive functions in survivors of primary central nervous system lymphoma. Neurology 62:548–555
28. Harder H, Holtel H, Bromberg JEC et al (2004) Cognitive status and quality of life after treatment for primary CNS lymphoma. Neurology 62:544–547

29. Meyers CA, Wefel JS (2003) The use of the mini-mental state examination to assess cognitive functioning in cancer trials: no ifs, ands, buts, or sensitivity. J Clin Oncol 21:3557–3558
30. Taphoorn MJB, Klein M (2004) Cognitive deficits in adult patients with brain tumours. Lancet 3:1–18
31. Wefel JS, Kayl AE, Meyers CA (2004) Neuropsychological dysfunction associated with cancer and cancer therapies: a conceptual review of an emerging target. Br J Cancer 90:1691–1696
32. Correa DD, Maron L, Harder H et al (2007) Cognitive functions in primary central nervous system lymphoma: literature review and assessment guidelines. Ann Oncol 18: 1145–1151
33. Hertzberg H, Huk WJ, Ueberall MA et al (1997) CNS late effects after ALL therapy in childhood. Part I: neuroradiological findings in long-term survivors of childhood ALL – an evaluation of the interferences between morphology and neuropsychological performance. The German Late Effects Working Group. Med Pediatr Oncol 28:387–400
34. Pels H, Deckert-Schulter M, Glasmacher A et al (2000) Primary central nervous system lymphoma: a clinicopathological study of 28 cases. Hematol Oncol 18:21–32
35. Correa DD, Rocco-Donovan M, DeAngelis LM et al (2009) Prospective cognitive follow-up in primary CNS lymphoma patients treated with chemotherapy and reduced-dose radiotherapy. J Neuro-Oncol 91:315–321
36. Butler RW, Copeland DR (1993) Neuropsychological effects of central nervous system prophylactic treatment in childhood leukemia: methodological considerations. J Pediatr Psychol 18:319–338
37. Waber DP, Turek J, Catania L et al (2007) Neuropsychological outcomes from a randomized trial of triple intrathecal chemotherapy compared with 18 Gy cranial radiation as CNS treatment in acute lymphoblastic leukemia: findings from Dana-Farber Cancer Institute ALL Consortium Protocol 95-01. J Clin Oncol 25:4914–4921
38. Tucker J, Prior PF, Green CR et al (1989) Minimal neuropsychological sequelae following prophylactic treatment of the central nervous system in adult leukaemia and lymphoma. Br J Cancer 60:775–780
39. Giglio P, Gilbert MR (2003) Cerebral radiation necrosis. Neurology 9:180–188
40. Wong ET, Huberman K, Lu X-Q et al (2008) Bevacizumab reverses cerebral radiation necrosis. J Clin Oncol 26:5649–5650
41. Ghering K, Sitskoorn MM, Aaronson NK et al (2008) Interventions for cognitive deficits in adults with brain tumours. Lancet Neurol 7:548–560
42. Meyers CA, Weitzner MA, Valentine AD (1998) Methylphenidate therapy improves cognition, mood, and function of brain tumor patients. J Clin Oncol 16:2522–2527
43. Weitzner MA, Meyers CA, Valentine AD (1995) Methylphenidate in the treatment of neurobehavioral slowing associated with cancer and cancer treatment. J Neuropsychiatry Clin Neurosci 7:347–350
44. Kaleita TA, Wellisch DK, Graham CA et al (2006) Pilot study of modafinil for treatment of neurobehavioral dysfunction and fatigue in adult patients with brain tumors. J Clin Oncol 24:1503
45. Shaw EG, Rosdhal R, D'Agostino RB et al (2006) Phase II study of donepezil in irradiated brain tumor patients: effect on cognitive function, mood and quality of life. J Clin Oncol 24:1415–1420

Chapter 22
Neurological Complications of Chemotherapy in Lymphoma and Leukemia Patients

Eudocia C. Quant, David C. Fisher, and Patrick Y. Wen

Introduction

In recent decades, important progress in the treatment of leukemia and lymphoma has resulted in patients surviving longer, thus increasing the likelihood that they will develop long-term neurologic complications from their therapy. These neurologic sequelae significantly affect the quality of life of patients with hematologic malignancies. Many of these complications were previously attributable to cranial irradiation. However, this modality is increasingly being replaced by intensive systemic and intrathecal chemotherapy regimens. The balance between efficacy and toxicity is a major focus of recent clinical trials. In patients with primary central nervous system lymphoma (PCNSL), neurologic complications also play a major role in limiting potential therapies. This chapter will review the most common neurologic complications of chemotherapy in leukemia and lymphoma.

Treatment for Leukemia and Lymphoma

Detailed discussion of the treatment regimens used in hematologic malignancies is beyond the scope of this chapter. These therapies are reviewed in Chapters 1 and 2, as well as in a number of other sources [1–7].

Leukemia

Patients with acute lymphocytic leukemia (ALL) or acute myelogenous leukemia (AML) may be treated with chemotherapy alone or with high dose chemotherapy

P.Y. Wen (✉)
Division of Neuro-Oncology, Department of Neurology, Dana Farber Cancer Institute, Center for Neuro-Oncology, Brigham and Women's Hospital, Boston, MA 02115, USA
e-mail: pwen@partners.org

T. Batchelor, L.M. DeAngelis (eds.), *Lymphoma and Leukemia of the Nervous System*, DOI 10.1007/978-1-4419-7668-0_22,

followed by hematopoietic stem cell transplantation, depending on age and risk factors. Chemotherapy regimens for ALL include high-dose methotrexate, cytarabine, cyclophosphamide, steroids, vincristine, L-asparaginase and/or an anthracycline, such as daunorubicin [1]. Patients with Philadelphia-chromosome (bcr-abl) positive ALL are also treated with imatinib, nilotinib, or dasatinib. The leptomeninges are a common site of extramedullary involvement in ALL, and therefore treatments are often administered to prevent or eradicate CNS leukemia [8]. CNS involvement is identified at the time of diagnosis in less than 10% of adults with ALL [8], and in these patients, CNS toxicity from aggressive systemic and CNS-directed regimens is often the dose limiting side effect of treatment. In patients without CNS involvement, CNS prophylaxis may include potentially neurotoxic treatments, such as intrathecal chemotherapy, high-dose systemic chemotherapy and/or cranial irradiation.

In adult AML, standard induction regimens include cytarabine and an anthracycline [2]. Postremission therapy may include more chemotherapy, such as high-dose cytarabine (HiDAC), autologous or allogeneic stem cell transplantation. Since CNS involvement is less common in AML, prophylactic therapy is usually not indicated. However, examination of the cerebrospinal fluid should be considered in subtypes with an increased risk of leptomeningeal leukemia or brain myeloid sarcoma, such as monocytic subtypes, patients with extramedullary disease, inversion of chromosome 16 and t(8:21) genotypes, CD7- and CD56-positive immunophenotypes, and patients with very high blast counts [9]. Therapies for patients with CNS involvement include high-dose cytarabine or methotrexate, intrathecal chemotherapy and/or cranial irradiation.

Chronic myeloid leukemia (CML) is characterized by a reciprocal translocation of chromosomes 9q and 22q, leading to the formation of the fusion oncogene bcr-abl [5]. Imatinib, a small molecule inhibitor of bcr-abl, is first-line therapy for newly diagnosed CML. Despite high rates of complete cytogenetic response on imatinib, the only proven curative treatment is an allogeneic hematopoietic stem cell transplant. CNS involvement is rare in CML, but may occur during blast crisis [10, 11].

Chronic lymphocytic leukemia (CLL) follows a more indolent course. Treatment may be withheld until a patient becomes symptomatic, although early treatment is justified in patients with poor prognosis [4, 12]. First line therapies for CLL often contain a nuceloside analog, such as fludarabine in combination with rituximab. CLL rarely involves the nervous system [13].

Primary CNS Lymphoma

As discussed Chapters 7, 8, and 9, the treatment of primary CNS lymphoma (PCNSL) generally involves chemotherapy, with or without whole-brain radiation therapy. The precise chemotherapeutic agents vary, but most regimens contain high-dose methotrexate [3, 14]. This may be given alone [15] or in combination with chemotherapeutic agents, such as procarbazine, cytosine arabinoside and vincristine [3]. Other regimens include high-dose chemotherapy with autologous stem cell support [16], blood-brain barrier disruption [17], or anti-CD20 immunotherapies, such as rituximab [18]. Intrathecal chemotherapy was previously standard treatment for patients with proven leptomeningeal disease. However, more recent regimens have generally excluded intrathecal chemotherapy since high-dose methotrexate penetrates the blood-brain-barrier sufficiently to achieve therapeutic levels in the CSF [19–21].

Almost all the drugs used to treat PCNSL and whole brain radiation therapy may result in neurotoxicity. In a retrospective review of 194 patients with PCNSL, the 5-year cumulative incidence of neurotoxicity was 24% [22]. Of particular importance is the leukoencephalopathy that occurs with high-dose methotrexate and radiation therapy. Since this complication tends to be much more severe when methotrexate is administered during or after radiation therapy, most regimens attempt to reduce this complication by administering the chemotherapy before radiation therapy [3, 14]. However, patients may develop leukoencephalopathy, even when they receive methotrexate before radiation therapy [14]. In one of the largest series, 32% of patients receiving combined modality treatment developed delayed neurotoxicity [23]. This complication was especially common in patients over the age of 60 [24]. To avoid this complication, there has been a trend towards treating patients, especially the elderly, with chemotherapy alone, and deferring radiation therapy until the time of relapse. Retrospective analysis suggests that this approach may decrease the incidence of neurotoxicity, but at the cost of an increase rate of relapse [25]. The challenge for future treatments for PCNSL is to optimize tumor control, while limiting the incidence of delayed neurotoxicity.

Systemic Lymphoma

Hodgkin disease (HD) rarely involves the central nervous system; so CNS-specific therapy is not required. Therefore, treatment-induced CNS toxicity, as seen in patients with PCNSL, is unusual. Most of the neurologic complications in HD patients result from indirect involvement of the nervous system included in a radiation field or as a result of the neurotoxic effects of chemotherapeutic agents. Patients with Stage I and II HD are generally treated with ABVD chemotherapy (doxorubicin, bleomycin, vinblastine and dacarbazine) alone or combined with radiation therapy, while Stage III and IV patients generally receive chemotherapy alone [usually ABVD, which has largely supplanted the more toxic MOPP regimen (mechlorethamine, vincristine, procarbazine and prednisone)] [6, 26]. Other commonly used regimens for advanced stage patients include Stanford V (doxorubicin, vinblastine, mechlorethamine, vincristine, bleomycin, etoposide, and prednisone) and BEACOPP (bleomycin, etoposide, doxorubicin, cyclophosphamide, vincristine, procarbazine and prednisone). For refractory and relapsed HD, most patients receive high-dose therapy using regimens, such as CBV (Cytoxan, BCNU and etoposide) or BEAM (BCNU, etoposide, cytosine arabinoside and melphalan), and autologous hematopoietic stem cell transplantation [27, 28].

Non-Hodgkin lymphomas (NHL) have a greater propensity to involve the CNS than HD. The treatment regimens for PCNSL are often used for NHL involving the

CNS, and as a result, the neurologic complications are also similar to those observed in patients with PCNSL.

Patients with indolent lymphomas generally have a good prognosis and may be observed for a period of time before therapy is instituted [29, 30]. Patients with limited stage disease are generally treated with radiation, while advanced stage patients receive single-agent chemotherapy such as chlorambucil, bendamustine or fludarabine, or combination chemotherapies, such as CVP (cyclophosphamide, vincristine, prednisone) and CHOP (cyclophosphamide, doxorubicin, vincristine and prednisone). These chemotherapeutic regimens may be combined with the monoclonal anti-CD20 antibody rituximab. Other treatment options with activity in indolent NHL include alpha-interferon, single-agent rituximab, and radioimmunotherapy with ^{131}I tositumomab or ^{90}Y ibritumomab.

Therapy for aggressive NHL is complex. In general, localized and advanced stage aggressive NHL (e.g., diffuse large B cell lymphoma) is treated with rituximab added to CHOP chemotherapy (R-CHOP) [31]. There is interest in autologous stem cell transplantation as consolidation after CHOP-based therapy for patients with high-risk disease, but studies on this treatment approach are ongoing [32, 33]. Therapy for highly aggressive NHL, such as Burkitt's lymphoma and lymphoblastic lymphoma, is complicated by their tendency to involve the CNS. The risk of CNS involvement in these highly aggressive forms of NHL is 30–50% [34]. As a result, most regimens include some form of CNS prophylaxis. Current treatment regimens are comprised of multiple, dose-intensive agents and incorporate high-dose systemic methotrexate or cytosine arabinoside for CNS prophylaxis or therapy [7]. These regimens are often supplemented with intrathecal chemotherapy, but the use of cranial irradiation has been largely abandoned to reduce the risk of neurotoxicity. Nonetheless, chemotherapy-induced neurotoxicity still remains a concern. An example of a regimen commonly used in Burkitt's lymphoma is CODOX-M (cyclophosphamide, vincristine, doxorubicin and high-dose methotrexate), alternating with IVAC (ifosfamide, etoposide and high-dose cytarabine). Patients on CODOX-M/IVAC also receive intrathecal cytarabine and methotrexate. The risk of severe neurologic toxicity from clinical trials of CODOX-M/IVAC ranged from 3 to 27% in patients with high-risk disease, with sensory, motor, cortical, and cerebellar toxicities all reported [35, 36].

Neurologic Complications of Chemotherapy

Chemotherapeutic Agents that Commonly Cause Neurologic Complications

Methotrexate

Methotrexate is a dihydrofolate reductase inhibitor, preventing the conversion of folic acid to tetrahydrofolate, which is required for purine and thymidine synthesis (Table 22.1). It inhibits DNA synthesis in the S-phase of the cell cycle and is used in

Table 22.1 Neurologic complications of chemotherapy for patients with leukemia or lymphoma

Acute encephalopathy		
Cisplatin	Fludarabine	Procarbazine (HD)
Cyclophosphamide	GM-CSF	Thalidomide
Cytosine arabinoside (HD)	Ifosfamide	Thiotepa (HD)
Denileukin	Interferons	Vinca alkaloids
Doxorubicin (IT)	Mechloramine	
Etoposide (HD)	Methotrexate	
Mood/Personality Change		
Cladribine	Interferons	Thalidomide
Corticosteroids	Mechlorethamine	Procarbazine
Headache		
ATRA	Ibritumomab	Fludarabine
Cisplatin	Interferons	Rituximab
Cladribine	Mechlorethamine	Thalidomide
Corticosteroids	Methotrexate (IT)	Tositumomab
Cytosine arabinoside	Oprelvekin (Neumega)	
Denileukin		
Seizures		
Busulphan (HD)	Erythropoietin	Mechloramine
BCNU	Fludarabine	Methotrexate
Chlorambucil (HD)	GM-CSF	Thalidomide
Cytosine arabinoside (HD or IT)	Ifosfamide	Vinca alkaloids
Dementia		
Cytosine arabinoside	Fludarabine	Methotrexate
	Interferon-alpha	Procarbazine
Peripheral neuropathy		
Cisplatin	Oprelvekin	Thalidomide
Cladribine	Procarbazine	Vinca alkaloids
Etoposide		
Cranial neuropathy		
Cisplatin	Methotrexate	Vincristine
Hearing loss		
Cisplatin	Mechlorethamine	
Visual disturbance		
Chlorambucil	Cytosine arabinoside	Interleukin-2
Corticosteroids	Etoposide	Vincristine
Cyclophosphamide	Fludarabine	
Cortical blindness		
Cisplatin	Fludarabine	Methotrexate (HD)
Erythropoietin	GM-CSF	Vinca alkaloids
Myelopathy		
BCNU (HD)	Cytosine arabinoside (IT)	Mitoxantrone (IT)
Cisplatin	Interferon-alpha	Thiotepa (IT)
Corticosteroids	Methotrexate (IT)	Vincristine (IT)

Table 22.1 (continued)

Extrapyramidal syndromes		
Ifosfamide	Interferon-alpha	Vincristine
Cerebellar syndrome		
Cytosine arabinoside (HD)	Procarbazine	Thalidomide
Ifosfamide		Vinca alkaloids
Dizziness		
Cladribine	Rituximab	Tositumomab
Cyclophosphamide		
Vasculopathy and stroke		
Bleomycin	Doxorubicin	Methotrexate
Cisplatin	Erythropoietin	
Aseptic meningitis		
Cytosine arabinoside (IT)	Etoposide (IT)	Thiotepa (IT)
	Methotrexate (IT)	

HD, high-dose; IT, intrathecal.

the treatment of leukemias, lymphomas, and leptomeningeal disease. Methotrexate crosses the blood-brain barrier relatively poorly, but significant CNS concentrations can be achieved when the drug is administered intrathecally, or when high intravenous doses are used [19, 37]. The clinical expression of its neurotoxicity is determined by the dosage, route of administration, and the use of other therapeutic modalities with overlapping neurotoxicities, such as irradiation.

Intrathecal methotrexate toxicity: Aseptic meningitis is the most common neurotoxicity associated with intrathecal methotrexate [38–40]. This occurs in approximately 10% of patients, although some series have reported incidences as high as 50% [39, 41]. Symptoms usually begin 2–4 h after the drug is injected and may last for 12–72 h. It is characterized by headache, nuchal rigidity, back pain, nausea, vomiting, fever, and lethargy, and is indistinguishable from other types of chemical meningitis. Cerebrospinal fluid (CSF) analysis shows a lymphocytic pleocytosis and an elevated protein, but cultures are negative. The symptoms are usually self-limited and require no specific treatment. Most patients have no sequelae, although rarely it may lead to delayed leukoencephalopathy [42]. Aseptic meningitis can be prevented to some extent by injecting methotrexate with hydrocortisone or using oral corticosteroids. Some patients who developed aseptic meningitis have been retreated with methotrexate without problems.

Transverse myelopathy, a much less common complication of intrathecal methotrexate, is characterized by back or leg pain followed by paraplegia, sensory loss, and sphincter dysfunction [41, 43, 44]. The symptoms usually occur between 30 min and 48 h after treatment, but may occur up to 2 weeks later [41, 44]. The majority of cases show clinical improvement, but the extent of recovery is variable [45]. The pathogenesis is unknown. Pathologically, there is vacuolar demyelination and necrosis in the spinal cord, without inflammatory or vascular changes [46].

If present, abnormalities on magnetic imaging resonance (MRI) tend to be non-specific with spinal cord swelling, hyperintensity on T2-weighted sequences and contrast enhancement [47]. Initial imaging is often normal. This complication is more common in patients receiving concurrent radiotherapy or frequent treatments of intrathecal methotrexate.

Rarely, intrathecal methotrexate produces an acute encephalopathy [42], especially if CSF outflow is obstructed, or if the methotrexate is injected directly into cerebral white matter as a result of a misplaced ventricular catheter [48]. Intrathecal methotrexate can also cause delayed leukoencephalopathy [49, 50], posterior reversible encephalopathy syndrome [51], seizures [52], subacute focal neurologic deficits [53], cranial nerve palsies, lumbosacral polyradiculopathy [54–56], noncardiogenic pulmonary edema [57], and sudden death [41, 58–60].

Accidental overdosage of intrathecal methotrexate (particularly doses > 500 mg) may result in myelopathy, encephalopathy, seizures, and death [61]. Prompt recognition and early treatment are essential to improve outcomes [62]. The use of rapid CSF drainage by lumbar puncture, CSF exchange, ventriculolumbar perfusion [63], carboxypeptidase G2 [64], high-dose intravenous leucovorin, and alkaline diuresis have allowed occasional patients to survive [59, 60].

Weekly low-dose methotrexate neurotoxicity: Up to 25% of patients receiving weekly, low dose methotrexate may experience headaches, dizziness, and subtle cognitive impairment [65]. These symptoms resolve when the methotrexate is discontinued.

High-dose methotrexate neurotoxicity: High-dose methotrexate may cause acute, subacute or chronic neurotoxicity. Renal function, hydration and alkalization, use of leucovorin rescue, coadminstration of other antineoplastic agents and pharmacogenomics may significantly influence the risk of toxicity from high-dose methotrexate [66].

Acute high-dose methotrexate neurotoxicity is characterized by somnolence, confusion, and seizures within 24 h of treatment. Symptoms usually resolve spontaneously without sequelae, and patients can often continue to receive this drug [41, 60, 67]. Although more commonly described with intrathecal methotrexate, an acute syndrome with symptoms and imaging findings similar to posterior reversible encephalopathy syndrome has also been described in patients receiving high-dose methotrexate [68, 69]. In one series, however, the patients also had hypomagnesemia, raising the possibility that the electrolyte abnormality may have been a contributing factor.

Weekly or biweekly treatments with moderate to high-dose methotrexate may produce a subacute stroke-like syndrome characterized by transient focal neurologic deficits, confusion, and occasionally seizures [70, 71]. Typically, the disorder develops 6 days after high-dose methotrexate, lasts 15 min to 72 h, and resolves spontaneously without sequelae. Neuroimaging studies are usually normal, although areas of restricted diffusion [72] and non-enhancing hyperintense T2 lesions in the white mater have been observed on MRI [73]. CSF is normal, but the EEG demonstrates diffuse slowing. Methotrexate may be administered subsequently without the encephalopathy recurring. The pathogenesis of this syndrome is unknown, but may be related to reduced cerebral glucose metabolism [74], reduced biogenic amine synthesis [75], excess adenosine release through inhibition of AICAR-formyltransferase by methotrexate [76], or increased levels of homocysteine [66].

Chronic leukoencephalopathy has been reported in a number of patients following high-dose methotrexate and is discussed further below.

Leukoencephalopathy: The major delayed complication of methotrexate therapy is leukoencephalopathy, which refers to white matter damage in the CNS identified on MRI as T2-weighted hyperintensities [77–80]. Although this syndrome may be produced by methotrexate alone, it is exacerbated by radiotherapy, especially if radiotherapy is administered before or during methotrexate therapy. The leukoencephalopathy usually occurs following repeated administration of intrathecal methotrexate or high-dose intravenous methotrexate, but has also been described after standard dose intravenous methotrexate [78]. The development of acute methotrexate neurotoxicity usually does not increase the likelihood of leukoencephalopathy. However, there has been a report of leukoencephalopathy developing in patients with methotrexate-induced aseptic meningitis [42]. The severity can range from mild asymptomatic leukoencephalopathy to irreversible and possibly fatal disseminated necrotizing leukoencephalopathy. The degree of neurotoxicity is difficult to predict and does not clearly correlate with imaging findings. For patients who are symptomatic, the clinical features are characterized by the gradual development of cognitive impairment months or years after treatment with methotrexate. This ranges from mild learning disabilities to severe progressive dementia together with somnolence, seizures, ataxia, and hemiparesis. The IQs in children treated with intrathecal methotrexate and radiation therapy or high-dose methotrexate deteriorate in excess of 15 points [41, 81]. Computed tomography (CT) and MRI scans show cerebral atrophy and diffuse white matter lesions. On CT, these are characteristically hypodense, nonenhancing lesions in the periventricular white matter, while on MRI, areas of high signal intensity are noted on T2-weighted/FLAIR images (Fig. 22.1). Disseminated necrotizing

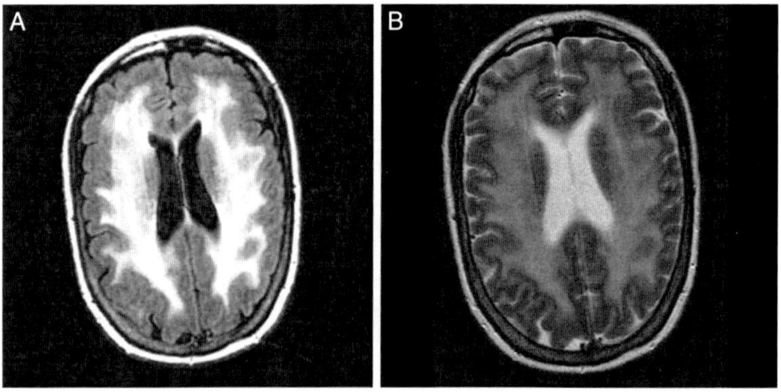

Fig. 22.1 Axial FLAIR (**a**) and T2-weighted (**b**) MRI showing diffuse increased signal in the periventricular white matter in a patient who received high-dose methotrexate and cranial irradiation for PCNSL 3 years previously

leukoencephalopathy produces a more rapid neurologic decline, and the MRI shows more extensive white matter damage [82]. Pathologic lesions range from loss of oligodendrocytes and gliosis to a necrotizing leukoencephalopathy [78]. There is demyelination, axonal swelling, dystrophic mineralization of axonal debris, and fibrinoid necrosis of small blood vessels [41]. Occasionally, children may have a mineralizing microangiopathy, characterized by calcification of capillaries and venules, especially in the basal ganglia [83]. The clinical course is variable. Many patients stabilize, but the course is progressive in some patients and may lead to death, particularly in disseminated necrotizing leukoencephalopathy. No effective treatment is available.

The cause of the leukoencephalopathy is unknown. Possibilities include injury to cerebral vascular endothelium, increasing blood-brain barrier permeability, depletion of reduced folates in the brain, inhibition of cerebral glucose or protein metabolism, inhibition of catecholamine synthesis [41, 74], or disturbance of myelin metabolism [84]. In addition, cranial irradiation may either potentiate the toxic effects of methotrexate or disrupt the blood-brain barrier, allowing higher concentrations of methotrexate to reach the brain.

Vinca Alkaloids: Vincristine (Oncovin), Vinblastine (Velban), Vindesine, and Vinorelbine (Navelbine)

Vincristine is a vinca alkaloid derived from the periwinkle plant, which is frequently used to treat leukemia, HD, and NHL. It binds to tubulin and prevents microtubule formation, thereby arresting cells in metaphase. Its main toxicity is an axonal neuropathy, resulting from disruption of the microtubules within axons and interference with axonal transport. The neuropathy involves both sensory and motor fibers, although small sensory fibers are especially affected [85, 86].

Virtually all patients receiving vincristine develop some degree of neuropathy. The clinical features resemble those of other axonal neuropathies, such as diabetic neuropathy. The earliest symptoms are usually paresthesias in the fingertips and feet, with or without muscle cramps. These symptoms often develop after several weeks of treatment, but they may occur after the first dose. Furthermore, symptoms may appear even after the drug has been discontinued, and progress for several months before improving. Initially, objective sensory findings tend to be relatively minor compared to the subjective complaints, but loss of ankle jerks is common. Occasionally, there may be profound weakness, with bilateral foot drop, wrist drop, and loss of all sensory modalities. Neurophysiologic studies are compatible with a primarily axonal neuropathy [87]. Severe neuropathies are particularly likely to develop in older or cachectic patients, those who have received prior irradiation to the peripheral nerves or concomitant hematopoietic colony-stimulating factors [88], patients with hepatic insufficiency [89], and those who have pre-existing neurologic conditions, such as Charcot-Marie-Tooth [90, 91]. There is generally no effective treatment. Patients with mild neuropathy can usually continue to receive full doses of vincristine, but when symptoms increase in severity and interfere with neurologic function, dose reduction or discontinuation of the drug may be necessary. The natural history following discontinuation of treatment is gradual improvement, which may take up to several months [86]. Children tend to recover more quickly than adults.

Autonomic neuropathies can also develop in patients receiving vincristine. Colicky abdominal pain and constipation occur in almost 50% of patients, and, rarely, a paralytic ileus may result [86]. Consequently, patients receiving vincristine should take prophylactic stool softeners or laxatives. Less commonly, patients may develop impotence, postural hypotension, or an atonic bladder.

Cranial neuropathies may occasionally be caused by vincristine [60]. The most common nerve to be involved is the oculomotor nerve, resulting in ptosis and ophthalmoplegia. Other nerves that may be involved include the optic [92], recurrent laryngeal, facial, and auditory. Vincristine may also cause retinal damage and night blindness. Some patients may experience jaw and parotid pain.

CNS complications are rare as vincristine poorly penetrates the blood-brain barrier. Accidental administration of vincristine into the CSF produces a rapidly ascending myelopathy, coma and usually, death [93]. Rarely, vincristine may cause SIADH, resulting in hyponatremia, confusion, and seizures [94]. CNS complications unrelated to SIADH may also occur, including seizures [95], encephalopathy, transient cortical blindness [96], ataxia, athetosis, tremor and parkinsonism [41, 60, 97].

The related vinca alkaloids vindesine, vinblastine, and vinorelbine tend to have less neurotoxicity. This may be related to differences in lipid solubility, plasma clearance, terminal half-life, and sensitivities of axoplasmic transport [41, 60]. Like vincristine, both vinblastine and vinorelbine inhibit microtubule assembly, but they have less affinity for neural tissue and are less neurotoxic. In fact, vinorelbine is associated with mild paresthesias in only about 20% of patients [59], and severe neuropathy is rare, occurring most often in patients treated previously with paclitaxel [98].

Chemotherapeutic Agents that Occasionally Cause Neurologic Complications

Cytosine Arabinoside (Cytarabine, Ara-C)

Cytosine arabinoside is a pyrimidine analogue converted by deoxycytidine kinase to its active metabolite Ara-CTP that inhibits DNA polymerase and incorporates itself into the DNA molecule resulting in premature chain termination. This agent has little neurotoxicity when used at conventional doses. High doses (3 g/m^2 every 12 h) cause an acute cerebellar syndrome in 10–25% of patients [99–101]. Patients above the age of 50 with abnormal liver or renal function, underlying neurologic dysfunction, or receiving more than 30 g of the drug are especially likely to develop cerebellar involvement [59, 60, 102]. Typically, the patients develop somnolence and occasionally encephalopathy 2–5 days after completing treatment.

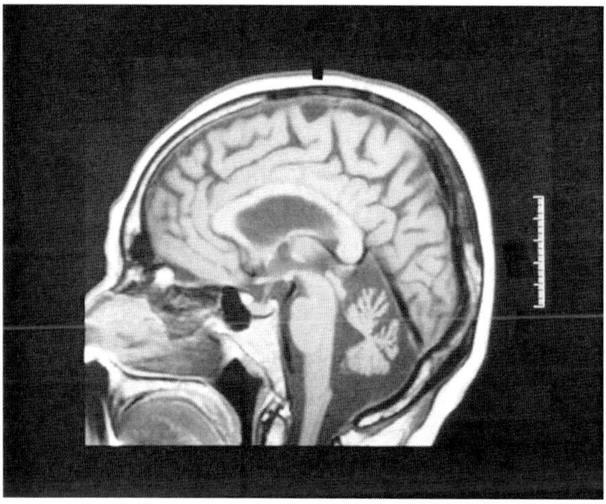

Fig. 22.2 Sagittal T1-weighted MRI of the brain of a 56 year old woman who developed cerebellar toxicity 7 years previously after receiving high-dose cytosine arabinoside. Although she improved with time, she was left with mild ataxia and severe dysarthria

Immediately afterwards, the patients develop cerebellar signs ranging from mild ataxia to inability to sit or walk unassisted. Rarely, patients experience seizures. Imaging studies may demonstrate white matter abnormalities, and later, cerebellar atrophy (Fig. 22.2). Cerebrospinal fluid is usually normal. The EEG may show slowing. The pathologic changes are localized to the cerebellum where there is widespread loss of Purkinje cells. No specific treatment is available, but the drug should be discontinued immediately at the first clinical indication of cerebellar dysfunction. In some patients, the cerebellar syndrome resolves spontaneously, but it is permanent in others. Avoidance of very high doses of the drug, especially in patients with renal impairment, has led to a decline in the incidence of this syndrome [103].

High-dose cytosine arabinoside rarely will cause peripheral neuropathies resembling Guillain-Barré syndrome [104], brachial plexopathy, encephalopathy, seizures, reversible ocular toxicity [105], lateral rectus palsy, bulbar and pseudobulbar palsy, Horner's syndrome, aseptic meningitis, anosmia, and an extrapyramidal syndrome [59, 60, 106, 107].

Intrathecal administration of cytosine arabinoside produces high levels of drug in the CSF for at least 24 h, and is used to treat leptomeningeal lymphoma and leukemia. In approximately 10% of patients, it causes an aseptic meningitis [60]. DepoCyt, a liposomal preparation of cytosine arabinoside that allows the drug to be released slowly over a 2-week period, is associated with a higher incidence of aseptic meningitis (40%). Concomitant administration of oral dexamethasone (4 mg twice a day × 5 days) significantly reduces the incidence of chemical meningitis and arachnoiditis associated with DepoCyt [39, 108].

Cytosine arabinoside rarely causes a transverse myelopathy similar to that observed with intrathecal methotrexate [109]. Occasionally, it can also lead to encephalopathy [110], headaches, seizures [111], pseudotumor cerebri [112], and a locked-in syndrome [113]. The risk of neurotoxicity is increased with higher doses and increased frequency of administration of cytosine arabinoside.

Ifosfamide (Ifex)

Ifosfamide is an analogue of cyclophosphamide occasionally used to treat lymphoma. The most common neurotoxicity associated with ifosfamide is encephalopathy [114, 115]. Decreased attention, sometimes with agitation, may develop within hours of administration and typically lasts 1–4 days. Estimations of incidence generally range from 10 to 25% without evidence of a dose-response curve. The pathophysiology of ifosfamide encephalopathy is unknown, but intoxication with chloracetaldehyde, a metabolic product of ifosfamide, is likely the critical factor. Small, non-randomized trials suggest that thiamine [116] or methylene blue [117] may prevent or treat the encephalopathy. Rarely, encephalopathy can progress to coma or death [118, 119]. Rarely, ifosfamide causes extrapyramidal signs, cerebellar signs, weakness, incontinence, or seizures [115, 119].

Chemotherapeutic Agents that Rarely Cause Neurologic Complications

Anthracycline Antibiotics (Doxorubicin [Adriamycin], Daunorubicin, Epirubicin, Idarubicin, Mitoxantrone)

Doxorubicin is an anthracycline antibiotic, which is frequently used to treat NHL as part of the CHOP regimen. It can cause arrhythmias and cardiomyopathies, which, in turn, can result in cerebrovascular complications [120]. Doxorubicin in combination with cyclosporine can lead to coma and death [60]. Accidental intrathecal injection can cause a myelopathy and encephalopathy [41, 121]. Idarubicin, epirubicin, and daunorubicin do not appear to be neurotoxic.

Bleomycin

Bleomycin is a mixture of polypeptide antibiotics that cuts DNA strands. Rarely, cardiovascular and cerebrovascular ischemia has been associated with multi-drug regimens including bleomycin. A causal link between bleomycin and stroke remains speculative.

Chlorambucil

This is an alkylating agent used for the treatment of HD and NHL. It usually has little neurotoxicity, but can cause encephalopathy, myoclonus [122, 123], and seizures when taken in very high doses [124]. Ocular toxicity, including keratitis, retinal edema, and hemorrhages have also been described following oral administration of chlorambucil [125].

Cladribine (2-Chlordeoxyadenosine)

This drug inhibits DNA polymerase and ligase and ribonucleotide reductase, resulting in DNA strand breakage. It is used for low-grade NHL. It has little neurotoxicity at conventional doses, but can produce a paraparesis [126], reversible blurred vision [127], or confusion [128] at high doses.

Cyclophosphamide (Cytoxan)

This is an alkylating agent used in the treatment of NHL and refractory leukemia. Standard dose cyclophosphamide has little neurotoxicity. High-dose cyclophosphamide can cause reversible visual blurring, dizziness, and confusion [41].

Etoposide (VP-16)

This is a topoisomerase II inhibitor used in the treatment of refractory lymphoma. It does not readily penetrate the blood-brain barrier and generally has little neurotoxicity, even in high doses. Rarely, it can cause a peripheral neuropathy, mild disorientation, seizures, transient cortical blindness, or optic neuritis [41, 129]. Intrathecal etoposide is associated with a mild transient arachnoiditis appearing within 1–5 days of treatment [130].

Fludarabine (Fludara)

Fludarabine, an inhibitor of DNA polymerase and ribonucleotide reductase, is used to treat indolent lymphomas. Neurotoxicity is uncommon, and appears to be dose-related. Over one-third of patients receiving more than 96 mg/m^2/day of intravenous fludarabine develop severe neurotoxicity, while less than 0.5% of patients receiving standard doses of fludarabine (< 40 mg/m^2/day) develop neurologic complications [131]. At low doses, fludarabine can cause headaches, somnolence, confusion, and paresthesias [41, 131–133]. Patients with mild neurologic complications usually improve when the drug is discontinued, but some patients have permanent deficits [134]. At high doses, fludarabine can cause a delayed progressive encephalopathy with visual loss, tremor, ataxia, seizures, paralysis, and coma [131, 135, 136]. Some of these patients progress to a persistent vegetative state and occasionally, death. A few cases have been attributed to progressive multifocal leukoencephalopathy due to JC virus [137–140]. Patients may also develop a severe myelopathy, leading to quadriparesis. MRI may show diffuse or multifocal areas of non-enhancing, increased T2 signal in the white matter and brainstem [131, 132]. Pathologically, there is multifocal demyelination and necrosis [133].

Mechlorethamine (Nitrogen Mustard)

This is an alkylating agent used to treat HD. Rarely, it causes sleepiness, headaches, weakness, hearing loss, and encephalopathy [41]. At high doses used for hematopoietic stem cell transplantation, it has been reported to cause confusion and seizures [141]. Intra-carotid administration produces a uveitis and cerebral necrosis [41, 134]. Older age and concomitant use of cyclophosphamide or procarbazine are associated with an increased risk of neurotoxicity.

Pentostatin

This is an inhibitor of adenosine deaminase and is used for the treatment of cutaneous T-cell lymphomas. At low doses, lethargy and fatigue are common. Higher doses can cause a severe encephalopathy, seizures, and coma [59, 131].

Nitrosoureas (Carmustine, Lomustine)

Carmustine is the prototype for this group of drugs and is used in the treatment of lymphomas. At conventional doses, carmustine does not cause neurotoxicity. However, patients who receive high dose intravenous carmustine can develop a profound encephalopathy, with or without a myelopathy that may progresses to coma and death [142].

Procarbazine (Matulane)

This is a weak monoamine oxidase inhibitor that probably acts as an alkylating agent. It is used to treat both HD and NHL. At standard oral doses, it can cause a mild reversible encephalopathy and neuropathy, and rarely psychosis and stupor [41, 143]. The incidence of encephalopathy may be increased in patients receiving "high dose" procarbazine [144]. Seventeen percent of patients develop a peripheral neuropathy with paresthesias and loss of deep tendon reflexes, which is usually reversible [145]. Other rare side effects include ataxia, orthostatic hypotension, and weakness of the intrinsic hand muscles. Procarbazine also potentiates the sedative effects of narcotics, phenothiazines, and barbiturates. Intravenous and intracarotid procarbazine produces a severe encephalopathy.

Thiotepa (Thioplex)

This is an alkylating agent occasionally used to treat leptomeningeal lymphoma. Intrathecal thiotepa can cause aseptic meningitis, and very rarely, a myelopathy [146]. Both thiotepa and its metabolite, TEPA, are lipid soluble and readily cross the blood-brain barrier. High intravenous doses of thiotepa can produce an encephalopathy that can be fatal [59].

Neurologic Complications of Corticosteroids

Corticosteroids are used frequently in lymphoma patients. Corticosteroids have a direct cytolytic effect against neoplastic lymphocytes and are part of many treatment regimens. In addition, corticosteroids reduce peritumoral edema in patients with CNS lymphoma and spinal cord edema in patients with epidural spinal cord compression.

The side effects of prolonged steroid therapy are well known [147, 148]. The incidence of complications increases with higher doses and prolonged therapy, but individual susceptibility varies significantly. One of the most common complications of corticosteroids is a steroid myopathy [149, 150]. Proximal muscle weakness is initially apparent in the hip girdle, and patients may complain of difficulty getting up from a chair or climbing stairs. In severe cases, the pectoral girdle and neck muscles may also be involved. Electromyography (EMG) is usually normal and serum creatine kinase levels are typically not elevated.

CNS complications also occur frequently. Corticosteroids often produce alterations in mood [151]. An improved sense of well-being, anxiety, irritability, insomnia, difficulty concentrating, and depression are all relatively common. Occasionally, patients may develop steroid psychosis [152]. This usually takes the form of acute delirium, but the psychosis may resemble mania, depression, or schizophrenia.

Other common neurologic complications of corticosteroids include tremors, visual blurring, reduced sense of taste and smell, and cerebral atrophy on neuroimaging studies. Rare complications include hiccups [153], dementia, seizures, and cord compression as a result of epidural lipomatosis [154].

Steroid withdrawal can also produce a variety of symptoms, which can be quite disabling. These include headaches, lethargy, nausea, vomiting, anorexia, myalgia, arthralgia, and postural hypotension. Rarely pseudotumor may occur.

Neurologic Complications of Biologic Agents

Alpha Interferon

This is a glycoprotein cytokine with antiviral, cytotoxic, and immunomodulatory activities. It is used therapeutically in patients with leukemia. Systemic toxicities include flu-like symptoms and myelosuppression. The flu-like symptoms, which include lethargy and headaches, tend to be worse at the onset of therapy, and usually improve with time. Neurotoxicity tends to be dose-related. It is generally mild when low doses of alpha-interferon are used [155]. At higher doses, alpha-interferon can cause headaches, dizziness, confusion, lethargy, hallucinations, and seizures [156–158]. These effects are more common in older patients [159] and in patients with prior psychiatric histories [160]. Neuroimaging studies are usually normal. EEG may show diffuse slowing [161] and rarely, epileptiform activity [162]. These neurotoxicities are usually reversible, but occasionally a permanent dementia or a persistent vegetative state may result [156, 157]. Rarely, alpha interferon has been associated with oculomotor palsy, visual hallucinations, retinopathy [163], parkinsonism [134] and spastic diplegia [164].

A high incidence of neuropsychiatric toxicity has been noted in patients treated with recombinant interferon alpha-2b (rIFNα2b). In one study of CML patients receiving rIFNα2b and low dose cytarabine, 24% of patients experienced grade 3 or 4 neuropsychiatric toxicity that affected daily functioning [160]. All patients recovered upon withdrawal of interferon alpha-2b. Patients with a psychiatric history were more likely to develop severe neuropsychiatric toxicity than patients without a psychiatric history. The mechanism of interferon neurotoxicity is unknown, but may include induction of proinflammatory cytokines, hyperactivity of corticotropin-releasing hormone-mediated stress pathway, and competition with naturally occurring neurotrophic hormones and opioids [134, 165].

Intrathecal administration of alpha interferon produces an acute reaction within hours of the first injection, consisting of headache, nausea, vomiting, fever, and dizziness. The symptoms usually resolve over the next 12–24 h. A severe encephalopathy develops in a significant number of patients within several days of the onset of treatment. This is dose dependent and tends to be worse in patients who have received cranial irradiation [156].

Pegylated rIFN-α2b (PEG Intron) has similar toxicities as rIFN-α2b [166].

All-Trans Retinoic Acid (ATRA, Vesanoid)

This is a biologic agent used to treat acute promyelocytic leukemia. ATRA differentiates promyelocytes into mature cells. Pseudotumor cerebri is an uncommon complication, but headache is seen frequently [167, 168].

Monoclonal Antibodies

Rituximab (Rituxan)

This is a genetically engineered chimeric murine/human monoclonal antibody directed against the CD20 antigen found on the surface of normal and malignant B lymphocytes. It is used for the treatment of NHL. Neurologic complications are uncommon, but some patients complain of headaches, myalgia, dizziness [169], or paresthesias [170].

Iodine-131 Tositumomab (Bexxar)

This is a radiolabeled immunoglobulin G-2a murine monoclonal antibody directed against the CD20 antigen. In addition to the cytotoxic effects induced by the antibody, the presence of iodine-131 results in focused targeting of beta radiation to the tumor and surrounding tissue. Iodine-131 tositumomab is used to treat NHL and is well tolerated. A minority of patients experience headache or myalgia and a few develop hypothyroidism [171, 172].

Yttrium-90 Ibritumomab Tiuxetan (Zevalin)

This is also a radiolabeled murine monoclonal antibody directed against CD20 used to treat NHL. It is well tolerated, but a few patients may complain of headaches or dizziness [173, 174].

Denileukin difitox (Ontak)

This is a fusion toxin used to treat cutaneous T-cell lymphoma, expressing the CD25 component for the IL-2 receptor. The most common complication is a vascular leak syndrome, but some patients experience myalgias, dizziness, paresthesias, nervousness, confusion, and insomnia [175, 176].

Targeted Agents

Imatinib (Gleevec)

This is an oral tyrosine kinase inhibitor of the fusion protein bcr-abl found in Philadelphia chromosome-positive leukemias. The most common neurotoxities are muscle cramping and myalgias, although symptoms are typically mild and respond to treatment with calcium, magnesium, or quinine [177, 178]. Other rare complications include muscle edema, rhabdomyolysis with myoglobinuria [179], and subdural hematomas [180]. Related tyrosine kinase inihibitors, dasatinib and nilotinib, do not seem to cause neurotoxicity as frequently as imatinib [181].

References

1. Onciu M (2009) Acute lymphoblastic leukemia. Hematol Oncol Clin North Am 23: 655–674
2. Shipley JL, Butera JN (2009) Acute myelogenous leukemia. Exp Hematol 37: 649–658
3. Morris PG, Abrey LE (2009) Therapeutic challenges in primary CNS lymphoma. Lancet Neurol 8:581–592
4. Hsi ED (2009) The leukemias of mature lymphocytes. Hematol Oncol Clin North Am 23:843–871
5. Milojkovic D, Apperley J (2008) State-of-the-art in the treatment of chronic myeloid leukaemia. Curr Opin Oncol 20:112–121
6. Evens AM, Hutchings M, Diehl V (2008) Treatment of Hodgkin lymphoma: the past, present, and future. Nat Clin Pract Oncol 5:543–556
7. Sweetenham JW (2008) Highly aggressive lymphomas in adults. Hematol Oncol Clin North Am 22:965–978, ix
8. Thomas X, Le QH (2008) Central nervous system involvement in adult acute lymphoblastic leukemia. Hematology 13:293–302
9. Liesveld JL, Lichtman MA (2006) Acute myelogenous leukemia. In: Lichtman MA, Beutler E, Kipps TJ, Seligsohn U, Kaushansky K, Prchal JT (eds) Williams hematology, 7th edn. McGraw-Hill Medical, New York, NY, pp 1183–1236
10. Pfeifer H, Wassmann BJ, Hofmann WK (2003) Risk and prognosis of central nervous system leukemia in patients with Philadelphia chromosome-positive acute leukemias treated with imatinib mesylate. Clin Cancer Res 9:4674–4681
11. Rytting ME, Wierda WG (2004) Central nervous system relapse in two patients with chronic myelogenous leukemia in myeloid blastic phase on imatinib mesylate therapy. Leuk Lymphoma 45:1623–1626
12. Chiorazzi N, Rai KR, Ferrarini M (2005) Chronic lymphocytic leukemia. N Engl J Med 352:804–815

13. Denier C, Tertian G, Ribrag V et al (2009) Multifocal deficits due to leukemic meningoradiculitis in chronic lymphocytic leukemia. J Neurol Sci 277:130–132
14. Batchelor T, Loeffler JS (2006) Primary CNS lymphoma. J Clin Oncol 24:1281–1288
15. Batchelor T, Carson K, O'Neil A et al (2003) Treatment of primary CNS lymphoma with methotrexate and deferred radiotherapy: a report of NABTT 96-07. J Clin Oncol 21(6):1044–1049
16. Ferreri AJ, Crochhiolo R, Assanelli A et al (2008) High-dose chemotherapy supported by autologous stem cell transplantation in patients with primary central nervous system lymphoma: facts and opinions. Leuk Lymphoma 49:2042–2047
17. McAllister LD, Doolittle ND, Guastadisegni PE et al (2000) Cognitive outcomes and long-term follow-up results after enhanced chemotherapy delivery for primary central nervous system lymphoma. Neurosurgery 46:51–60; discussion 60–1
18. Shah GD, Yahalom J, Correa DD et al (2007) Combined immunochemotherapy with reduced whole-brain radiotherapy for newly diagnosed primary CNS lymphoma. J Clin Oncol 25:4730–4735
19. Glantz MJ, Cole BF, Recht L et al (1998) High-dose intravenous methotrexate for patients with nonleukemic leptomeningeal cancer: is intrathecal chemotherapy necessary? J Clin Oncol 16:1561–1567
20. Tetef ML, Margolin KA, Doroshow JH et al (2000) Pharmacokinetics and toxicity of high-dose intravenous methotrexate in the treatment of leptomeningeal carcinomatosis. Cancer Chemother Pharmacol 46:19–26
21. Vassal G, Valteau D, Bonnay M et al (1990) Cerebrospinal fluid and plasma methotrexate levels following high-dose regimen given as a 3-hour intravenous infusion in children with non-Hodgkin's lymphoma. Pediatr Hematol Oncol 7:71–77
22. Omuro AM, Ben-Porat LS, Panageas KS et al (2005) Delayed neurotoxicity in primary central nervous system lymphoma. Arch Neurol 62:1595–1600
23. Abrey LE, DeAngelis LM, Yahalom J (1998) Long-term survival in primary CNS lymphoma. J Clin Oncol 16(3):859–863
24. Abrey LE, Yahalom J, DeAngelis LM et al (2000) Treatment for primary CNS lymphoma: the next step. J Clin Oncol 18(17):3144–3150
25. Gavrilovic IT, Hormigo A, Yahalom J et al (2006) Long-term follow-up of high-dose methotrexate-based therapy with and without whole brain irradiation for newly diagnosed primary CNS lymphoma. J Clin Oncol 24:4570–4574
26. Seam P, Janik JE, DeAngelis LM et al (2009) Role of chemotherapy in Hodgkin's lymphoma. Cancer J 15:150–154
27. Brice P (2008) Managing relapsed and refractory Hodgkin lymphoma. Br J Haematol 141: 3–13
28. Quddus F, Armitage JO (2009) Salvage therapy for Hodgkin's lymphoma. Cancer J 15: 161–163
29. Gribben JG (2007) How I treat indolent lymphoma. Blood 109:4617–4626
30. Feuerlein K, Zucca E, Ghielmini M et al (2009) First-line treatment of follicular lymphoma: a patient-oriented algorithm. Leuk Lymphoma 50:325–334
31. Michallet AS, Coiffier B (2009) Recent developments in the treatment of aggressive non-Hodgkin lymphoma. Blood Rev 23:11–23
32. Friedberg JW, Fisher RI (2008) Diffuse large B-cell lymphoma. Hematol Oncol Clin North Am 22:941–952, ix
33. Wrench D, Gribben JG (2008) Stem cell transplantation for non-Hodgkin's lymphoma. Hematol Oncol Clin North Am 22:1051–1079, xi
34. Lim HY, Thiel E, Glantz MJ (2008) To protect and defend: central nervous system prophylaxis in patients with non-Hodgkin's lymphoma. Curr Opin Oncol 20:495–501
35. Mead GM, Sydes MR, Walewski J et al (2002) An international evaluation of CODOX-M and CODOX-M alternating with IVAC in adult Burkitt's lymphoma: results of United Kingdom lymphoma group LY06 study. Ann Oncol 13:1264–1274

36. Magrath I, Adde M, Shad A et al (1996) Adults and children with small non-cleaved-cell lymphoma have a similar excellent outcome when treated with the same chemotherapy regimen. J Clin Oncol 14:925–934
37. Lippens RJ, Winograd B (1988) Methotrexate concentration levels in the cerebrospinal fluid during high-dose methotrexate infusions: an unreliable prediction. Pediatr Hematol Oncol 5:115–124
38. Geiser CF, Bishop Y, Jaffe N et al (1975) Adverse effects of intrathecal methotrexate in children with acute leukemia in remission. Blood 45:189–195
39. Glantz MJ, Jaeckle KA, Chamberlain MC et al (1999) A randomized controlled trial comparing intrathecal sustained-release cytarabine (DepoCyt) to intrathecal methotrexate in patients with neoplastic meningitis from solid tumors. Clin Cancer Res 5:3394–3402
40. Phillips PC (1991) Methotrexate toxicity. In: Rottenberg DA (ed) Neurological complications of cancer treatment. Butterworth-heinemann, Boston, MA, pp 115–134
41. DeAngelis LM, Posner JB (2009) Side effects of chemotherapy: Neurologic complications of cancer. Oxford University Press, New York, NY, pp 447–510
42. Boogerd W, vd Sande JJ, Moffie D et al (1988) Acute fever and delayed leukoencephalopathy following low dose intraventricular methotrexate. J Neurol Neurosurg Psychiatry 51(10):1277–1283
43. Bates S, McKeever P, Masur H et al (1985) Myelopathy following intrathecal chemotherapy in a patient with extensive Burkitt's lymphoma and altered immune status. Am J Med 78: 697–702
44. McLean DR, Clink HM, Ernst P et al (1994) Myelopathy after intrathecal chemotherapy. A case report with unique magnetic resonance imaging changes. Cancer 73:3037–3040
45. Gagliano RG, Costanzi JJ (1976) Paraplegia following intrathecal methotrexate: report of a case and review of the literature. Cancer 37:1663–1668
46. Clark AW, Cohen SR, Nissenblatt MJ et al (1982) Paraplegia following intrathecal chemotherapy: neuropathologic findings and elevation of myelin basic protein. Cancer 50:42–47
47. Counsel P, Khangure M (2007) Myelopathy due to intrathecal chemotherapy: magnetic resonance imaging findings. Clin Radiol 62:172–176
48. Lemann W, Wiley RG, Posner JB (1988) Leukoencephalopathy complicating intraventricular catheters: clinical, radiographic and pathologic study of 10 cases. J Neurooncol 6: 67–74
49. Baehring JM, Fulbright RK (2008) Delayed leukoencephalopathy with stroke-like presentation in chemotherapy recipients. J Neurol Neurosurg Psychiatry 79:535–539
50. Riva D, Giorgi C, Nichellli F et al (2002) Intrathecal methotrexate affects cognitive function in children with medulloblastoma. Neurology 59:48–53
51. Dicuonzo F, Salvati A, Palma M et al (2009) Posterior reversible encephalopathy syndrome associated with methotrexate neurotoxicity: conventional magnetic resonance and diffusion-weighted imaging findings. J Child Neurol 24:1013–1018
52. Winick NJ, Bowman WP, Kamen BA et al (1992) Unexpected acute neurologic toxicity in the treatment of children with acute lymphoblastic leukemia. J Natl Cancer Inst 84:252–256
53. Yim YS, Mahoney DH Jr, Oshman DG (1991) Hemiparesis and ischemic changes of the white matter after intrathecal therapy for children with acute lymphocytic leukemia. Cancer 67:2058–2061
54. Anderson SC, Baquies GD, Jackson A et al (2002) Ventral polyradiculopathy with pediatric acute lymphocytic leukemia. Muscle Nerve 25(1):106–110
55. Koh S, Nelson MD Jr, Kovanlikaya A et al (1999) Anterior lumbosacral radiculopathy after intrathecal methotrexate treatment. Pediatr Neurol 21:576–578
56. Pascual AM, Coret F, Casanova B et al (2008) Anterior lumbosacral polyradiculopathy after intrathecal administration of methotrexate. J Neurol Sci 267(1-2):158–161
57. Bernstein ML, Sobel DB, Wimmer RS (1982) Noncardiogenic pulmonary edema following injection of methotrexate into the cerebrospinal fluid. Cancer 50:866–868

58. Shore T, Barnett MJ, Phillips GL (1990) Sudden neurologic death after intrathecal methotrexate. Med Pediatr Oncol 18:159–161
59. Paleologos N (1998) Complications of chemotherapy. In: Biller J (ed) Iatrogenic neurology. Butterworth-heinemann, Boston, MA, pp 439–460
60. Dietrich J, Wen PY (2008) Neurologic complications of chemotherapy. In: Schiff D, Kesari S, Wen PY (eds) Cancer neurology in clinical practice, Humana Press, Totowa, NJ, pp 287–326
61. Ettinger LJ (1982) Pharmacokinetics and biochemical effects of a fatal intrathecal methotrexate overdose. Cancer 50:444–450
62. Finkelstein Y, Zevin S, Heyol J et al (2004) Emergency treatment of life-threatening intrathecal methotrexate overdose. Neurotoxicology 25:407–410
63. Spiegel RJ, Cooper PR, Blun RH et al (1984) Treatment of massive intrathecal methotrexate overdose by ventriculolumbar perfusion. N Engl J Med 311:386–388
64. Widemann BC, Balis FM, Shalabi A et al (2004) Treatment of accidental intrathecal methotrexate overdose with intrathecal carboxypeptidase G2. J Natl Cancer Inst 96(20):1557–1559
65. Wernick R, Smith DL (1989) Central nervous system toxicity associated with weekly low-dose methotrexate treatment. Arthritis Rheum 32:770–775
66. Schmiegelow K (2009) Advances in individual prediction of methotrexate toxicity: a review. Br J Haematol 146:489–503
67. Rubnitz JE, Relling MV, Harrison PL et al (1998) Transient encephalopathy following high-dose methotrexate treatment in childhood acute lymphoblastic leukemia. Leukemia 12:1176–1181
68. Sanchez-Carpintero R, Narbona J, Lopez de Mesa R et al (2001) Transient posterior encephalopathy induced by chemotherapy in children. Pediatr Neurol 24:145–148
69. Erbetta A, Salmaggi A, Sghirlanzoni A et al (2008) Clinical and radiological features of brain neurotoxicity caused by antitumor and immunosuppressant treatments. Neurol Sci 29:131–137
70. Martino RL, Benson AB, 3rd, Merritt JA et al (1984) Transient neurologic dysfunction following moderate-dose methotrexate for undifferentiated lymphoma. Cancer 54:2003–2005
71. Walker RW, Allen JC, Rosen G et al (1986) Transient cerebral dysfunction secondary to high-dose methotrexate. J Clin Oncol 4:1845–1850
72. Inaba H, Khan RB, Laninghan FH et al (2008) Clinical and radiological characteristics of methotrexate-induced acute encephalopathy in pediatric patients with cancer. Ann Oncol 19:178–184
73. Borgna-Pignatti C, Battisti L, Marradi P et al (1992) Transient neurologic disturbances in a child treated with moderate-dose methotrexate. Br J Haematol 81:448
74. Phillips PC, Dhawan Y, Strother SC et al (1987) Reduced cerebral glucose metabolism and increased brain capillary permeability following high-dose methotrexate chemotherapy: a positron emission tomographic study. Ann Neurol 21:59–63
75. Millot F, Dhondt JL, Hayte JM et al (1992) Impairment of cerebral biogenic amine synthesis in a patient receiving high-dose methotrexate. Am J Pediatr Hematol Oncol 14:276–278
76. Chabner BA, Allegra CJ, Curt GA et al (1985) Polyglutamation of methotrexate. Is methotrexate a prodrug? J Clin Invest 76:907–912
77. Pizzo PA, Poplack DG, Blyer WA et al (1979) Neurotoxicities of current leukemia therapy. Am J Pediatr Hematol Oncol 1:127–140
78. Rubinstein LJ, Herman MM, Long TF et al (1975) Disseminated necrotizing leukoencephalopathy: a complication of treated central nervous system leukemia and lymphoma. Cancer 35:291–305
79. Shuper A, Stark B, Kornreich L et al (2000) Methotrexate treatment protocols and the central nervous system: significant cure with significant neurotoxicity. J Child Neurol 15:573–580
80. Lai R, Abrey LE, Rosenblum MK et al (2004) Treatment-induced leukoencephalopathy in primary CNS lymphoma: a clinical and autopsy study. Neurology 62:451–456

81. Ochs J, Mulhern R, Fairclough D et al (1991) Comparison of neuropsychologic functioning and clinical indicators of neurotoxicity in long-term survivors of childhood leukemia given cranial radiation or parenteral methotrexate: a prospective study. J Clin Oncol 9: 145–151
82. Oka M, Terae S, Kobayashi R et al (2003) MRI in methotrexate-related leukoencephalopathy: disseminated necrotising leukoencephalopathy in comparison with mild leukoencephalopathy. Neuroradiology 45:493–497
83. Price RA, Birdwell DA (1978) The central nervous system in childhood leukemia. III. Mineralizing microangiopathy and dystrophic calcification. Cancer 42:717–728
84. Davidson A, Payne G, Leach MO et al (2000) Proton magnetic resonance spectroscopy ((1)H-MRS) of the brain following high-dose methotrexate treatment for childhood cancer. Med Pediatr Oncol 35:28–34
85. Casey EB, Jellife AM, Le Quesne PM et al (1973) Vincristine neuropathy. Clinical and electrophysiological observations. Brain 96:69–86
86. Legha SS (1986) Vincristine neurotoxicity. Pathophysiology and management. Med Toxicol 1:421–427
87. McLeod JG, Penny R (1969) Vincristine neuropathy: an electrophysiological and histological study. J Neurol Neurosurg Psychiatry 32:297–304
88. Weintraub M, Adde MA, Venzon DJ et al (1996) Severe atypical neuropathy associated with administration of hematopoietic colony-stimulating factors and vincristine. J Clin Oncol 14:935–940
89. Sandler SG, Tobin W, Henderson ES et al (1969) Vincristine-induced neuropathy. A clinical study of fifty leukemic patients. Neurology 19:367–374
90. Nishikawa T, Kawakami K, Kumamoto T et al (2008) Severe neurotoxicities in a case of Charcot-Marie-Tooth disease type 2 caused by vincristine for acute lymphoblastic leukemia. J Pediatr Hematol Oncol 30:519–521
91. Naumann R, Moham J, Reuner U et al (2001) Early recognition of hereditary motor and sensory neuropathy type 1 can avoid life-threatening vincristine neurotoxicity. Br J Haematol 115:323–325
92. Munier F, Perentes E, Herbort CP et al (1992) Selective loss of optic nerve beta-tubulin in vincristine-induced blindness. Am J Med 93:232–234
93. Gaidys WG, Dickerman JD, Walters CL et al (1983) Intrathecal vincristine. Report of a fatal case despite CNS washout. Cancer 52:799–801
94. Robertson GL, Bhoopalam N, Zelkowitz LJ (1973) Vincristine neurotoxicity and abnormal secretion of antidiuretic hormone. Arch Intern Med 132:717–720
95. Hurwitz RL, Mahoney DH Jr, Armstrong DL et al (1988) Reversible encephalopathy and seizures as a result of conventional vincristine administration. Med Pediatr Oncol 16: 216–219
96. Byrd RL, Rohrbaugh TM, Raney RB Jr et al (1981) Transient cortical blindness secondary to vincristine therapy in childhood malignancies. Cancer 47:37–40
97. Boranic M, Raci F (1979) A Parkinson-like syndrome as side effect of chemotherapy with vincristine and adriamycin in a child with acute leukaemia. Biomedicine 31:124–125
98. Fazeny B, Zifko U, Meryn S et al (1996) Vinorelbine-induced neurotoxicity in patients with advanced breast cancer pretreated with paclitaxel – a phase II study. Cancer Chemother Pharmacol 39:150–156
99. Herzig RH, Hines JD, Herzig GP et al (1987) Cerebellar toxicity with high-dose cytosine arabinoside. J Clin Oncol 5(6):927–932
100. Hwang TL, Yung WK, Estey EH et al (1985) Central nervous system toxicity with high-dose Ara-C. Neurology 35:1475–1479
101. Winkelman MD, Hines JD (1983) Cerebellar degeneration caused by high-dose cytosine arabinoside: a clinicopathological study. Ann Neurol 14:520–527
102. Gottlieb D, Bradstock K, Koutts J et al (1987) The neurotoxicity of high-dose cytosine arabinoside is age-related. Cancer 60:1439–1441

103. Smith GA, Damon LE, Rugo HS et al (1997) High-dose cytarabine dose modification reduces the incidence of neurotoxicity in patients with renal insufficiency. J Clin Oncol 15:833–839
104. Johnson NT, Crawford SW, Sargur M (1987) Acute acquired demyelinating polyneuropathy with respiratory failure following high-dose systemic cytosine arabinoside and marrow transplantation. Bone Marrow Transplant 2:203–207
105. Ritch PS, Hansen RM, Heuer DK (1983) Ocular toxicity from high-dose cytosine arabinoside. Cancer 51:430–432
106. Baker WJ, Royer GL Jr, Weirs RB (1991) Cytarabine and neurologic toxicity. J Clin Oncol 9:679–693
107. Luque FA, Selhorst JB, Petruska P (1987) Parkinsonism induced by high-dose cytosine arabinoside. Mov Disord 2:219–222
108. Glantz MJ, LaFollette S, Jaeckle KA et al (1999) Randomized trial of a slow-release versus a standard formulation of cytarabine for the intrathecal treatment of lymphomatous meningitis. J Clin Oncol 17:3110–3116
109. Dunton SF, Nitschke R, Spruce WE et al (1986) Progressive ascending paralysis following administration of intrathecal and intravenous cytosine arabinoside. A pediatric oncology group study. Cancer 57:1083–1088
110. Resar LM, Phillips PC, Kastan MB et al (1993) Acute neurotoxicity after intrathecal cytosine arabinoside in two adolescents with acute lymphoblastic leukemia of B-cell type. Cancer 71:117–123
111. Eden OB, Goldie W, Wood T et al (1978) Seizures following intrathecal cytosine arabinoside in young children with acute lymphoblastic leukemia. Cancer 42:53–58
112. Fort JA, Smith LD (1999) Pseudotumor cerebri secondary to intermediate-dose cytarabine HCl. Ann Pharmacother 33:576–578
113. Kleinschmidt-DeMasters BK, Yeh M (1992) "Locked-in syndrome" after intrathecal cytosine arabinoside therapy for malignant immunoblastic lymphoma. Cancer 70: 2504–2507
114. Watkin SW, Husband DJ, Green JA et al (1989) Ifosfamide encephalopathy: a reappraisal. Eur J Cancer Clin Oncol 25:1303–1310
115. Zalupski M, Baker LH (1988) Ifosfamide. J Natl Cancer Inst 80:556–566
116. Buesa JM, Garcia-Teijido P, Losa R et al (2003) Treatment of ifosfamide encephalopathy with intravenous thiamin. Clin Cancer Res 9:4636–4637
117. Pelgrims J, De Vos F, Van den Brande J et al (2000) Methylene blue in the treatment and prevention of ifosfamide-induced encephalopathy: report of 12 cases and a review of the literature. Br J Cancer 82:291–294
118. Gieron MA et al (1988) Severe encephalopathy associated with ifosfamide administration in two children with metastatic tumors. J Neurooncol 6(1):29–30
119. Shuper A, Stein J, Goshen J et al (2000) Subacute central nervous system degeneration in a child: an unusual manifestation of ifosfamide intoxication. J Child Neurol 15:481–483
120. Schachter S, Freeman R (1982) Transient ischemic attack and adriamycin cardiomyopathy. Neurology 32:1380–1381
121. Arico M, Nespoli L, Porta F et al (1990) Severe acute encephalopathy following inadvertent intrathecal doxorubicin administration. Med Pediatr Oncol 18:261–263
122. Vandenberg SA, Kulig K, Spoerke DG et al (1988) Chlorambucil overdose: accidental ingestion of an antineoplastic drug. J Emerg Med 6:495–498
123. Wyllie AR, Bayliff CD, Kovacs MJ (1997) Myoclonus due to chlorambucil in two adults with lymphoma. Ann Pharmacother 31:171–174
124. Salloum E, Khan KK, Cooper DL (1997) Chlorambucil-induced seizures. Cancer 79: 1009–1013
125. Burns LJ (1992) Ocular toxicities of chemotherapy. Semin Oncol 19:492–500
126. Chabner BA, Longo DL (1996) Cancer chemotherapy and biotherapy: principles and practice, Lippincott-Raven, Philadelphia, PA

127. Kende G, Sirkin SR, Thomas PR et al (1979) Blurring of vision: a previously undescribed complication of cyclophosphamide therapy. Cancer 44:69–71
128. Tashima CK (1975) Immediate cerebral symptoms during rapid intravenous administration of cyclophosphamide (NSC-26271). Cancer Chemother Rep 59:441–442
129. Leff RS, Thompson JM, Daly MB et al (1988) Acute neurologic dysfunction after high-dose etoposide therapy for malignant glioma. Cancer 62:32–35
130. Chamberlain MC, Tsao-wei DD, Groshen S (2006) Phase II trial of intracerebrospinal fluid etoposide in the treatment of neoplastic meningitis. Cancer 106:2021–2027
131. Cheson BD, Vena DA, Foss FM et al (1994) Neurotoxicity of purine analogs: a review. J Clin Oncol 12:2216–2228
132. Cohen RB, Abdsallah JM, Gray JR et al (1993) Reversible neurologic toxicity in patients treated with standard-dose fludarabine phosphate for mycosis fungoides and chronic lymphocytic leukemia. Ann Intern Med 118:114–116
133. Spriggs DR, Stopa E, Mayer RJ et al (1986) Fludarabine phosphate (NSC 312878) infusions for the treatment of acute leukemia: phase I and neuropathological study. Cancer Res 46:5953–5958
134. Hammack JE, Cascino TL (1998) Chemotherapy and other common drug-induced toxicities of the central nervous system in patients with cancer. In: Vecht CJ (ed) Handbook of clinical neurology. Elsevier Science, Amsterdam, pp 481–514
135. Chun HG, Leyland-Jones BR, Caryk SM et al (1986) Central nervous system toxicity of fludarabine phosphate. Cancer Treat Rep 70:1225–1228
136. Warrell RP Jr, Berman E (1986) Phase I and II study of fludarabine phosphate in leukemia: therapeutic efficacy with delayed central nervous system toxicity. J Clin Oncol 4:74–79
137. Cid J, Revilla M, Cervera A et al (2000) Progressive multifocal leukoencephalopathy following oral fludarabine treatment of chronic lymphocytic leukemia. Ann Hematol 79:392–395
138. Kiewe P, Seyfert S, Korper S et al (2003) Progressive multifocal leukoencephalopathy with detection of JC virus in a patient with chronic lymphocytic leukemia parallel to onset of fludarabine therapy. Leuk Lymphoma 44:1815–1818
139. Rodriguez L, Ribera JM, Batlle M et al (2002) Progressive multifocal leukoencephalopathy shortly after the diagnosis of follicular lymphoma in a patient treated with fludarabine. Haematologica 87:ECR26
140. Saumoy M, Castells G, Escoda L et al (2002) Progressive multifocal leukoencephalopathy in chronic lymphocytic leukemia after treatment with fludarabine. Leuk Lymphoma 43: 433–436
141. Sullivan KM, Storb R, Shulman HM et al (1982) Immediate and delayed neurotoxicity after mechlorethamine preparation for bone marrow transplantation. Ann Intern Med 97:182–189
142. Burger PC, Kamenar E, Schold SC et al (1981) Encephalomyelopathy following high-dose BCNU therapy. Cancer 48:1318–1327
143. Weiss HD, Walker MD, Wiernik PH (1974) Neurotoxicity of commonly used antineoplastic agents (second of two parts). N Engl J Med 291:127–133
144. Postma TJ, van Groenigen CJ, Witjes RJ et al (1998) Neurotoxicity of combination chemotherapy with procarbazine, CCNU and vincristine (PCV) for recurrent glioma. J Neurooncol 38(1):69–75
145. Spivack SD (1974) Drugs 5 years later: procarbazine. Ann Intern Med 81:795–800
146. Gutin PH, Levi JA, Wiernik PH et al (1977) Treatment of malignant meningeal disease with intrathecal thioTEPA: a phase II study. Cancer Treat Rep 61:885–887
147. Drappatz J, Schiff D, Kesaru S et al (2007) Medical management of brain tumor patients. Neurol Clin 25:1035–1071
148. DeAngelis LM, Posner JB (2009b) Supportive care and its complications: Neurologic complications of cancer. Oxford University Press, New York, NY, pp 95–140
149. Batchelor TT, Taylor LP, Thaler HT et al (1997) Steroid myopathy in cancer patients. Neurology 48:1234–1238

150. Dropcho EJ, Soong SJ (1991) Steroid-induced weakness in patients with primary brain tumors. Neurology 41:1235–1239
151. Stiefel FC, Breitbart WS, Holland JC (1989) Corticosteroids in cancer: neuropsychiatric complications. Cancer Invest 7:479–491
152. Lewis DA, Smith RE (1983) Steroid-induced psychiatric syndromes. A report of 14 cases and a review of the literature. J Affect Disord 5:319–332
153. Baethge BA, Lidsky MD (1986) Intractable hiccups associated with high-dose intravenous methylprednisolone therapy. Ann Intern Med 104:58–59
154. Haddad SF, Hitchon PW, Godersky JC (1991) Idiopathic and glucocorticoid-induced spinal epidural lipomatosis. J Neurosurg 74:38–42
155. Caraceni A, Gangeri L, Martini C et al (1998) Neurotoxicity of interferon-alpha in melanoma therapy: results from a randomized controlled trial. Cancer 83:482–489
156. Meyers CA, Obbens EA, Scheibel RS et al (1991) Neurotoxicity of intraventricularly administered alpha-interferon for leptomeningeal disease. Cancer 68:88–92
157. Meyers CA, Scheibel RS, Forman AD (1991) Persistent neurotoxicity of systemically administered interferon-alpha. Neurology 41:672–676
158. Rohatiner AZ, Prior PF, Burton AC et al (1983) Central nervous system toxicity of interferon. Br J Cancer 47:419–422
159. Spiegel RJ (1987) The alpha interferons: clinical overview. Semin Oncol 14:1–12
160. Hensley ML, Peterson B, Silver RT et al (2000) Risk factors for severe neuropsychiatric toxicity in patients receiving interferon alfa-2b and low-dose cytarabine for chronic myelogenous leukemia: analysis of Cancer and Leukemia Group B 9013. J Clin Oncol 18:1301–1308
161. Smedley H, Katrak M, Sikora K et al (1983) Neurological effects of recombinant human interferon. Br Med J (Clin Res Ed) 286:262–264
162. Suter CC, Westmoreland BF, Shabrough FW et al (1984) Electroencephalographic abnormalities in interferon encephalopathy: a preliminary report. Mayo Clin Proc 59:847–850
163. Hejny C, Sternberg P, Lawson DH et al (2001) Retinopathy associated with high-dose interferon alfa-2b therapy. Am J Ophthalmol 131:782–787
164. Vesikari T, Nuutila A, Cantell K (1988) Neurologic sequelae following interferon therapy of juvenile laryngeal papilloma. Acta Paediatr Scand 77:619–622
165. Raison CL, Demetrashvili M, Capuron L et al (2005) Neuropsychiatric adverse effects of interferon-alpha: recognition and management. CNS Drugs 19:105–123
166. Michallet M, Maloisel F, Delain M et al (2004) Pegylated recombinant interferon alpha-2b vs recombinant interferon alpha-2b for the initial treatment of chronic-phase chronic myelogenous leukemia: a phase III study. Leukemia 18:309–315
167. Adamson PC, Reaman G, Finklestein JZ et al (1997) Phase I trial and pharmacokinetic study of all-trans-retinoic acid administered on an intermittent schedule in combination with interferon-alpha2a in pediatric patients with refractory cancer. J Clin Oncol 15:3330–3337
168. Tallman MS, Andersen JW, Schiffer CA et al (1997) All-trans-retinoic acid in acute promyelocytic leukemia. N Engl J Med 337:1021–1028
169. Maloney DG, Press OW (1998) Newer treatments for non-Hodgkin's lymphoma: monoclonal antibodies. Oncology (Williston Park) 12:63–76
170. Foran JM, Rohatiner AZ, Cunninghan D et al (2000) European phase II study of rituximab (chimeric anti-CD20 monoclonal antibody) for patients with newly diagnosed mantle-cell lymphoma and previously treated mantle-cell lymphoma, immunocytoma, and small B-cell lymphocytic lymphoma. J Clin Oncol 18:317–324
171. Kaminski MS, Estes J, Zasadny KR et al (2000) Radioimmunotherapy with iodine (131)I tositumomab for relapsed or refractory B-cell non-Hodgkin lymphoma: updated results and long-term follow-up of the University of Michigan experience. Blood 96:1259–1266
172. Vose JM, Wahl RL, Saleh M et al (2000) Multicenter phase II study of iodine-131 tositumomab for chemotherapy-relapsed/refractory low-grade and transformed low-grade B-cell non-Hodgkin's lymphomas. J Clin Oncol 18:1316–1323

173. Dillman RO, Hendrix CS (2003) Unique aspects of supportive care using monoclonal antibodies in cancer treatment. Support Cancer Ther 1:38–48
174. Morschhauser F, Radford J, Van Hoof A et al (2008) Phase III trial of consolidation therapy with yttrium-90-ibritumomab tiuxetan compared with no additional therapy after first remission in advanced follicular lymphoma. J Clin Oncol 26:5156–5164
175. Apisarnthanarax N (2002) Treatment of cutaneous T cell lymphoma: current status and future directions. Am J Clin Dermatol 3:193–215
176. Olsen E, Duvic M, Frankal A et al (2001) Pivotal phase III trial of two dose levels of denileukin diftitox for the treatment of cutaneous T-cell lymphoma. J Clin Oncol 19:376–388
177. Deininger MW, O'Brien SG, Ford JM et al (2003) Practical management of patients with chronic myeloid leukemia receiving imatinib. J Clin Oncol 21:1637–1647
178. Kantarjian H, Sawyers C, Hochhaus A et al (2002) Hematologic and cytogenetic responses to imatinib mesylate in chronic myelogenous leukemia. N Engl J Med 346:645–652
179. Penel N, Blay JY, Adenis A et al (2008) Imatinib as a possible cause of severe rhabdomyolysis. N Engl J Med 358:2746–2747
180. Song KW, Rifkind J, Al-Beirouti B et al (2004) Subdural hematomas during CML therapy with imatinib mesylate. Leuk Lymphoma 45:1633–1636
181. Schiff D, Wen PY, van den Bent MJ et al (2009) Neurological adverse effects caused by cytotoxic and targeted therapies. Nat Rev Clin Oncol 6:596–603

Chapter 23
Neurological Complications of Bone Marrow Transplantation in Lymphoma and Leukemia Patients

Jacoline E.C. Bromberg and Warren P. Mason

Introduction

Hematopoietic stem-cell transplantation (HSCT) is increasingly being incorporated into standard management for patients with a variety of leukemias and lymphomas. This procedure refers to the reconstitution of a patient's depleted hematopoietic system by the intravenous infusion of progenitor cells obtained from bone marrow or peripheral blood. Hematopoietic stem-cell transplantation can be allogeneic (transfer of stem cells from one human leukocyte antigen-matched individual to another) or autologous (infusion of a patient's own stem cells following collection and storage).

In preparation for HSCT, patients are treated with myeloablative doses of chemotherapy, often in conjunction with total body irradiation (TBI), as a means of eliminating all cancerous cells. Following allogeneic HSCT patients must receive extended doses of immunosuppressive agents as a means of preventing graft versus host disease (GVHD). Neurologic complications of HSCT can occur during any stage of this procedure, and can relate to the underlying illness and its potential recurrence, the treatments and procedures used to prepare the patient for transplantation, and the drugs used following HSCT to control infections, prevent rejection, and treat other complications [1, 2]. Neurologic complications following HSCT are common, but the incidence varies somewhat from series to series, being higher in autopsy studies than retrospective reviews of clinical cases [3–7]. For instance, a recent autopsy series of 180 patients who died following HSCT reported neuropathological abnormalities in over 90% of cases [4]. Common postmortem findings included subarachnoid and intraparenchymal hemorrhage, and fungal infections. In contrast, clinical series have reported symptomatic neurologic complications in the range of 10–40%; common complications included

W.P. Mason (✉)
Department of Medicine, Princess Margaret Hospital and University of Toronto, Toronto, ON M5G 2M9, USA
e-mail: warren.mason@uhn.on.ca

T. Batchelor, L.M. DeAngelis (eds.), *Lymphoma and Leukemia of the Nervous System*, DOI 10.1007/978-1-4419-7668-0_23,

encephalopathy, seizures, psychiatric symptoms, and cerebral hemorrhage [8, 9]. Neurologic complications are somewhat different and possibly more frequent in series of allogeneic HSCT, due likely to toxicities of drugs used to prevent rejection, the risk of opportunistic infections during the protracted period of immunosuppression, and the high incidence of acute and chronic GVHD [9–12]. In particular, patients transplanted from an unrelated HLA-matched or related HLA-unmatched (alternative donor) donor appear to have an increased risk of neurologic complications [10]. However, a large retrospective series of 425 patients has challenged this assumption, reporting similar incidences of neurologic complications in allogeneic and autologous HSCT, although the frequency and spectrum of complications differed between these two groups [5] (Table 23.1). Not unexpectedly, intracranial hemorrhage was more common in autologous HSCT, being related to prolonged thrombocytopenia, and opportunistic infections were more common in allogeneic HSCT, in this instance a consequence of extended immunosuppression needed to prevent or control GVHD.

Table 23.1 Comparison of allogeneic and autologous transplants

	Allogeneic HSCT	Autologous HSCT
Source of SC	HLA-matched relative or unrelated donor	Patient
Conditioning Regimen	Chemotherapy and TBI	Chemotherapy TBI uncommon
Neurologic Complications	Drug Toxicity GVHD Opportunistic infections Metabolic encephalopathy Coagulopathy	Drug toxicity Infections Coagulopathy Metabolic encephalopathy
Mortality	≥40%	≤10%

Abbreviations: GVHD, graft versus host disease; SC, stem cells; TBI, total body irradiation

Neurologic complications of HSCT are frequently serious and affect survival in a detrimental way [3, 4, 13]. Patients who are admitted to an intensive care unit with neurologic complications generally have a poor prognosis [14]. Putative risk factors have been identified for the development of neurologic complications following HSCT. Increased risks for neurologic sequelae include prolonged immunosuppression, the development of GVHD, the incorporation of TBI or methotrexate into the conditioning regimen, and an underlying diagnosis of acute myelogenous leukemia [3, 11, 15, 16]. It is hypothesized that TBI damages endothelial cells within the CNS, potentially aggravating the neurotoxicity of many chemotherapeutic agents. It remains unclear why patients with acute myelogenous leukemia are at increased risk, but this association appears consistently in several case series. Prospective evaluation of patients undergoing HSCT may clarify risk factors, thereby serving as the basis for anticipating and possibly preventing disastrous neurologic complications of this resource-intensive therapy.

Neurologic Complications During Harvesting

Bone marrow or peripheral stem cell harvesting are very safe, and neurologic complications are altogether uncommon [17]. Occasionally, laceration of the lumbosacral meninges during bone marrow harvesting from the region of the iliac crest can create a CSF leak and the syndrome of intracranial hypotension, manifested by symptoms of headache, nausea, and vomiting [18]. Spontaneous closure of the defect and remission of symptoms is the usual course.

The insertion of jugular venous catheters has rarely been associated with neurologic complications, such as the development of a Horner's syndrome, brachial plexopathy or lower cranial nerve palsies [19]. Finally, rare cases of cerebral infarction have been related to air embolism during this procedure [20].

The use of growth factors, particularly recombinant granulocyte colony stimulating factor, has been implicated in the exacerbation of a variety of autoimmune diseases [21, 22]. While the mechanism underlying this observation remains unknown, empirical use of concurrent cyclophosphamide during stem cell mobilization can reduce the risk or minimize the severity of disease flares [21].

Neurologic Complications During Conditioning

During the period of conditioning, neurologic complications are typically due to toxicities from high-dose chemotherapy and TBI [23]. A variety of chemotherapeutic agents are used as part of conditioning regimens designed to deplete the bone marrow in preparation for HSCT, and common neurologic toxicities of these drugs are listed in Table 23.2. Conditioning regimens vary according to the underlying disease and source of the stem cells, and often include TBI for the management

Table 23.2 Neurotoxicity of common chemotherapeutic agents used in HSCT conditioning regimens

Busulfan	Encephalopathy with headaches, confusion, seizures, impaired consciousness
Ifosphamide	Encephalopathy with hallucinations, confusion, seizures, impaired consciousness, myoclonus
Cytosine arabinoside	Encephalopathy with seizures, cerebellar syndrome, peripheral neuropathy
Carboplatin	Sensorineural hearing loss
Carmustine	Optic disc and retinal disease, encephalopathy with high doses
Etoposide	Encephalopathy with confusion, somnolence and seizures
Thiotepa	Encephalopathy
Methotrexate	Meningitis and myeloradicular syndrome after intrathecal administration, leukoencephalopathy

Abbreviations: HSV, herpes simplex virus; HHV, human herpes virus; MOF, multi-organ failure; aGVHD, acute graft versus host disease; CMV, cytomegalovirus; SDH, subdural hematoma; PTLD, post-transplant lymphoproliferative disease; VZV, varicella zoster virus; PML, progressive multifocal leukoencephalopathy; JCV, JC virus of acute leukemia. Recently, the recognition of the beneficial impact of controlled GVHD on prognosis and the increasing use of HSCT in elderly and frail patients, have resulted in the development of reduced-intensity conditioning regimens [24]. These regimens are likely to be associated with fewer and less severe neurologic complications.

Busulfan and ifosphamide are amongst the most neurotoxic of agents used in HSCT conditioning regimens [25]. Both agents can frequently cause reversible encephalopathies with alteration in consciousness, confusion, seizures, hallucinations, myoclonus, and tremors. Patients receiving busulfan are usually treated prophylactically with anticonvulsants. Cytosine arabinoside can cause a variety of neurologic toxicities, including the development of a pancerebellar syndrome, a diffuse encephalopathy with confusion and seizures, and a peripheral neuropathy. These toxicities are usually reversible. Occasionally, intrathecal methotrexate can cause chemical meningitis with headache and neck stiffness, and a reversible myeloradicular syndrome. Intrathecal methotrexate can contribute to a leukoencephalopathy with white matter changes on MR scans [26].

During the infusion of cryopreserved bone marrow or stem cells, neurologic symptoms are rare, but have been reported. In one series, three out of 179 patients developed neurologic complications during infusion of cryopreserved stem cells: transient global amnesia in one, and cerebral infarction in the absence of hypotension or cardiac events in two [27]. However, the strokes in both circumstances could not clearly be attributed to the infusions, as thrombocytopenia and cerebral aspergillosis were pre-existing conditions. Rarely, seizures and a reversible posterior leukoencephalopathy syndrome have been reported during stem cell transfusions [28, 29].

Neurologic Complications During Pancytopenia (Pre-engraftment)

The risk of specific neurologic complications varies with time after transplantation and the status of the patient's immune system (Table 23.3). Distinct phases are defined by the time interval from the day of the infusion of the transplanted cells to the onset of neurologic symptoms [30]. Neurologic complications in the pancytopenic phase (<30 days) after transplantation may be due to metabolic abnormalities as a result of organ failure, coagulopathies and infections resulting from pancytopenia, and drug toxicity [1, 2, 12].

Infections

Prolonged neutropenia and frequent breaks in the mucocutaneous barrier due to the preparative regimens, as well as indwelling lines and catheters lead to heightened susceptibility to infections in the pancytopenic phase [30]. When the CNS

Table 23.3 CNS complications of HSCT

	Phase I – Pancytopenia (< 30 days)	Phase II – Engraftment (day 30–100)	Phase III – Late complications (>100 days)
Infectious	Fungi: aspergillus, candida; Viruses: HSV, HHV 6; Bacteria: gram negative bacteria; Protozoa	If GVHD or graft failure: Candida/aspergillus CMV, HHV-6, Gram positive bacteria toxoplasmosis	VZV, PML (JCV) Encapsulated bacteria (hemophilus, streptococcus), Toxoplasmosis
Vascular		Hemorrhage, SDH, infarction	Vasculitis
Metabolic	MOF, aGVHD Wernicke encephalopathy		
Toxic		Cyclosporine or tacrolimus encephalopathy antibiotic-induced seizures	
Post HSCT carcinogenesis		PTLD	PTLD solid tumors

Abbreviations: HSV, herpes simplex virus; HHV, human herpes virus; MOF, multi-organ failure; aGVHD, acute graft versus host disease; CMV, cytomegalovirus; SDH, subdural hematoma; PTLD, post-transplant lymphoproliferative disease; VZV, varicella zoster virus; PML, progressive multifocal leukoencephalopathy; JCV, JC virus

is infected, classic findings of fever and meningismus may be absent due to the inability of the patient to generate an inflammatory response. Meningitis due to gram-negative bacteria or *Listeria monocytogenes* and fungal infections, such as *Aspergillus* and *Candida*, may occur during this phase. Additionally, viral infections, such as adenovirus or coxsackievirus may be acquired from the donor, and herpes simplex virus (HSV) reactivation may occur [1, 30]. Prophylactic use of antiviral agents has reduced the incidence of HSV and cytomegalovirus (CMV) meningoencephalitis. Patients undergoing autologous or allogeneic transplantation are at risk for infections during this phase.

Cerebral aspergillosis may occur in the first weeks after transplantation, especially in recipients of allogeneic transplantation, but it is observed more frequently several months after transplantation [31, 32]. Nevertheless, most patients are neutropenic when aspergillosis is diagnosed and most have experienced prior acute GVHD. Symptoms include seizures, focal deficits, and mental alteration. Septic infarctions, frequently associated with hemorrhage and abscess formation may cause single or multiple lesions, with or without ring-enhancement on cranial CT or MRI imaging [31, 33]. Definitive diagnosis is frequently difficult; examination of the CSF has a low diagnostic yield, but is useful for differential diagnosis of other pathogens or recurrent malignancy in the CNS. Cerebral aspergillosis is usually associated with pulmonary aspergillosis and prognosis is dismal with most patients dying within 1–2 weeks despite treatment [31]. Limited data suggest that treatment with voriconazole may be superior to amphotericin B [34].

Vascular Disease

Intracranial hemorrhage has been reported in 2–4% of HSCT patients. Subdural hematoma is most common and is related to persistent thrombocytopenia and acute myeloid leukemia (AML) [1, 2, 5]. Intraparenchymal or subarachnoid hemorrhage may also occur, with the former being strongly associated with AML (Fig. 23.1). Occasionally, patients with prolonged thrombocytopenia develop a mononeuropathy or even plexopathy due to intraneural hemorrhage [5]. Ischemic strokes are less frequent, not associated with pancytopenia and may be caused by disseminated intravascular coagulation (DIC), bacterial endocarditis or infection with *Aspergillus* or varicella zoster virus (VZV) [5, 7, 35]. Additionally, a hypercoagulable state as a result of deficiencies in anticoagulant proteins has been postulated to play a role in the etiology of early ischemic strokes [36, 37].

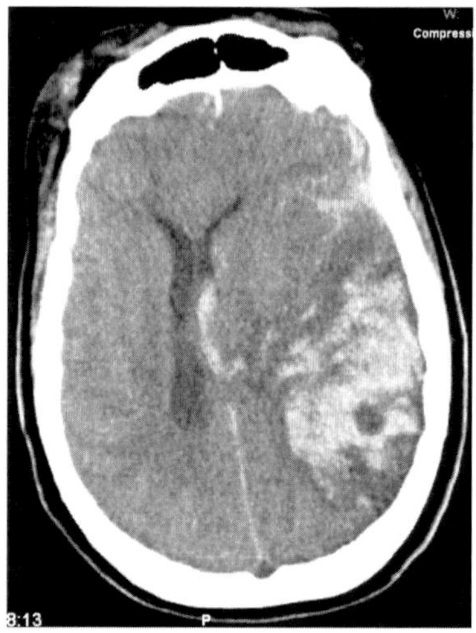

Fig. 23.1 Intracerebral hemorrhage in an AML patient. A 47-year old woman was treated with chemotherapy followed by an HLA-matched allogeneic HSCT. Ten weeks after transplantation, she was found unconscious. CT scan showed a large intracerebral hematoma in the left hemisphere

Thrombotic Microangiopathy

Thrombotic microangiopathy (TMA), presenting as hemolytic uremic syndrome (HUS), or thrombotic thrombocytopenic purpura (TTP) is a well recognized complication of HSCT. It occurs in 8% of recipients of allogeneic transplantation within 3 months, and has a mortality rate of 75%. The classic presentation is relatively acute onset of anemia and thrombocytopenia with concomitant acute renal dysfunction. Neurologic deficits, such as confusion, seizures and focal signs occur in up to 50% of patients [38]. While the etiology of this syndrome remains elusive, it is associated with advanced age, unrelated or mismatched donor grafts, acute GVHD, viral or fungal infections, and use of calcineurin inhibitors such as cyclosporine. Treatment is withdrawal of calcineurin inhibitors; other interventions have uncertain efficacy, but immunosuppressive agents and plasma exchange have been used.

Metabolic Encephalopathy

Clinical signs of a diffuse encephalopathy, either with or without seizures, are the most frequent reason for neurological consultation in the first 3 months after transplantation. Causes include infections, drug toxicity, hepatic or renal dysfunction, or multi-organ failure, frequently as a result of acute GVHD [3, 5, 39, 40]. A subdural hematoma may present without focal signs, which is one reason brain imaging should always be performed, preferably with MRI. Wernicke encephalopathy has been reported in up to 1% of patients and should be considered in those with severe diarrhea as a result of acute GVHD [15, 40]. Most metabolic encephalopathies in HSCT patients have multifactorial etiologies.

Toxic Encephalopathy

Encephalopathy and seizures may be caused by a variety of drugs used in patients after transplantation. Cyclosporine and tacrolimus are the most neurotoxic frequently used agents, but antibiotics, such as cefepime or imipenem may cause seizures and amphotericin B has been reported to cause tremor, confusion, and parkinsonism.

Cyclosporine, a calcineurin inhibitor, is commonly used for the prevention of GVHD after allogeneic transplantation. It causes neurologic side effects in up to 40% of patients. A posterior reversible encephalopathy syndrome (PRES) is the most serious complication, with headache, confusion, seizures, visual disturbances, and motor symptoms as classical manifestations [41]. PRES is frequently associated with hypertension, hypomagnesemia, and a high serum cyclosporine concentration, although the latter may be within the normal range. Neuroimaging is remarkable for reversible symmetric white matter edema most commonly, but not exclusively in the parietooccipital regions [41] (Fig. 23.2). Dose reduction or withdrawal of cyclosporine usually results in resolution of symptoms. Although tacrolimus is also a calcineurin inhibitor and has a similar neurotoxicity profile, substituting tacrolimus is an option if continued use of GVHD-prevention is required. Other frequent side effects of calcineurin inhibitors are postural tremor and headache [1, 41].

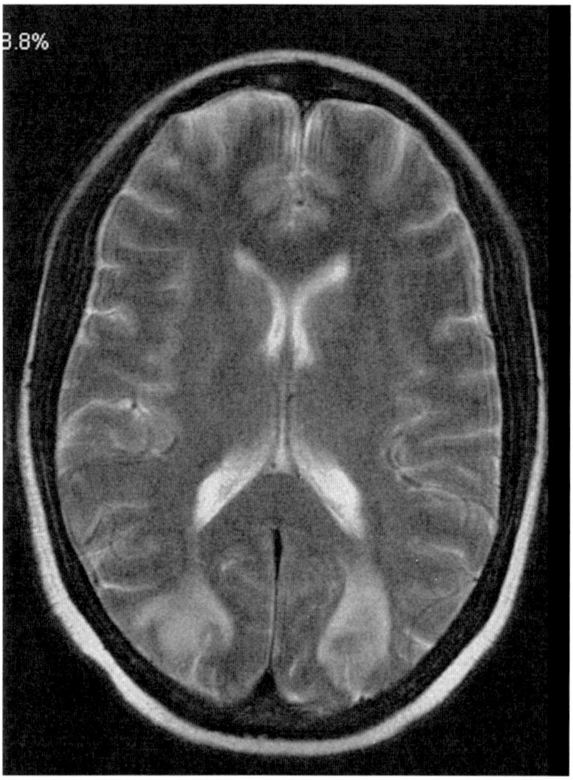

Fig. 23.2 Posterior reversible encephalopathy syndrome (PRES). A 39 year-old woman was treated for AML with allogeneic cord blood transplantation and cyclosporine for immunosuppression. She presented with a generalized tonic-clonic seizure, headache, and hypertension. T2-weighted MR images revealed bilateral hyperintense, white matter abnormalities in the occipital lobes consistent with PRES related to cyclosporine. Dose reduction of cyclosporine resulted in complete resolution of symptoms and disappearance of MR abnormalities

Neurologic Complications After Engraftment

Complications Due to Chronic Immunosuppression

The first months after engraftment are dominated by impaired cell-mediated immunity, generally caused by incomplete reconstitution and use of immunosuppressive agents. The herpesviruses, particularly cytomegalovirus (CMV), and human herpes virus 6 (HHV-6) are major pathogens in this period. Other dominant pathogens during this phase include fungi, especially *Aspergillus* species, *Toxoplasma*, and to a lesser extent gram-positive bacteria. such as *Staphylococcus* species and *Listeria* [30, 33]. The frequency of opportunistic infections is greatest in the second to fourth month after transplantation. After this period, autologous HSCT patients usually

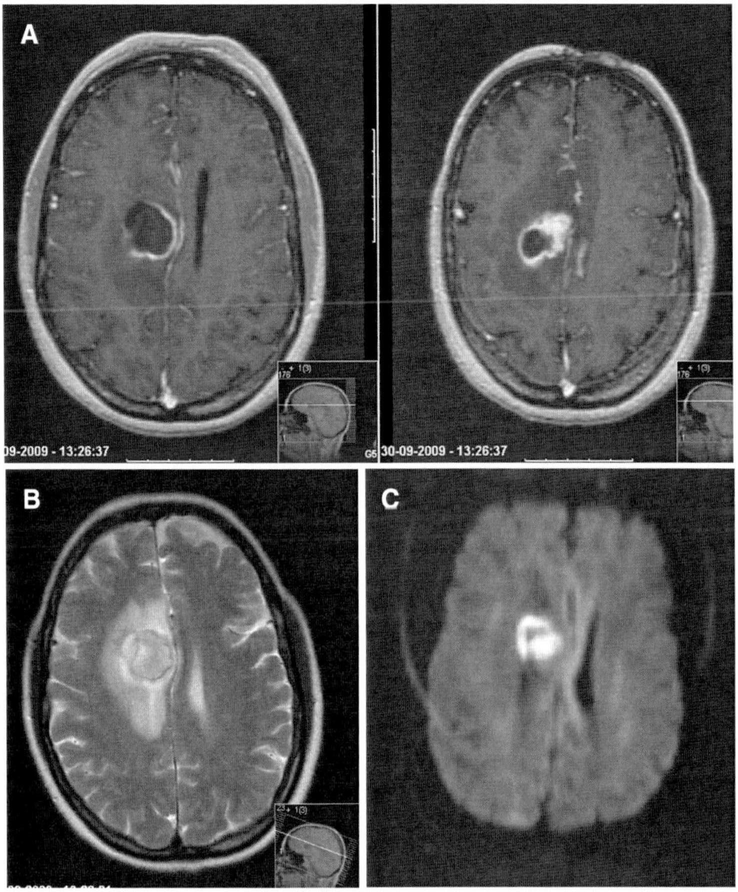

Fig. 23.3 One year after undergoing an allogeneic stem cell transplant for chronic lymphocytic leukemia a 47 year-old female presented with gait disturbance and mild headache. Her medication included mycophenolate mofetil and prednisone for suppression of chronic graft versus host disease. On post-contrast T1-weighted sequences a ring-enhancing mass lesion was identified in the right frontal (**a**). The lesion was further characterized by increased signal intensity on T2-weighted sequences (**b**) and restricted water mobility on diffusion-weighted imaging sequences (**c**). A nocardia abscess was identified after emergency surgical decompression

have more rapid recovery of immune function and therefore, a lower risk of opportunistic infections than do allogeneic HSCT patients. Allogeneic HSCT patients with chronic GVHD who require continued immunosuppression are still at risk for various opportunistic infections including CMV, varicella zoster virus (VZV) reactivation, nocardia abscess formation, and progressive multifocal leukoencephalopathy (PML) after the fourth month post-HSCT [30, 33] (Fig. 23.3). In addition to these infectious complications, direct neurotoxic effects of immunosuppressive medication may occur.

Human herpes virus 6 (HHV-6) encephalitis has been reported in 3–12% of patients after allogeneic HSCT, with the higher incidence reported after treatment with alemtuzumab [42, 43]. Encephalitis presents, most characteristically, after engraftment with an acute limbic encephalitis with confusion, amnesia, seizures, a syndrome of inappropriate ADH secretion (SIADH), mild CSF pleocytosis, and temporal EEG abnormalities. More atypical features such as fever, headache, and coma have also been reported. MR imaging reveals hyperintensities on T2-weighted, FLAIR or DWI images in the temporal lobes, although imaging may be normal initially. CSF PCR can establish the diagnosis of HHV-6 encephalitis; serum PCR is occasionally negative in confirmed cases. Prophylaxis against HHV-6 with valciclovir or valganciclovir is not necessarily protective; however, prompt treatment with intravenous foscarnet may be beneficial [42–44].

Toxoplasma encephalitis is reported to occur weeks to months after transplantation [32]. Patients may present with seizures, cognitive disturbances, focal symptoms and signs, and impairment of consciousness. Gadolinium enhanced T1-weighted MR imaging shows either multiple ring-enhancing lesions with frequent hemorrhagic transformation, or multiple non-enhancing lesions that are hyperintense on T2-weighted images and hypointense, or isointense on T1-weighted images with minimal mass effect [32, 45]. The latter group appears to have a shorter latency from HSCT and a more fulminant clinical course. Prophylaxis with cotrimoxazole prevents some, but not all cases. Treatment with pyrimethamine and sulfadiazine results in improvement in some patients, but mortality is high.

PML is rare after HSCT, but can occur after either autologous or allogeneic transplantation [46, 47]. It is caused by reactivation of the JC virus, which has a high community seroprevalence, thus all patients are potentially at risk. JC virus is trophic for renal epithelium and also infects oligodendrocytes where reactivation leads to cell death and neurologic symptoms [1]. Patients typically present with slowly progressive focal deficits or a subacute dementia; rarely, a brainstem syndrome arises. MR imaging shows multiple subcortical white matter lesions with FLAIR and T2 prolongation in the frontal and parietooccipital regions. These lesions lack mass effect and rarely enhance on post-contrast images [1, 33]. Diagnosis depends on demonstrating the JC virus in the CNS by CSF PCR, which is reported to have a sensitivity of 74% and a specificity of 96% [47]. Treatment is frequently ineffective, but recovery of CD4 counts by stimulation with IL-2 has led to resolution of symptoms in anecdotal cases [47].

Complications Due to Chronic GVHD

Acute GVHD occurs in the first 3 months after transplantation and affects primarily skin, liver, and GI tract with neurologic symptoms, resulting from metabolic disturbances or immunosuppression. Chronic GVHD more closely resembles an autoimmune collagen vascular disease with multisystem involvement and can present months to years after transplantation. Neurologic complications appear to affect the peripheral nervous system primarily, but more recently CNS complications have also been described.

Peripheral Nervous System

Polymyositis, with an acute or subacute onset of myalgia and proximal muscle weakness, elevated creatine kinase, and typical pathology on electromyography and muscle biopsy is an infrequent manifestation of GVHD [48–51]. Patients generally, but not always, have prior or concurrent systemic manifestations of GVHD, and a majority respond within days to increased immunosuppression with corticosteroids, with or without cyclosporine [50, 51]. Myasthenia gravis has also been reported as a rare manifestation of GVHD, usually during the taper of immunosuppressive agents. It is usually associated with elevated anti-acetylcholine receptor antibodies [1, 52, 53].

Peripheral neuropathies in the setting of GVHD, although infrequent, may cause motor disability with significant morbidity. The neuropathy is demyelinating and similar to chronic idiopathic demyelinating polyneuropathy (CIDP) [49]. It may respond to treatment with immunosuppressive drugs, intravenous IgG or plasma exchange, like CIDP. The differential diagnosis includes axonal neuropathies, which are more frequently toxic, and a critical illness polyneuropathy that may occur in patients who have protracted ICU admissions. Another rare and severe, predominantly motor, demyelinating polyneuropathy has been described 2–3 weeks after high dose cytarabine. This syndrome is unresponsive to immunosuppressive treatments. Primary sensory neuropathies may also occur, are generally axonal, and are presumed to result from direct toxic effects of chemotherapeutic agents [49].

Central Nervous System

Involvement of the CNS in GVHD is rare, but a CNS vasculitis-like syndrome with acute to subacute, frequently multifocal, neurological deficits, encephalopathy, or cognitive deficits has been described. Patients may have progressive or remitting symptoms coinciding with exacerbations of the GVHD. MR imaging reveals ischemic or white matter lesions, and in a few patients, a vasculitis has been confirmed at autopsy [54, 55].

Mild neurologic and cognitive deficits, and MRI abnormalities, consisting mainly of cerebral atrophy and white matter lesions have been described in up to 54% of patients surviving 3 years after HSCT [56]. These neurologic and MR abnormalities have been attributed to chronic GVHD, cyclosporine, and other immunosuppressive agents and age. However, most patients retain normal cognition following HSCT, and carefully conducted longitudinal neuropsychological studies of long-term HSCT patients have demonstrated no appreciable changes or only minor decreases in attention, executive function, and psychomotor function [15, 57, 58].

Late Complications – Carcinogenesis

In a large multicenter series, the cumulative incidence of post-transplant lymphoproliferative disease (PTLD) after HSCT was 1.0% at 10 years. Incidence was highest 1–5 months post-transplant with a peak incidence at 3 months, and a steep decline in incidence after 5 months [59]. In 82% of PTLD patients, the tumor was EBV-related, arose within 1 year of HSCT, and was rapidly fatal. In contrast, patients who develop late onset PTLD rarely have EBV-driven neoplasms [59]. CNS localization of the PTLD is seldom reported [60]. The cumulative incidence of solid tumors after HSCT is similar to that of PTLD. However, it is uncommon for solid tumors to develop within 10 years of HSCT, with most arising after at least 15 years [59, 61]. Primary brain tumors, including glioblastoma, astrocytoma, and primitive neuroectodermal tumors, are the most common solid tumors post-HSCT; these neoplasms are likely induced by conditioning regimens that included cranial radiotherapy or TBI [61].

References

1. Rosenfeld MR, Pruitt A (2006) Neurologic complications of bone marrow, stem cell, and organ transplantation in patients with cancer. Semin Oncol 33:352–361
2. Saiz A, Graus F (2004) Neurological complications of hematopoietic cell transplantation. Semin Neurol 24:427–434
3. Antonini G, Ceschin V, Morino S et al (1998) Early neurologic complications following allogeneic bone marrow transplant for leukemia: a prospective study. Neurology 50:1441–1445
4. Bleggi-Torres LF, de Medeiros BC, Werner B et al (2000) Neuropathological findings after bone marrow transplantation: an autopsy study of 180 cases. Bone Marrow Transplant 25:301–307
5. Graus F, Saiz A, Sierra J et al (1996) Neurologic complications of autologous and allogeneic bone marrow transplantation in patients with leukemia: a comparative study. Neurology 46:1004–1009
6. Mohrmann RL, Mah V, Vinters HV (1990) Neuropathologic findings after bone marrow transplantation: an autopsy study. Hum Pathol 21:630–639
7. Patchell RA, White CL III, Clark AW et al (1985) Neurologic complications of bone marrow transplantation. Neurology 35:300–306
8. Guerrero A, Perez-Simon JA, Gutierrez N et al (1999) Neurological complications after autologous stem cell transplantation. Eur Neurol 41:48–50
9. Snider S, Bashir R, Bierman P (1994) Neurologic complications after high-dose chemotherapy and autologous bone marrow transplantation for Hodgkin's disease. Neurology 44:681–684
10. de Brabander C, Cornelissen J, Smitt PA et al (2000) Increased incidence of neurological complications in patients receiving an allogenic bone marrow transplantation from alternative donors. J Neurol Neurosurg Psychiatry 68:36–40
11. Faraci M, Lanino E, Dini G et al (2002) Severe neurologic complications after hematopoietic stem cell transplantation in children. Neurology 59:1895–1904
12. Krouwer HGJ, Wijdicks EFM (2003) Neurologic complications of bone marrow transplantation. Neurol Clin 21:319–352
13. Gordon B, Lyden E, Lynch J et al (2000) Central nervous system dysfunction as the first manifestation of multiple organ dysfunction syndrome in stem cell transplant patients. Bone Marrow Transplant 25:79–83
14. Jackson SR, Tweeddale MG, Barnett MJ et al (1998) Admission of bone marrow transplant recipients to the intensive care unit: outcome, survival and prognostic factors. Bone Marrow Transplant 21:697–704
15. Sostak P, Padovan CS, Yousry TA et al (2003) Prospective evaluation of neurological complications after allogeneic bone marrow transplantation. Neurology 60:842–848

16. Uckan D, Cetin M, Yigitkanli I et al (2005) Life-threatening neurological complications after bone marrow transplantation in children. Bone Marrow Transplant 35:71–76
17. Bain BJ (2005) Bone marrow biopsy morbidity: review of 2003. J Clin Pathol 58:406–408
18. Lieberman F, Gulati S (1996) Headaches after inadvertent lumbar puncture during bone marrow harvest. Neurology 46:268–269
19. Sylvestre DL, Sandson TA, Nachmanoff DB (1991) Transient brachial plexopathy as a complication of internal jugular vein cannulation. Neurology 41:760
20. Heckmann JG, Lang CJ, Kindler K et al (2000) Neurologic manifestations of cerebral air embolism as a complication of central venous catheterization. Crit Care Med 28:1621–1625
21. Burt RK, Fassas A, Snowden JA et al (2001) Collection of hematopoietic stem cells from patients with autoimmune diseases. Bone Marrow Transplant 28:1–12
22. Openshaw H, Stuve O, Antel JP et al (2000) Multiple sclerosis flares associated with recombinant granulocyte colony-stimulating factor. Neurology 54:2147–2150
23. DeAngelis LM, Posner JB (2008) Side effects of chemotherapy. In: Neurologic complications of cancer, 2nd edn. Oxford University Press, New York, NY
24. Kassim AA, Chinratanalab W, Ferrara JLM et al (2005) Reduced-intensity allogeneic hematopoietic stem cell transplantation for acute leukemias: "what is the best recipe?" Bone Marrow Transplant 36:565–574
25. DiMaggio JR, Brown R, Baile WF et al (1994) Hallucinations and ifosfamide-induced neurotoxicity. Cancer 73:1509–1514
26. Tahsildar HI, Remler BF, Creger RJ et al (1996) Delayed, transient encephalopathy after marrow transplantation: case reports and MRI findings in four patients. J Neurooncol 27:241–250
27. Hoyt R, Szer J, Grigg A (2000) Neurological events associated with the infusion of cryopreserved bone marrow and/or peripheral blood progenitor cells. Bone Marrow Transplant 25:1285–1287
28. Ferrucci PF, Martinoni A, Cocorocchio E et al (2000) Evaluation of acute toxicities associated with autologous peripheral blood progenitor cell reinfusion in patients undergoing high-dose chemotherapy. Bone Marrow Transplant 25:173–177
29. Higman MA, Port JD, Beauchamp NJ Jr. et al (2000) Reversible leukoencephalopathy associated with re-infusion of DMSO preserved stem cells. Bone Marrow Transplant 26:797–800
30. Dykewicz CA (2001) Summary of the guidelines for preventing opportunistic infections among hematopoietic stem cell transplant recipients. Clin Infect Dis 33:139–144
31. Jantunen E, Volin L, Salonen O et al (2003) Central nervous system aspergillosis in allogeneic stem cell transplant recipients. Bone Marrow Transplant 31:191–196
32. Maschke M, Dietrich U, Prumbaum M et al (1999) Opportunistic CNS infection after bone marrow transplantation. Bone Marrow Transplant 23:1167–1176
33. Yoshida S, Hayakawa K, Yamamoto A et al (2008) The central nervous system complications of bone marrow transplantation in children. Eur Radiol 18:2048–2059
34. Herbrecht R, Denning DW, Patterson TF et al (2002) Voriconazole versus amphotericin B for primary therapy of invasive aspergillosis. N Engl J Med 347:408–415
35. Coplin WM, Cochran MS, Levine SR et al (2001) Stroke after bone marrow transplantation: frequency, aetiology and outcome. Brain 124:1043–1051
36. Gordon B, Haire W, Kessinger A et al (1991a) High frequency of antithrombin 3 and protein C deficiency following autologous bone marrow transplantation for lymphoma. Bone Marrow Transplant 8:497–502
37. Gordon BG, Saving KL, McCallister JA et al (1991b) Cerebral infarction associated with protein C deficiency following allogeneic bone marrow transplantation. Bone Marrow Transplant 8:323–325
38. Ho VT, Cutler C, Carter S et al (2005) Blood and marrow transplant clinical trials network toxicity committee consensus summary: thrombotic microangiopathy after hematopoietic stem cell transplantation. Biol Blood Marrow Transplant 11:571–575
39. Denier C, Bourhis JH, Lacroix C et al (2006) Spectrum and prognosis of neurologic complications after hematopoietic transplantation. Neurology 67:1990–1997

40. Teive HAG, Funke V, Bitencourt MA et al (2008) Neurological complications of hematopoietic stem cell transplantation (HSCT): a retrospective study in a HSCT center in Brazil. Arq Neuropsiquiatr 66:685–690
41. Gijtenbeek JMM, van den Bent MJ, Vecht CJ (1999) Cyclosporine neurotoxicity: a review. J Neurol 246:339–346
42. Seeley WW, Marty FM, Holmes TM et al (2007) Post-transplant acute limbic encephalitis: clinical features and relationship to HHV6. Neurology 69:156–165
43. Vu T, Carrum G, Hutton G et al (2007) Human herpesvirus-6 encephalitis following allogeneic hematopoietic stem cell transplantation. Bone Marrow Transplant 39:705–709
44. Singh N, Paterson DL (2000) Encephalitis caused by human herpesvirus-6 in transplant recipients: relevance of a novel neurotropic virus. Transplantation 69:2474–2479
45. Ionita C, Wasay M, Balos L et al (2004) MR imaging in toxoplasmosis encephalitis after bone marrow transplantation: paucity of enhancement despite fulminant disease. Am J Neuroradiol 25:270–273
46. Coley SC, Jager HR, Szydlo RM et al (1999) CT and MRI manifestations of central nervous system infection following allogeneic bone marrow transplantation. Clin Radiol 54:390–397
47. Kharfan-Dabaja MA, Ayala E, Greene J et al (2007) Two cases of progressive multifocal leukoencephalopathy after allogeneic hematopoietic cell transplantation and a review of the literature. Bone Marrow Transplant 39:101–107
48. Couriel R, Beguelin GZ, Giralt S et al (2002) Chronic graft-versus-host disease manifesting as polymyositis: an uncommon presentation. Bone Marrow Transplant 30:543–546
49. Openshaw H (1997) Peripheral neuropathy after bone marrow transplantation. Biol Blood Marrow Transplant 3:202–209
50. Parker PM, Openshaw H, Forman SJ (1997) Myositis associated with graft-versus-host disease. Curr Opin Rheumatol 9:513–519
51. Stevens AM, Sullivan KM, Nelson JL (2003) Polymyositis as a manifestation of chronic graft-versus-host disease. Rheumatology (Oxford) 42:34–39
52. Grau JM, Casademont J, Monforte R et al (1990) Myasthenia gravis after allogeneic bone marrow transplantation: report of a new case and pathogenetic considerations. Bone Marrow Transplant 5:435–437
53. Tse S, Saunders EF, Silverman E et al (1999) Myasthenia gravis and polymyositis as manifestations of chronic graft-versus-host-disease. Bone Marrow Transplant 23:397–399
54. Kamble R, Chang CC, Sanchez S et al (2007) Central nervous system graft-versus-host disease: report of two cases and literature review. Bone Marrow Transplant 39:49–52
55. Padovan CS, Bise K, Hahn J et al (1999) Angiitis of the central nervous system after allogeneic bone marrow transplantation? Stroke 30:1651–1656
56. Padovan CS, Yousry TA, Schleuning M et al (1998) Neurological and neuroradiological findings in long-term survivors of allogeneic bone marrow transplantation. Ann Neurol 43:627–633
57. Harder H, Van Gool AR, Duivenvoorden HJ et al (2007) Case-referent comparison of cognitive functions in patients receiving haematopoietic stem-cell transplantation for haematological malignancies: two-year follow-up results. Eur J Cancer 43:2052–2059
58. Schulz-Kindermann F, Mehnert A, Scherwath A et al (2007) Cognitive function in the acute course of allogeneic hematopoietic stem cell transplantation for hematological malignancies. Bone Marrow Transplant 39:789–799
59. Curtis RE, Travis LB, Rowlings PA et al (1999) Risk of lymphoproliferative disorders after bone marrow transplantation: a multi-institutional study. Blood 94:2208–2216
60. Nozzoli C, Bartolozzi B, Guidi S et al (2006) Epstein-Barr virus-associated post-transplant lymphoproliferative disease with central nervous system involvement after unrelated allogeneic hematopoietic stem cell transplantation. Leuk Lymphoma 47:167–169
61. Socie G, Curtis RE, Deeg HJ et al (2000) New malignant diseases after allogeneic marrow transplantation for childhood acute leukemia. J Clin Oncol 18:348–357

Index

Note: The letters ‘f’ and ‘t’ following the locators refer to figures and tables respectively.

T. Batchelor, L.M. DeAngelis (eds.), *Lymphoma and Leukemia of the Nervous System*, DOI 10.1007/978-1-4419-7668-0,

N

O

P

MIX
Papier aus verantwortungsvollen Quellen
Paper from responsible sources
FSC® C105338

Printed by Books on Demand, Germany